RISK AND HEALTH COMMUNICATION IN AN EVOLVING MEDIA ENVIRONMENT

Broadcast media has a particular fascination with stories that involve risk and health crisis events—disease outbreaks, terrorist acts, and natural disasters—contexts where risk and health communication play a critical role. An evolving media landscape introduces both challenges and opportunities for using communication to manage extreme events and hazardous contexts.

Risk and Health Communication in an Evolving Media Environment addresses issues of risk and health communication with a collection of chapters that reflect state-of-the-art discussion by top scholars in the field. The authors in this volume develop unique and insightful perspectives by employing the best available research on topics such as brand awareness in healthcare communication, occupational safety, climate change communication, local broadcasts of weather emergencies, terrorism, and the Ebola outbreak, among many other areas. It features analysis of new and traditional media that connects disasters, crises, risks, and public policy issues into a coherent fabric. This book bridges a substantial, but sometimes disconnected body of literature, and by doing so asks how contexts related to risk and health communication are best approached, how researchers balance scientific findings with cultural issues, and how scholars study an increasingly media-savvy society with traditional research methods.

H. Dan O'Hair is Dean of the College of Communication and Information and Professor of Communication at the University of Kentucky. He received his PhD in communication from the University of Oklahoma. In 2006, he served as the president of the National Communication Association, the world's largest and oldest professional association devoted to the study of communication. He has published over 100 research articles and scholarly chapters in risk and health communication, media management, and psychology journals and volumes, and has authored and edited 18 books in the areas of communication, risk management, health, and terrorism. He has been the principal investigator or Co-PI for several grants from business, nonprofit, and government institutions totaling more than $11 million. O'Hair has served on the editorial boards of over 30 research journals and is a past editor of the *Journal of Applied Communication Research*. In April 2013, he was honored by the Broadcast Education Association with their Lifetime Achievement Award for Scholarship.

ELECTRONIC MEDIA RESEARCH SERIES
Sponsored by the Broadcast Education Association
Robert K. Avery and Donald G. Godfrey, Series Editors

MEDIA MANAGEMENT AND ECONOMICS RESEARCH IN A
TRANSMEDIA ENVIRONMENT
Edited by Alan B. Albarran

MEDIA AND THE MORAL MIND
Edited by Ron Tamborini

MEDIA AND SOCIAL LIFE
Edited by Mary Beth Oliver, Arthur A. Raney

DIGITAL TECHNOLOGY AND THE FUTURE
OF BROADCASTING
Edited by John V. Pavlik

RACE AND GENDER IN ELECTRONIC MEDIA:
CONTENT, CONTEXT, CULTURE
Edited by Rebecca Ann Lind

RISK AND HEALTH COMMUNICATION IN AN EVOLVING MEDIA ENVIRONMENT

Edited by
H. Dan O'Hair

Assistant Editors
Heather Chapman
Megan Sizemore

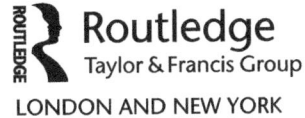

Routledge
Taylor & Francis Group

LONDON AND NEW YORK

First published 2018 by Routledge

2 Park Square, Milton Park, Abingdon, Oxon OX14 4RN
605 Third Avenue, New York, NY 10017

Routledge is an imprint of the Taylor & Francis Group, an informa business

First issued in paperback 2021

Publisher's Note

The publisher has gone to great lengths to ensure the quality of this reprint but points out that some imperfections in the original copies may be apparent.

Library of Congress Cataloging in Publication Data
Names: O'Hair, Dan, editor.
Title: Risk and health communication in an evolving media environment / [edited by] H. Dan O'Hair.
Description: New York : Routledge, 2018. | Series: Electronic media research series
Identifiers: LCCN 2017037145 | ISBN 9781138050273 (hardback)
Subjects: LCSH: Communication in crisis management. | Communication in medicine. | Crisis management.
Classification: LCC RA423.2 .R445 2018 | DDC 610—dc23
LC record available at https://lccn.loc.gov/2017037145

ISBN: 978-1-138-05027-3 (hbk)
ISBN: 978-1-03-217881-3 (pbk)
DOI: 10.1201/9781315168821

Typeset in Sabon
by Swales & Willis Ltd, Exeter, Devon, UK

CONTENTS

CONTENTS

CONTENTS

ACKNOWLEDGMENTS

The symposium director and book editor would like to thank the following people for their help in making this process competitive, productive, and scholarly. First, Robert Avery, who served as the chair of BEA's Research Committee when this idea was launched, was both visionary and conscientious as he worked to secure a strong program of research for the symposium. Louise Benjamin carried on the work of the committee after Robert's tenure as chair with professionalism and enthusiasm for the project. Linda Bathgate, Ross Wagenhofer, and Nicole Salazar, editors for Routledge, were superb in providing timely information about the book's publishing deadlines and handling contracts with the editor and authors. Megan Sizemore served as Associate Director of the Research Symposiums and as an editorial assistant for the book. Also serving as editorial assistant and copy editor was Heather Chapman.

CONTRIBUTORS

Jordan Alpert received his PhD in Communication from George Mason University and shortly thereafter completed his postdoctoral training in behavioral and health services cancer control research in the National Cancer Institute R25 training program at Virginia Commonwealth University School of Medicine. He is currently an assistant professor at the University of Florida in the Department of Advertising, College of Journalism and Communications.

Paula K. Baldwin is an associate professor of Communication at Western Oregon University in Monmouth, Oregon. Her current research focuses on the interpersonal challenges in a variety of communication contexts including nonverbal communication and disabilities, and end of life communication. At Western, she facilitates Death Cafes for students, staff, and faculty to further discussion around end of life issues. Paula is the new Managing Editor for Western's undergraduate journal, PURE Insights as well as being a founding board member for Western's student and community food pantry. At Western, she teaches courses in interpersonal, health, nonverbal, family, relational, small group, end of life, and dark side communication. Paula has authored over 20 peer-reviewed publications and presented over 40 conference papers.

Shannon A. Bowen is an elected member of the Board of Trustees of the Arthur W. Page Society, and sits on the Board of Directors of the International Public Relations Research Conference. Until 2012, Shannon Bowen was tenured in the S. I. Newhouse School of Public Communications at Syracuse University, but was happy to return home to South Carolina. Her PhD is from the University of Maryland; her dissertation on Kantian ethics won the Robert Heath Outstanding Dissertation Award. Her master's degree is from the University of South Carolina (so she is a double Gamecock), and her bachelor's degree is from the University of North Carolina at Chapel Hill.

Michael D. Bruce is an associate professor teaching sports broadcasting in the Department of Journalism and Creative Media. His scholarship is a mix of creative activity and research. Bruce's research focuses on risk and crisis communication with an emphasis on terrorism, conflict and violence, health, and natural disasters. Prior to coming to UA, he taught courses in communication, advertising, broadcasting, and sports media for 13 years at his alma mater, Oklahoma Baptist University. His professional experience includes various video/television production positions at television stations, corporate communications, and in sports media.

Katheryn Christy is a postdoctoral research associate, University of Utah.

Chandra Clark is an assistant professor at the University of Alabama in the Department of Journalism and Creative Media. She teaches electronic news and new media marketing classes. Chandra started in a television station when she was 16 years old as a volunteer and her passion for broadcast journalism has developed following a career as a senior producer at the ABC affiliate in Birmingham, a freelance producer, and a broadcast media marketing specialist for the University of Alabama. Chandra has produced a series of award-winning videos relating to how broadcast television and radio played a role in the deadly April and May 2011 tornadoes in Tuscaloosa and Joplin plus Hurricane Sandy's devastation along the East Coast. Chandra believes in learning in action and enjoys working with nonprofits, companies, cities, and community leaders in Central Alabama. She and her students have helped more than 40 clients learn to take control of their message and use traditional and social media to help brand themselves better to the community.

Ligia Cohen received her MA in Communication degree from George Mason University in 2012. After serving in the U.S. Navy as a Public Affairs Officer in a variety of assignments around the world for 20 years, she retired and founded VetSPARK Energy, a minority and veteran-owned company dedicated to solving our nation's energy security challenges by expanding access to clean solar energy. Cohen also holds an MA early education from Old Dominion University and BS in Mass Communication from the University Externate of Bogota, Colombia. She is an active advocate for veterans and the environment. She can be reached at li.cohen@vetSPARK.net

Kaylee Crossley has experience in public health and health promotion, with a particular interest in oral health education. She has partnered with the Oral Health Program at the Utah Department of Health on several projects to better meet the oral health needs of residents in

Utah. She will be pursuing her doctorate degree in the communication program at the University of Utah in the fall of 2017.

Laura Crosswell is an assistant professor of health communication at the University of Nevada, Reno. She holds a joint appointment with the Reynolds School of Journalism and the University of Nevada, Reno School of Medicine. Crosswell also serves as the assistant director of the Center for Advanced Media Studies at the Reynolds School. Her research focuses on the cultural implications of consumerism and persuasive texts, as well as the physiological and psychosocial influences of media content. Specifically, she concentrates on the politicized and commercialized mechanisms of public health messaging. Much of her work highlights the shifting nature of health communication and new messaging models in the digital age. Crosswell earned her doctorate in media and public affairs from the Manship School of Mass Communication at Louisiana State University. She has a master's degree in communication from the College of Charleston and a bachelor's degree in communication and media studies from Clemson University.

Thomas R. Cunningham is a behavioral scientist and the Chief of the NIOSH Training Research and Evaluation Branch in the Education and Information Division. He also coordinates the NIOSH Small Business Assistance Program and Translation Research Program. His research addresses intervention development and research translation for safety and health applications in construction, health care, and several small business sectors. He received his MS and PhD in clinical psychology from Virginia Tech.

Lifeng Deng is an associate professor of communication with the School of Communication and Design at Sun Yat-sen University, Guangzhou, China. His research interests include science communication, risk governance, and communication in China. He has published several research papers on nuclear science communication, trust and distrust in risk communication, and a book, *Competing Voices? Deconstructing the Mechanism of Corporate Public Relations' Impacts on News Production* (Communication University of China Press, 2014).

Lindsay L. Dillingham (PhD, University of Kentucky, 2014) is an assistant professor of marketing in the College of Business at Lipscomb University in Nashville, Tennessee. Her research foci include social influence, resistance to persuasion, and risk and crisis communication.

Laura C. Farrell, PhD, is president and founder of Unbridled Communication Research Inc., a 501(c)3 that studies human communication through interaction with horses. She also currently works as a special service associate at Home Depot. Farrell previously served as an Assistant Professor at Longwood University where she directed the undergraduate senior theses, taught a variety of public relations, media, theory, and research courses, and helped mold citizen leaders. She served under Robert Littlefield as Assistant Editor for the regional journal, Communication Studies, an opportunity that emerged during her graduate career at North Dakota State University. It was at NDSU that Farrell developed her strong passion and research foundation in media, interpersonal/relational communication, health communication, and crisis/risk communication, which she complimented with professional experience in broadcast, journalism, public relations, marketing, finance, and equine science.

Christy L. Forrester is a health scientist in the NIOSH Research to Practice Office (r2p). She leads the NIOSH r2p team in developing and adapting innovative strategies and solutions to bridge gaps in the translation of research findings into practical use to improve the safety and health of workers. Her research interests include organizational and risk communication, as well as the role partnerships play in the successful transfer of research into effective workplace safety and health policy and practice. She received her BA in psychology and MS in epidemiology from the University of Cincinnati, and is currently completing her doctorate in communication at George Mason University.

Morgan Getchell, PhD, is an assistant professor of strategic communication and convergent media at Morehead State University in Morehead, Kentucky. Getchell recently completed her PhD at the University of Kentucky where she focused her scholarship on the areas of risk and crisis communication. Her dissertation, which examined emergent organizations in the 2014 West Virginia water contamination crisis, was funded by a grant from the National Center for Food Protection and Defense, a Department of Homeland Security center of excellence. She has also worked on funded projects through the Centers for Disease Control and Prevention and the United States Department of Agriculture. Her research is published in several refereed journals and has been presented at regional, national, and international conferences.

Michel M. Haigh, Texas State University (PhD, University of Oklahoma) is a professor in the School of Journalism and Mass Communication at Texas State University. She spent 11 years working in the Donald P. Bellisario College of Communications at Penn State before joining the faculty at Texas State. Haigh has taught public relations writing, campaign, and research methods courses. Haigh has more than six years as a public relations writer, editor, and designer. She has co-authored more than 40 conference presentations, seven of which have been recognized with a "Top Paper" award. She has published more than 35 articles in journals such as *Journalism & Mass Communication Quarterly*, *Journal of Broadcasting & Electronic Media*, *Communication Monographs*, *Communication Research*, *Journal of Social and Personal Relationships*, *Newspaper Research Journal*, *Corporate Communications: An International Journal*, and *Communication Quarterly*. The author would like to thank Kaylen Chung, Yiling Feng, Sarah Kim, Brooke Koller, and Melissa Payne, undergraduates in the Donald P. Bellisario College of Communications at Penn State when this study was conducted, for their assistance in coding. Coders were compensated thanks to an Undergraduate Research Fund grant. Thanks to the Arthur W. Page Center for Integrity in Public Communication for funding the travel to the 2016 Broadcast Education Association's annual conference to present the study.

Michael Hecht is interested in the theory and practice of health, intercultural, and interpersonal communication. His work has produced new theoretical approaches, such as the Communication Theory of Identity and the Principal of Cultural Grounding. He has also been involved in many different community-based research programs and collaborations on drug abuse intervention, crime prevention, and mental health support. Michael Hecht has taught courses on interpersonal communication, interpersonal communication theory, and nonverbal communication. He has won numerous awards, including the Gerald R. Philips Award for Distinguished Applied Communication Scholarship, two Distinguished Scholarship Awards for the International and Intercultural Division of the National Communication Association, and the Article of the Year Award for SIETAR.

Erin Hester provides health communication expertise for the Obesity Prevention Program with the Kentucky Department for Public Health. She specializes in developing meaningful communication strategies for behavior change, interpreting complex health information and reframing messages that promote health equity in the areas of obesity and chronic disease prevention. Her background in public health communication campaigns has been applied to numerous statewide nutrition and physical activity efforts, including 5-2-1-0 Healthy Numbers for Kentucky Families and Step It Up, Kentucky! Hester holds a master's degree in communication from the University of Kentucky and a bachelor's degree in psychology from Wittenberg University.

Douglas Blanks Hindman is Chair of the Journalism and Media Production Department in the Edward R. Murrow College of Communication.

He teaches News and Society, New Communication Technologies, and Media, Social Control, and Social Change. Hindman conducts research on social structural impacts on news content, news organizations, news distribution, and news production. Recent work focuses on belief gaps, which are widening differences in beliefs about verifiable knowledge among groups with different political or social identities that result primarily from misinformation propagated by political elites.

Scott Hodgson is a professor at the University of Oklahoma at the Gaylord College of Journalism and Mass Communication. He is a producer/director and also began teaching after being invited to teach for one semester. He says, "Creating media with a message is my passion. Making a difference is my mission. Working with students is my joy. For over 30 years I served dual roles as both a producer/director and an educator. Since 2006 I have been at the University of Oklahoma where I teach video production and run a contract unit called Gaylord Hall Productions."

Bobi Ivanov (PhD, University of Oklahoma) is Associate Dean for Graduate Programs in Communication and Professor of Integrated Strategic Communication in the Department of Integrated Strategic Communication at the University of Kentucky. He studies strategic message design, consumer behavior, and strategic communications. He has primarily taught marketing, communication, research, and strategic communication related courses in a number of different departments/units. His main research interests concern social influence (persuasion and resistance) and message design, processing, and retention. Ivanov's theoretical work focuses on the study of inoculation theory, images, and attitudes and their composition, hierarchical structure, and function as applied in various contexts including commercial, health, inter-cultural, instructional/educational, interpersonal, political, and risk/crisis management. His scholarship has appeared in numerous presentations (five top paper awards), books, book chapters, and journal publications such as *Communication Monographs*, *Communication Research*, *Human Communication Research*, *the International Journal of the Image*, *Communication Reports*, *Journal of Communication*, *Iowa Journal of Communication*, *The Global Studies Journal*, *Health Communication*, *Journal of Public Relations Research*, *Western Journal of Communication*, *Communication Yearbook*, *Journal of Applied Communication Research*, *Central Business Review*, *Communication Research Reports*, and *Atlantic Marketing Journal*, among others.

Jakob D. Jensen is an expert in health communication. His research focuses on the strategic communication of health information to the public, with a special focus on cancer. He routinely works with public health departments to design and evaluate their campaigns, interventions, and programs. Most recently, he has worked with the Utah Department of Health on the design and evaluation of colorectal and breast cancer screening campaigns.

Barry A. Klinger is an associate professor in the Atmospheric, Oceanic, and Earth Sciences Department at George Mason University. He studies large-scale ocean circulation and its impact on climate, and is interested in science communication and the global warming debate.

John Kotcher is a research assistant professor in the Center for Climate Change Communication at George Mason University. His research explores ways to reduce political polarization and increase public engagement with climate change.

Melinda Krakow is a public health communication researcher currently serving as a postdoctoral cancer prevention fellow at the National Cancer Institute, investigating social and behavioral aspects of population-based cancer prevention. She completed her doctorate in the Department of Communication at the University of Utah (PhD, May 2015), where she worked on a variety of projects with the Health Communication and Technology (HCAT) research lab led by Jakob D. Jensen.

Gary L. Kreps is a University Distinguished Professor and Director of the Center for Health and Risk Communication in the Department of Communication at George Mason University. His research examines dissemination of relevant health information in society, especially to vulnerable populations. He teaches undergraduate and graduate courses in communication research, health communication, risk communication, communication campaigns, and e-health communication. He received his BA and his MA in Communication from the University of Colorado, Boulder, and his PhD from the University of Southern California. Prior to joining the faculty at GMU he served as Chief of the Health Communication and Informatics Research Branch at the National Cancer Institute, where he introduced major national health communication research initiatives, such as the Health Information National Trends Survey (HINTS) and the Centers of Excellence in Cancer Communication Research. He recently launched the HINTS-China research program and is working to establish HINTS-Germany. His work is reported in more than 400 widely cited books, articles, and chapters.

Jo-Yun Li is a doctoral student in the School of Journalism and Mass Communications at the University of South Carolina. She is also currently enrolled in the Certificate of Graduate Study in Health Communication. She is a former journalist for an ethnic news media, covering politics and health news in New York City. It was her prior professional experience in one of the most diverse places in the world that inspired her research. Li's primary research interest is health communication in diverse populations. One aspect of her research focus is about how mass communication can be used to promote beneficial changes in behavior among members of different populations.

Robert Littlefield is Professor and Director of the Nicholson School of Communication. Formerly a professor of communication at North Dakota State University, Littlefield is the author or co-author of over 85 refereed publications and several books, receiving recognition from state, regional, and national organizations for his scholarly activity. His recent co-edited book, *Risk and Crisis Communication: Navigating the Tensions Between Organizations and the Public*, reflects his current focus on identifying the micro-processes at work when decision-makers are faced with a risk or crisis situation and must determine how best to develop and respond to prevent or mitigate the situation.

Kevin J. Macy-Ayotte received his PhD in rhetoric and communication from the University of Pittsburgh in 2003 and is currently a professor of communication at California State University, Fresno. Although his research interests range from classical Greek rhetoric to post-structuralist rhetorical criticism, Macy-Ayotte's primary area of inquiry involves the examination of language and power in public argumentation concerning international security threats and foreign policy intended to address those threats. His recent work explores the ways in which government and media discourses about terrorism and weapons of mass destruction shape public understanding of these problems and support for various counter-terrorism and counter-proliferation policies. He has published articles in journals such as *The Quarterly Journal of Speech*, *Rhetoric Society Quarterly*, and *Argumentation and Advocacy*; he is a co-editor of the book, *Terrorism: Communication and Rhetorical Perspectives*.

Edward W. Maibach is a university professor at George Mason University, and director of Mason's Center for Climate Change Communication. Ed's research—funded by NSF, NASA, and private foundations—focuses on public engagement in climate change. Ed co-chaired the Engagement & Communication Working Group for the third National Climate Assessment. He earned his PhD in communication science at Stanford University and his MPH at San Diego State University, and has previously served as associate director of the National Cancer Institute, worldwide director of social marketing at Porter Novelli, and board chairman for Kidsave International.

Michelle Miller-Day (PhD, Arizona State University) is a professor of communication studies at Chapman University in Orange, California. Prior to joining Chapman in the fall of 2012, Miller-Day occupied a faculty position at Penn State University at University Park as an associate professor of communication arts and sciences and biobehavioral health and faculty affiliate with the Penn State Center for Health Care and Policy Research.

H. Dan O'Hair is Dean of the College of Communication and Information and Professor of Communication at the University of Kentucky. In 2006, he served as the president of the National Communication Association. He has published over 90 research articles and scholarly chapters in risk and health communication journals and volumes, and has authored and edited 18 books in the areas of communication, risk management, health, and terrorism. O'Hair has served on the editorial boards of over 30 research journals and is a past editor of the *Journal of Applied Communication Research*. In 2013, he was honored by the Broadcast Education Association with their Lifetime Achievement Award for Scholarship.

Kimberly A. Parker (PhD, 2004, University of Oklahoma) is an associate professor in the College of Communication and Information. Parker has over 20 years' experience working with nonprofits in the area of social change campaigns. Kimberly's research has appeared in *Communication Monographs, Journal of Communication, Human Communication Research, Journal of Public Relations Research, Communication Quarterly, Communication Research Reports*, and *Health Communication*.

Lance Porter, with more than 19 years of marketing experience, has focused on digital media since 1995, when he built his first commercial website. Before coming to LSU, Porter spent four years as executive director of Internet marketing for Disney. There he oversaw the creative and media strategies for more than 80 films and won a Clio Award for excellence in advertising. He currently teaches advertising creative strategy and campaigns. His research focuses on digital media effects. He holds a joint appointment with the Center for Computation and Technology (CCT). He won the 2009 LSU Alumni Faculty Excellence

Award and was the 2010 American Advertising Federation Donald G. Hileman Memorial Educator of the Year in the seventh district.

Chelsea L. Ratcliff is a graduate student in the Department of Communication at University of Utah. Her research interests include cancer communication, message effects, news coverage of health/medical research, and ethical issues in health and risk communication. Ratcliff worked as a health journalist prior to graduate school and was a contributor to major national health news outlets.

Deborah Sellnow-Richmond is an assistant professor in the Department of Communication at Columbus State University where she teaches courses in the public relations track. She researches the efficacy and unforeseen effects of public relations messages in health and organizational crisis context, and the emerging role of social media in creating and resolving organizational crises. Her research appears in a number of communication journals including the *Journal of Applied Communication, the Journal of Risk Research*, and *Communication Studies*. Debbie holds a PhD in communication from Wayne State University in Detroit, Michigan, a master's degree in public service from the University of Arkansas Clinton School of Public Service, and a bachelor's degree from the University of Minnesota. She has conducted community-centered campaigns at the state, national, and international levels.

Katherine E. Rowan is a professor of communication at George Mason University in Fairfax, Virginia. Her research concerns the challenges of earning trust and explaining complexities in risk and crisis communication contexts. At Mason, she teaches courses in public relations, science communication, risk communication, and crisis communication. She has authored or edited over 70 scholarly and governmental publications. A Fellow of the American Association for the Advancement of Science, her work has been funded by the National Science Foundation and Virginia Sea Grant. She directs Mason's graduate certificate program in science communication.

Meghan Sanders is an associate professor in the Manship School of Mass Communication at Louisiana State University. Her research focuses on the psychological effects of mass media, as they pertain to psychological and subjective well-being, and enjoyment and appreciation of entertainment. Her work has been published in journals such as *Communication Theory, Mass Communication and Society*, and *Psychology of Popular Media Culture*, and she has presented at national and international conferences including the National Communication Association, the Broadcast Education Association, and the International Communication Association. Sanders also serves as director of the Media Effects Lab where she educates and trains undergraduate and graduate students and faculty on the theory and technology behind some of the most cutting-edge media effects measures (i.e. reaction time, skin conductance, eye tracking, etc.). From 2008 to 2012, she served as the associate dean for research and strategic planning for the Manship School. In this position, she promoted, fostered, and assisted with extramural funding for faculty research and teaching while providing oversight to the school's research professorship program. Sanders managed the unit's role in the university's SACSCOC reaccreditation process and the reaccreditation of the unit by the Accrediting Council of Education in Journalism and Mass Communication. Sanders continues to direct the Scripps Howard Academic Leadership Academy—a program aimed at mentoring new and would-be administrators by providing four days of leadership training and professional networking. She earned her undergraduate degree in mass communication at Dillard University, her master's degree in media studies from the Pennsylvania State University, and her doctorate in mass communication from the Pennsylvania State University.

Juliann C. Scholl is Health Communication Fellow and Co-Director of the National Center for Productive Aging and Work (NCPAW) within NIOSH. In addition to co-directing NCPAW, Scholl conducts translation research with an emphasis on the reduction of musculoskeletal disorders among workers of different age groups. She also examines workplace intergenerational tensions and does survey research in assessing stakeholder satisfaction and impact. She received her MA (University of Alabama) and PhD (University of Oklahoma) in Communication Studies.

Matthew Seeger (PhD, 1982, Indiana University) is Dean of the College of Fine, Performing, and Communication Arts and a professor of communication. Seeger's research interests concern crisis and risk communication, crisis response and agency coordination, health communication, the role of media in crisis, crisis and communication ethics, failure of complex systems, and post-crisis renewal. He has worked closely with the United States Centers for Disease Control and Prevention on communication and anthrax attack and on pandemic influenza preparedness. He is also an affiliate of the World Health Organization. Seeger has also worked with issues of food and water safety, including with the Flint, Michigan water crisis. His recent book is *Narratives of Crisis: Telling Stories of Ruin and Renewal* (Stanford University Press, 2016).

Timothy Sellnow joined the University of Central Florida in 2015 as professor at the Nicholson School of Communication. Sellnow's research focuses on bioterrorism, pre-crisis planning, and strategic communication for risk management and mitigation in organizational and health settings. He has conducted funded research for the Department of Homeland Security, the United States Department of Agriculture, the Centers for Disease Control and Prevention, the Environmental Protection Agency, and the United States Geological Survey. He has also served in an advisory role for the National Academy of Sciences and the World Health Organization. He has published numerous refereed journal articles on risk and crisis communication and has co-authored five books on risk and crisis communication. Sellnow's most recent book is entitled *Theorizing Crisis Communication.*

YoungJu Shin is an assistant professor in the Hugh Downs School of Human Communication at Arizona State University. In 2012, she received her PhD in Health Communication from Pennsylvania State University. Some of her academic interests are health communication, youth substance use prevention, intervention, and family communication.

Zixue Tai is an associate professor in the School of Journalism and Media at the University of Kentucky. His primary area of research pertains to the social, political, and cultural ramifications of the new media sector in China.

Jagadish Thaker is a senior lecturer at the School of Communication, Journalism and Marketing at Massey University, New Zealand. His research examines ways to understand and enhance vulnerable communities' adaptive capacity to climate change impacts, and he specializes in the fields of science and climate change communication, health communication, and strategic communication campaigns.

Candice Tresch has been a public affairs officer with the US Navy since 2007, and a military officer since 2002. Her passion is centered in helping people find their voice to stimulate positive change in their lives and organizations. Grounded in military and government communication, she is experienced in sharing how the few can connect with the many. Candice holds an MA in Communication from George Mason University.

Janey Trowbridge received her PhD in Communication from George Mason University where she was a presidential research fellow, instructor, and postgraduate research associate. Her research, reflected in published articles and book chapters and conference presentations, focuses on the application of strategic communication in environmental conflict management and public health. Recently she was a lecturer in the McCoy College of Business and Communication Studies Department at Texas State University in San Marcos.

Donna M. Van Bogaert is a researcher and consultant in the field of cognitive styles, health communication, and organizational communication and behavior. Her business, Van Bogaert & Associates, Inc., specializes in cognitive-based coaching, management consulting, and leadership development. She leads the Information Resources and Dissemination Branch of the Education Information Dissemination Division at the National Institute for Occupational Safety and Health.

Jenell Walsh-Thomas holds an MS in earth systems science and a PhD in environmental science and public policy, both from George Mason University, Fairfax, Virginia. She graduated with her PhD in 2016, and was selected for a 2017 Mirzayan Science and Technology Policy Graduate Fellowship at the National Academies of Sciences, Engineering, and Medicine and assigned to work with the Board on Environmental Change and Society. During her doctoral studies, Jenell coordinated the Center for Climate Change Communication and the National Park Service Partnership where she mentored undergraduates as well as graduate student interns in developing a variety of informative climate change communication materials for park staff and visitors.

Ruoxu Wang is an assistant professor at the University of Memphis. Her research focuses on the intersection of media effects and persuasion under the context of communication technology and strategic communication. Her research has been published in peer-reviewed journals such as *Journal of Interactive Advertising, Computers in Human Behavior, Telematics and Informatics, Social Media + Society, Mass Communication and Society*, and *American Behavioral Scientist*. Wang holds a PhD from Penn State University (2017) and an MS from North Dakota State University (2013).

Greg Williams (MA, Southern Illinois University Edwardsville) is currently a data coordinator in the Department of Surgery at Washington University in St. Louis. His research interests include clinical outcomes, patient education, and health communication. His work has appeared in Journal of the American College of Surgeons, Health Communication, and Communication Studies. Mr. Williams forthcoming work focuses on improving outcomes among patients with hepatobiliary and pancreatic cancer.

H. Joe Witte is an outreach specialist (Climate Science) at Aquent/JPL-NASA, Pasadena, California. After 4 decades as a network and local TV meteorologist (MS, University of Washington), Joe switched careers, acquired an MA from George Mason University in communication, emphasizing science communication, and now works on climate science outreach to the 2,000 TV meteorologists in the United States. He produces short visual science stories for use on television and in social media.

Chelsea Woods (PhD, University of Kentucky) is an assistant professor in the Department of Communication at Virginia Tech where she teaches public relations. Her research interests include strategic crisis management, post-crisis discourse, issues management, and anti-corporate activism. She has assisted on projects funded by the Center for Risk and Economic Analysis of Terrorism Events (CREATE) and the National Science Foundation. Her research has presented at national and international conferences and published in several journals.

Nan Yu is an associate professor at University of Central Florida. Her research focuses on health communication and communication technology with an emphasis on health promotion using digital technologies. Yu currently serves as the associate editor of *Asian Journal of Communication*. Her research has been published in premier peer-reviewed journals such as *Health Communication, Information Sciences, International Journal of Human-Computer Studies*, and *Journal of Immigrant and Minority Health*. Yu holds a PhD from Penn State University (2009) and an MS from Ohio University (2005).

Zhian Zhang is a professor and Dean of the School of Communication and Design, and Deputy Director of the Institute of Research on National Governance, and Deputy Director of the Institute of Hong Kong and Macau Studies, at Sun Yat-sen University, Guangzhou, China. He also serves on the advisory board on China's State Council Information Office. His main area of expertise is sociology of news.

Part I

ADVANCES IN HEALTH COMMUNICATION RESEARCH

1

PRELUDE

Advancing Media Research in Risk and Health Communication Contexts

H. Dan O'Hair

Disease outbreaks, terrorist acts, and natural disasters are obvious examples of contexts in which risk and health communication play a critical role. Broadcast media have found risk and health crisis events to be particularly seductive as stories that fascinate their audiences. Moreover, with digital media evolving at such a rapid rate, many audience members have taken on the role of newsmaker or reporter (Kim, Brossard, Scheufele, & Xenos, 2016)—we are not entirely certain to what effect. Digital media has proven to serve many useful functions such as operating as a conduit for warnings to the public and acting as a gauge for how messages are received and acted upon (Fraustino & Ma, 2015). On top of these dynamic conditions, many in the risk and health communication research communities find extreme events and hazardous contexts to be on the increase, and an evolving media landscape introduces both challenges and opportunities for using communication to manage these situations.

This book will address these issues as well as the research implications inherent in risk and health communication contexts. For example, how are these contexts best approached—inductively or deductively? How do researchers balance scientific finding with social and cultural issues? To what extent can media (legacy and digital) play a role in mitigating the effects of risk and adverse health events? How are potential ethical repercussions of communication disentangled from unfolding and unpredictable events? How do we study an increasingly media-savvy society with traditional research methods?

This book features chapters with leading-edge discussion by authors who offer the best available thinking and analysis on the topics of risk and health communication. To do so, the authors have selected the most salient issues associated with these contexts. Each chapter isolates a particular issue or concern and peels away the surface to expose the difficult choices and subsequent processes facing participants in the communication of risks and health issues. In addition, this book will feature analyses of new and traditional media that connect disasters, crises, risks, and public policy issues into a coherent fabric.

How the Book Evolved

The research committee of the Broadcast Education Association approached the editor about developing one of the annual research symposiums that is held in conjunction with the annual convention. Routledge has been an important and consistent partner in publishing essays from the symposium. A review team was recruited and empaneled to help the symposium director (and the book's editor) make competitive selections to appear at the convention. Approximately 80 percent of the essays presented at BEA were invited to be part of the book, and additional chapters were commissioned by the editor from known scholars in the areas of risk and health communication.

The unique perspectives of each author was invaluable in characterizing these contexts and their accompanying challenges. Each chapter represents the best available research in these areas with insightful notions of where current research and best practices should move in the future. In most chapters, original research findings are offered from ongoing research programs. In others, original models and frameworks are presented, capturing a wide array of constituent elements of complex processes and casting them into discernable designs worthy of consideration by researchers, practitioners, and policy makers.

To ensure that the aforementioned goals were met and that the book presents a consistent feel throughout the chapters, each author was asked to adhere to suggestions for conceptualizing and organizing chapter contents. Exceptions and modifications were attended to on an individual basis, but in general authors were asked to address the following issues in their chapters.

- What is the best available media research in risk and health communication?
- What communication and media theories are most relevant and applicable in this context?
- What new ideas are offered in this area (framework, model, theory)?
- What are specific research directions that should be pursued for this context of risk and health communication research?
- What pragmatic implications can you offer practitioners in this area of risk and health communication?

Thus, the importance of this work is its ability to bring together the best minds on the topics of risk and health communication. These are vital topics that each merit the treatment that is typical of scholarly books. For several years, scholarly books have been one of the featured ways in which academics collect and organize chapters by leading scholars. These works help to establish milestones and may even serve as benchmarks for the development of literature in specific sub-disciplines.

We hope this work will be a capstone for current work in risk and health communication, and serve as a text for an increasing number of undergraduate and graduate courses in crisis communication. It can foster additional interest in risk communication and offer connections between health communication and others engaged in discussing risk and crisis. This book would bridge a substantial but sometimes disconnected body of literature.

Each chapter was reviewed with the following issues in mind.

- Theoretical Grounding (sufficient, appropriate)?
- Risk/Health (significant issue/problem)?
- Connection to "an Evolving Media Environment"?
- Practical and Impactful Implications?
- Theoretical Implications (going forward)?
- Future Directions?
- Unique Contribution to Media Research?

Risk and Health Communication in an Evolving Media Environment is intended for multiple audiences, although each overlap to a large extent. The primary audience is one quite familiar to scholarly publishers and academic researchers. The book should attract interest among those communication scholars and researchers focusing on media and communication, but also those with specialties in particular aspects of disasters, risk, and crisis addressed in one of the chapters. In addition, it is expected that graduate seminars in risk communication, crisis management, policy management, and even political science will find *Risk and Health Communication in an Evolving Media Environment* attractive as a primary or secondary text. A third audience is likely to be found in main campus libraries and public libraries as well as libraries situated at health sciences centers. By involving multiple disciplines, it is expected that a large audience for the volume will be realized.

This volume will follow in the footsteps of other applied scholarly books that have become a vital part of the academic and professional contributions of the communication disciplines. These volumes not only offer the opportunity to capture the best thinking on a well-defined topic, but they have been extremely influential in sparking subsequent discussion and fostering the relevant research agendas. Their individual and collective impact on the field is inestimable.

Introduction to the Chapters

In the following paragraphs, O'Hair sets the stage for the remaining theory and research presentations by previewing the content of the chapters in the sections to follow. In Part I: Advances in Health Communication Research, four chapters address contexts that are both new and problematic for media professionals.

In Chapter 2, Shin, Miller-Day, and Hecht focus on how alcohol is handled in the media. "Media Literacy and Parent–Adolescent Communication About Alcohol in Media: Effects on Adolescent Alcohol Use" characterizes how media literacy and parent-adolescent communication can affect how young people interpret media portrayals of alcohol use. These effects lead to reports of lower lifetime use of alcohol. The study offers important implications for how messages among family members can influence key behavioral decision-making in essential life choices.

In Chapter 3, Hindman discusses legalized marijuana and unravels the uncertainty often associated with various users. In his chapter, "College Students and Legalized Marijuana: Knowledge Gaps and Belief Gaps Regarding the Law and Health Effects," Hindman builds theoretical scaffolding from the knowledge gap hypothesis and his own work—termed the belief gap hypothesis—in order to test claims about how students (potential users of marijuana) may be affected in their thinking and knowledge about the health effects of using marijuana during the initial phases following the legalization of marijuana in Washington state. Social media and an evolving media environment play a role in how social media portrayals are linked with social identity expression and potential and the use of marijuana.

The fourth chapter, authored by Crosswell, Porter, and Sanders, "Out of Sight, Out of Mind? Addressing Unconscious Brand Awareness in Healthcare Communication," approaches the context of pharmaceutical advertising as a means of shedding light on the visual elements used during message campaigns by pharmaceutical companies. By focusing on how potential consumers perceive the prominence of branding and how it is used to promote awareness of the message, the authors discover that study participants who fixated more on the visual elements of branding had more skeptical views of the communication campaign. Importantly, the idea of "unconscious awareness" was introduced as a critical variable to be considered in future work of this kind, particularly as researchers attempt to make sense of the divide between conscious versus unconscious brand awareness in communication campaigns.

Tai, Zhang, and Deng wrap up Part I with their chapter, which focuses on a national context. In "Communicating Health-Related Risk and Crisis in China: State of the Field and Ways Forward," the authors provide a critique to the image of China as a country with unparalleled growth and prosperity for the past 30 years. Attendant to these changes are the presence of natural disasters and hazards, environmental degradation such as water and air pollution and the depletion of natural resources that bring diseases, significant risk, and health issues. This chapter, different from those in this section or elsewhere in the book, first describes an overview of the field of risk communication in China and offers some paths moving forward. In subsequent sections, Tai et al. illuminate many of the challenges facing risk and health communication, in particular nuclear power. Their proposed general strategy for risk and health communication management involves an integrated approach melding research and perspectives from the natural and general sciences, government administrators, and the general public.

In Part II: Communicating and Educating the Public and Media About Risk and Science, four chapters take up issues dealing directly with how messages are formed, crafted, conveyed, and then evaluated for public use. In the first chapter of this section, Scholl, Bogaert, Forrester, and Cunningham, approach risk and health communication from focused and pragmatic viewpoints. As scientists from the National Institute for Occupational Safety and Health (NIOSH), the authors marry theory with innovative tactics to offer compelling methods for translating research into practice. In their chapter, "Risk Communication in Occupational Safety and Health: Reaching Diverse Audiences in an Evolving Communication Environment," they forward the argument that the workplace, like many other communicative contexts, is an evolving media home to multiple messages about risks and illnesses perpetrated by chemical and environmental hazards. The chapter takes care to focus attention on the influence of new and emerging media and offers suggestions for how best practices can be developed for use by risk and health communication professionals interested in the occupational safety context.

In the chapter that follows, Rowan and her colleagues present research that explores the influence of television weathercasters on ideas and impressions of climate change. Climate change is presented as a particularly difficult hazard given the slow onset of attendant problems (and contested scientific results). "Best Practices of 'Innovator' TV Metereologists Who Act as Climate Change Educators" extends our understanding of media as a tool for informing viewers about science as it affects our lives through weather and climate. In particular, the authors offer a number of different venues and platforms from which to send climate change messages (e.g., blogs, TV, parks, etc.) that would appeal to targeted audiences.

7

Extending the notion of how media plays a critical part of our education about risk and health, Ratcliff, Jensen, Christy, Crossley, and Krakow discuss how news coverage of serious diseases—in this case cancer—can influence viewership levels of uncertainty that can lead to decision-making about the disease. Their chapter, "News Coverage of Cancer Research: Does Disclosure of Scientific Uncertainty Enhance Credibility?", provides robust findings of the connection between what is presented as scientific news and how viewers are able to generate confidence in that which is reported.

In the last chapter of this section, Kreps and Alpert place emphasis on how online information is assessed in "Evaluating Online Health Information Systems." The authors organize their chapter according to three major evaluation programs: (a) formative evaluation (initial analysis often involving needs assessment and audience analysis); (b) process evaluation (message tracking and assessing user feedback); and (c) summative evaluation (tracking key indicators and costs associated with the ongoing program). The chapter explains how various methods can be used to provide the process for conducting evaluations for the various stages of a communication program or campaign.

In Part III: Situating Theory in Risk and Health Communication Contexts, the book places additional emphases on a number of theoretical frameworks that add clarity to risk and health communication contexts.

Haigh, in her chapter "Examining Print Coverage of the Keystone XL Pipeline: Using the Social Amplification of Risk Framework," investigated the newspaper coverage associated with the famous Keystone Pipeline in the critical period of its development, 2008–2015. Haigh used analytics techniques to determine tone, frame, and depiction of coverage of the two principal players in the environmental controversy: US government agencies and the energy industry. Her work discovered that different frames were used by the media in depicting the crisis, in particular a focus on environmental risk factors instead of spotlighting economic and human factors. Implications from the study offer compelling recommendations for investigating such environmental crises that are portrayed in the media.

In the following chapter, entitled "Terrorism, Risk Communication, and Pluralistic Inquiry," Macy-Ayotte argues for a more nuanced and tolerant approach to studying contexts involving terrorism. Macy-Ayotte challenges other scholars to consider "disciplinary pluralism" where multiple perspectives and disciplines are considered during analyses of risk contexts, especially that of terrorism. Macy-Ayotte asks for more recognition of rhetorical approaches that heretofore have been neglected in many risk analyses.

The authors of the next chapter, Bowen and Li, placed ethics and professionalism front and center during considerations of risk and health messages. In their chapter, entitled "Communication Ethics for Risk,

Crises, and Public Health Contexts," the authors make convincing arguments that ethical communication is a prerequisite for situations where communicators must provide information about circumstances where people are given choices as part of a decision-making context. Their chapter takes up the challenge of evolving media and how communication can take multiple paths. Grounded in three theoretical schools of thought, the authors suggest an integrated framework for decision-making that can be employed to investigate a risk or health problem.

In the final chapter of this section, Ivanov, Parker, and Dillingham explore inoculation theory as a means for understanding risk and health communication contexts. Aptly entitled "Inoculation as a Risk and Health Communication Strategy in an Evolving Media Environment," this chapter melds together two large bodies of work that have generally only existed independently. Specifically, the chapter offers special consideration for how risk and health communication scholars and practitioners can take advantage of the rich history and theoretical background of inoculation-based strategies in service of communication directed to risk and health circumstances.

In Part IV: Exploring Messages and Media During Extreme Events, the book explores the research associated with the challenging issues of communicating before, during, and after extreme events such as tornados, health emergencies, and outbreaks. Bruce, Clark, and Hodgson begin this section by examining the possible effects of weather broadcaster messages on viewers' perceptions, and potential cautionary behavior. The chapter, "First Alert Weather: Local Broadcasters' Communication During Weather Emergencies," takes a close look at the role meteorologists play in educating broadcast viewers about the nuances of severe weather. The authors note that the Federal Communication Commission has required broadcasters to serve their local communities in a forthright way in order to qualify for their license. In recent years, the channels and evolving media available to both broadcasters and their viewers has expanded significantly. Using the CDC's Crisis and Emergency Risk Communication model, the research reported in this chapter interviews broadcasters to determine the strategies they utilize during three severe weather outbreaks (two tornados and one hurricane).

In the following chapter, Yu, Littlefield, Farrell, and Wang explore the 2012 West Nile Outbreak as a context from which to investigate information and decision-making in an extreme event. The chapter, entitled, "It's Not Preventable, Yet You Are Responsible: Media's Risk and Attribution Assessment of the 2012 West Nile Outbreak," creates some interesting tensions that are not easily unpacked in this particular context. The authors present something of a conundrum where the media portrays the West Nile virus as unpreventable while at the same time recommending that individuals and communities take precautions to ward off potential infection. The chapter concludes with a series of practical implications for how the media can cover pandemic disease outbreaks in an evolving media environment.

In the final chapter in this section, Getchel and colleagues present the chapter "Competing and Complimentary Narratives in the Ebola Crisis," where narrative theory is the focus of the contextual analysis within the highly volatile Ebola crisis. Once the authors make the case for the critical importance of narrative theory for risk and health communication situations, they make a convincing argument for the literal competition that different players in the contexts engage in using narratives as the basis for their claims. The multifaceted nature of narratives becomes more problematic during lengthy crises, as possible interpretations become more plentiful. The authors recommend that a narrative convergence process be invoked in order to reduce uncertainty and move to a point of greater understanding for the different viewpoints being advanced.

These chapters paint a unique picture of how risk and health communication is studied in various contexts. One unmistakable trend is how online communities are forming rapidly to address risk and health issues. Increasingly, individuals are influencing one another through social media, and as a result, they are influencing public opinion (Kim et al., 2016). In a general sense, social networking services (SNS) have proven to be useful for improving health behaviors. One of the key reasons for this phenomenon, according to Namkoong, Nah, Record, and Stee (2017), is that online messages create space for participants to contribute personally to the risk and health management processes (especially campaigns). A slightly different perspective is how online health and risk communities rapidly form on the Internet in order to improve the understanding of the disease or the disaster the participants are facing; it gives people a chance to interact with like-minded individuals (Willis & Royne, 2017). A term has even been constructed—cybercoping—to describe how blogs are used as a form of dealing with issues (Donovan, Nelson, & Scheinfeld, 2017). Cybercoping involves online communication activities such as describing experiences, seeking information, gaining insight into coping strategies, and developing relationships with fellow online users.

Other uses of emerging media include personalized health records, which can become more useful when made more interactive with personalized alerts. When personalized health records included a communication dimension with a patient's provider, the context stimulated the patient to be more proactive with their healthcare provider (Rief Hamm, Zickmund, Nikola, . . . Roberts, 2017). Even physicians are getting in on the act. Research by Allport and Womble (2016) reported that more physicians are using Twitter as a means of communicating better with patients, reviewing new research, and connecting with colleagues. Physician tweeting is likely to increase even more as providers are able to overcome their concerns of privacy and time constraints. Emerging media has also created opportunities for physicians and patients to construct virtual visits through online communication. Jiang and Street (2017) reported that many more physicians would like to be involved in virtual visits with their patients, again, if they can overcome concerns about privacy, security, and the thought that they may be delivering less personalized care.

Taken together, the chapters in this book and the research reported above echo what Heath and O'Hair (2009) argued regarding the challenges of risk and health communication: It can be difficult to base judgments on science, values, and policy while crafting communication messages that are simultaneously competent and understandable. Emerging media is a key mechanism for surmounting these challenges.

References

Allport, J. M., & Womble, F. E. (2016). Just what the doctor tweeted: Challenges and rewards of using Twitter. *Health Communication, 31*, 824–832.

Donovan, E. E., Nelson, E. C., & Scheinfeld, E. (2017). Cyberframing cancer: An exploratory investigation of valenced cybercoping on cancer blogs. *Health Communication, 32*, 1–10.

Fraustino, J. D., & Ma, L. (2015). CDC's use of social media and humor in a risk, campaign—"Preparedness 101: Zombie Apocalypse." *Journal of Applied Communication Research, 43*, 222–241.

Heath, R. L., & O'Hair, H. D. (2009). The significance of risk and crisis communication. In R. Heath & H. D. O'Hair (Eds.), *Handbook of risk and crisis communication* (pp. 5–30). New York: Routledge.

Jiang, S., & Street, R. L. (2017). Factors influencing communication with doctors via the Internet: A cross-sectional analysis of 2014 HINTS survey. *Health Communication, 32*, 108–188.

Kim, J., Brossard, D., Scheufele, D. A., & Xenos, M. (2016). "Shared" information in the age of big data: Exploring sentiment expression related to nuclear energy on Twitter. *Journalism & Mass Communication Quarterly, 93*, 430–445.

Moon, T., Chih, M., Shah, D. V., Yoo, W., & Gustafson, D. H. (2017). Breast cancer survivors' contribution to psychosocial adjustment of newly diagnosed breast cancer patients in a computer-mediated social support group. *Journalism & Mass Communication Quarterly, 94*, 486–514.

Namkoong, K., Nah, S., Record, R. A., & Stee, S. K. V. (2017). Communication, reasoning, and planned behaviors: Unveiling the effect of interactive communication in an anti-smoking social media campaign. *Health Communication, 32*, 41–50.

Rief, J. J., Hamm, M. E., Zickmund, S. L., Jikolajski, C., Lesky, D., Hess, R., Fisdcher, G. S., Weimer, M., Clark, S., Zieth, C., & Roberts, M. S. (2017). Using health information technology to foster engagement: Patients' experiences with an active patient health record. *Health Communication, 32*, 310–319.

Willis, E., & Royne, M. B. (2017). Online health communities and chronic disease self-management. *Health Communication, 32*, 269–278.

2

MEDIA LITERACY AND PARENT–ADOLESCENT COMMUNICATION ABOUT ALCOHOL IN MEDIA

Effects on Adolescent Alcohol Use

YoungJu Shin, Michelle Miller-Day, and Michael Hecht

Introduction

During the developmental period of adolescence, the likelihood of engaging in risky behaviors dramatically increases (Griffin, Scheier, Botvin, & Diaz, 2000; Wong et al., 2006). A recent *Monitoring the Future* study (2015) reports that adolescent substance use in the United States drastically increases from 8th grade to 12th grade. In this national study, it is noted that among 8th grade students, alcohol (26 percent) is the most prevalent substance used, followed by illicit drugs (21 percent) and cigarettes (13 percent). When youth reach the 12th grade, lifetime alcohol, illicit drugs, and cigarettes increase to 64 percent, 49 percent, and 31 percent respectively.

While adolescent substance use is multi-determined, there has been an increasing interest in examining the influence of media on shaping adolescent perceptions of substance use (CAMY, 2009). Adolescents are increasingly exposed to media images of substance use by adults and underage youth in film, television, and print media in addition to social media (Banarjee & Greene, 2007). By portraying pro-use images of substances, mass media images tend to make substance use appealing and attractive, especially for adolescents (Kelly, Slater, & Karan, 2002b; Sargent, Wills, Stoolmiller, Gibson, & Gibbons, 2006) leading to increased substance use and abuse (Anderson, De Bruin, Angus, Gordon, & Hastings, 2009).

Fortunately, increased substance use is not an inevitable outcome of media exposure to pro-use messages because media influence can be mitigated.

One approach to reducing the potential risks associated with media exposure is protecting adolescents by increasing their media literacy (Greene et al., 2015b; Hindmarsh, Jones, & Kervin, 2015; Peek & Beresin, 2016; Potter, 2013). Adolescents who are high in media literacy are less likely to be persuaded by media depictions of positive substance use behavior than those with low media literacy (Draper et al., 2015; Scull, Kupersmidt, & Erausquin, 2014; Shensa Phelps-Tschang, Miller, & Primack, 2016). Therefore, it is plausible to argue that media literacy can be a protective factor for adolescent substance use. Yet, few studies to our knowledge have assessed the impact of media literacy on the lifetime substance use of adolescents.

In addition to the important role of media literacy, parent-adolescent communication about substances and substance use also serves as a protective factor to buffer risks. More importantly, past literature documents that parental communication about substance use in general affects adolescent attitudes, norms, and intentions to use substance use as well as actual substance use behaviors (Kam & Middleton, 2013; Miller-Day & Kam, 2010; Shin & Miller-Day, 2017; Shin Lee, Lu, & Hecht, 2016). The parent-adolescent communication characterized in the literature suggests conversations about expectations, rules, and knowledge (e.g., Miller-Day & Dodd, 2004), but little is known about what messages parents and adolescents exchange about *media portrayals* of substances and substance use and how these messages influence adolescents' actual substance use. Parents' discussion of media images of substance use may help students understand how marketing messages in advertisements and use of substances by characters in entertainment media can influence their attitudes toward drinking, and these discussions can correct erroneous beliefs about substance use that tend to be promoted by media (NIAAA, 2004/2005). Yet, there are few studies that examine the impact of parental discussions of media images on adolescents' actual substance use behavior.

To begin to fill this research gap, the present study examines the effects of adolescent media literacy and parent-adolescent communication about media portrayals of alcohol use on adolescents' lifetime alcohol use. The focus on alcohol is warranted when evaluating a young adolescent population since alcohol is the substance most commonly used and abused by adolescents (NIDA, 2016).

Media Literacy and Substance Use

There is evidence indicating that media portrayals of substance use make substance use appear normative and attractive (Cin et al., 2009; Heatherton & Sargent, 2009; Primack, Kraemer, Fine, & Dalton, 2009; Wills, Sargent, Stoolmiller, Gibbons, & Gerrard, 2008). Recent research from the Centers for Disease Control and Prevention (CDC, 2013) reports that adolescent exposure to alcohol advertisements on television exceeded the viewership of the industry threshold (24 percent) and the standard proposed by the National Research Council/Institute of Medicine (36 percent). The excessive exposure to positive portrayals of alcohol on mass media socializes adolescents to believe that drinking alcohol is common in adolescence and makes the drinker more attractive, which in turn leads youth to initiate and continue drinking alcohol (Anderson et al., 2009; Kelly et al., 2002b; McClure et al., 2016; Sargent et al., 2006; Wills, Sargent, Gibbons, Gerrard, & Stoolmiller, 2009).

Adolescents, however, are not the powerless victims of manipulative media moguls, submitting to pro-alcohol use images. Rather, adolescents with high levels of media literacy are fully capable of resisting these appeals, with media literacy referring to "the ability to access, analyze, evaluate, and produce media in a variety of forms" (Kupersmidt, Scull, & Austin, 2010, p. 526) and media literacy education results in counteracting negative impacts on adolescents (Greene et al., 2015b; Hindmarsh et al., 2015; Peek & Beresin, 2016; Potter, 2013). Beyond alcohol, evidence suggests that smoking media literacy intervention changed high school students' attitudes and normative beliefs about smoking (Primack et al., 2014; Shensa et al., 2016) and significantly reduced high school students' intention to smoke (Phelps-Tschang, Miller, Rice, & Primack, 2016). What is more, there is a promising result that adolescent media literacy has stronger relationships with intention and actual behavior of drinking and smoking (Chang et al., 2016). Kupersmidt et al. (2010) found that children who received a media literacy intervention reported higher levels of critical thinking and understanding of persuasive intent of media than those in the control condition. Moreover, children in the intervention condition were less likely to intend uses of alcohol and tobacco than others in the control condition. More evidence highlights that media literacy of elementary school students was significantly associated with normative beliefs and intention to use alcohol and tobacco (Austin & Johnson, 1997b; Scull et al., 2014). Despite the strong evidence supporting the claim that increasing media literacy in youth leads to changes in substance use related beliefs, attitudes, and intentions, few studies have measured adolescents' actual substance use behavior. Moreover, a majority of past studies focus on pre-adolescent children (K1–K6) and late adolescents (9th grade or above). Thus, more research needs to investigate media literacy on actual substance use behaviors of early adolescents (6th–8th grade).

Based on previous research, it is logical to assume that adolescents who score high in media literacy are less likely to be influenced by media portrayals of alcohol use than those who score low in media literacy. Therefore, the first research hypothesis we pose is:

RH1: Adolescent media literacy is negatively related to adolescent alcohol use.

Parent-Adolescent Communication about Media Portrayals of Substance Use

It is recognized that parents serve as anti-substance use socialization agents for adolescent behavioral health (Kam & Miller-Day, 2017; Miller-Day, 2008; Pettigrew et al., 2017a; Van der Vorst, Engels, Meeus, Dekovic, & Van Leeuwe, 2005). Primary socialization theory (Oetting & Donnermeyer, 1998) explains the important role of parents for adolescent developmental functioning; parental communication about substance use is key to socialize adolescent attitudes, norms, intentions, and actual use of substances (Choi et al., 2017; Kam, Potocki, & Hecht, 2014; Pettigrew, Shin, Stein, & Raalte, 2017b; Shin & Miller-Day, 2017). Past literature suggests that parental messages mitigate the negative impacts of media messages on children, adolescent media usage, and the risky behaviors of both children and adolescents (Dalton et al., 2006: Fisher et al., 2009; Nathanson, 1999). This effect is particularly strong on adolescents' intention to drink alcohol (Tanski, Cin, Stoolmiller, & Sargent, 2010). Furthermore, it was found that parental communication is an intervention that remains effective in reducing substance use for older adolescents and emerging adults (Chen & Austin, 2013).

Despite the protective effects of parental anti-substance socialization and the pervasiveness of exposure to pro-alcohol media content, little is known about the effects of parental communication about media content, specifically portrayals of alcohol use, and how this might impact adolescents' alcohol use. While it is evident that general openness in communicating about rules, expectations, and providing knowledge about substances seems to impact adolescent alcohol use (Kelly, Comello, & Hunn, 2002a), it is not clear if parents talk about pro-alcohol media content. If they do, are those messages effective in affecting adolescent alcohol use?

One would expect that parents, exposed to some of the same media influences, would address this with their children and such communication would have the same positive effects as communicating in general about substances and substance use. Based on the primary socialization theory (Oetting & Donnermeyer, 1998) and previous literature (Dalton et al., 2006: Fisher et al., 2009; Nathanson, 1999; Tanski et al., 2010), we postulate that adolescents who engage in parent-adolescent communication about media portrayals of substance use are less likely to drink alcohol than those with less communication. Thus, it is hypothesized that:

RH2: Parent-adolescent communication about media portrayals of alcohol use is negatively related to adolescent alcohol use.

15

Methods

Participants and Procedure

As part of a larger project that examined adaptation and implementation processes of a school-based drug prevention intervention (Colby et al., 2013; Pettigrew et al., 2015), cross-sectional survey data were collected in rural communities in two Midwestern states.[1] The 8th grade students participated in a paper and pencil, self-report survey. For the present study, we used a subsample (n = 603) of students in the control condition who had not received any substance use intervention. Prior to the survey, the university institutional review board approved the procedures of the current study and parental informed consents and student assents were obtained. The sample was comprised of (51 percent) male and (49 percent) female, with a European American majority (94 percent), African American (3 percent), Hispanic (2 percent), and Asian or Pacific Islander (1 percent), which matched the demographic distribution of the geographic location.

Measures

Media literacy. Six-items were adapted from Primack and Hobbs' (2009) scales to measure the degree of general adolescent media literacy. Using four-point scales, students answered questions such as "People are influenced by advertising" and "When people make movies and TV shows, every camera shot is very carefully planned." (1 = definitely no, 4 = definitely yes). Higher scores indicated higher levels of media literacy. Cronbach's alpha was 0.73 (mean = 2.83, SD = .64).

Parent-adolescent communication about alcohol portrayals in media. Students were asked to report how frequently their parent(s) discussed media portrayals of alcohol use with them. Three items with four-point scales were selectively chosen from the original measurement (Miller-Day & Kam, 2010). For example, items included "At least one of your parents ever makes comments about how drinking alcohol is bad if a character on TV is drinking or drunk?" and "At least one of your parents ever show you information on the Web, TV, or in the news about the dangers of drinking alcohol, smoking/chewing, or other drug use?" (1 = no, never; 4 = yes, all the time). Higher scores indicated frequent parent-adolescent communication. Cronbach's alpha was 0.90 (mean = 1.79, SD = .89).

Lifetime alcohol use. A single item was used to assess adolescent alcohol use in their lifetime (Hansen & Graham, 1991). Using a 9-point scale, a question was asked, "How many drinks of alcohol have you had in your entire life?" (A "drink" = 1 bottle or can of beer, 1 glass of wine, or 1 shot of hard liquor; 10 = more than 100 drinks) (mean = 3.23, SD = 2.51). Higher scores indicated more alcohol drinking. Due to the nature of a single item measure, no reliability test was available for the lifetime alcohol use.

16

There is ample evidence that using a single item measure for reporting substance use is effective and is commonly used in other studies (Elek et al., 2006; Pettigrew et al., 2017b; Shin et al., 2016).

Analysis Summary

A confirmatory factor analysis (CFA) was first conducted to test the measurement model of adolescent media literacy and parent-adolescent communication about alcohol portrayals in media, using *MPlus* 7.1 (Muthén & Muthén, 2012). Based on the model fit criteria [the root mean square error of approximation (RMSEA) < .08, the comparative fit index (CFI) > .95, and the standardized root mean square residual (SRMR) > .08)] (Kline, 2005; Hu & Bentler, 1999; Yu, 2002), the CFA model fit the data well [x^2 (19) = 125.94, p< .001, RMSEA = .07, CFI = .96, SRMR = .03].

Next, a regression analysis with the measurement model was performed. Adolescent media literacy and parent-adolescent communication about alcohol portrayals in media were entered as independent variables and lifetime alcohol use was entered as a dependent variable. The gender variable was also included as a controlling variable in the regression analysis. The test of skewness (–.42 for media literacy, .98 for parent-adolescent communication, 1.17 for lifetime alcohol use) and kurtosis (.06 for media literacy, –.90 for parent-adolescent communication, .46 for lifetime alcohol use) of the independent and dependent variables were considered as an acceptable range (Kline, 2005), maximum likelihood (ML) estimation method that deals with normally distributed data was used. It was also found that missing data was not a significant concern for the data analysis (.02 percent). Thus, it was handled as missing at random (Graham, Cumsille, & Elek-Fisk, 2003). The analysis yielded an appropriate model fit [x^2 (33) = 90.09, p < .001, RMSEA = 05, CFI = .97, SRMR = .04].

Results

Two research hypotheses were posited to test the significant relationships between adolescent media literacy and lifetime alcohol use, as well as between parent-adolescent communication about media portrayals of alcohol use and adolescents' lifetime alcohol use. Both research hypotheses were supported. It was found that media literacy was significantly associated with adolescent lifetime alcohol use (β = –0.149, SE = .049, p < .01). Parent-adolescent communication about media portrayals of alcohol use was also found to be a significant predictor for adolescent lifetime alcohol use (β = –0.092, SE = .043, p < .05). Approximately 4 percent of the variance was explained by the regression analysis with the measurement model while controlling for gender. See Figure 2.1 for the visual analysis model.

17

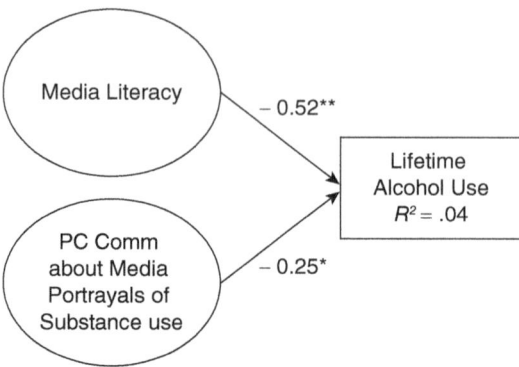

Figure 2.1 Regression Analysis with the Measurement Model

Note: Regression coefficients in the figure are standardized and only significant pathways and correlations are highlighted by boldface [χ^2 (33) =90.086; RMSEA = .05; CFI = .97; SRMR = 0.04]. Effect of gender was controlled but the pathways are not shown in the figure for reasons of clarity. * p < .05; ** p < .01; *** p < .001

Discussion

The present study seeks to investigate the effects of adolescent media literacy and parent-adolescent communication about media alcohol portrayals on adolescents' lifetime alcohol use. Results revealed that both media literacy and parent-adolescent communication were significant predictors of 8th graders' lifetime alcohol use. This is consistent with previous studies reporting that media literacy is negatively related to alcohol use intentions, and also extends these findings to actual alcohol use behavior. Higher levels of media literacy seemed to buffer the adolescents in this sample against drinking alcohol, likely by increasing their ability to analyze images and cognitively frame the media messages in a way that makes those messages less persuasive or glamorous. The findings of this study suggest that it may be critical to offer curricula in school settings to teach media literacy in the context of substance use. Previous intervention attempts have been reported, but these programs are targeted at improving media literacy among high school students to reduce alcohol use (Austin & Johnson, 1997a; Greene et al., 2015a; Greene et al., 2015b). Perhaps future research should investigate the important role of media literacy among early adolescents. More research is needed to examine the differential effects of various types of mass media and new communication technology on attitudes about substance use and testing the effects of media literacy in all forms of media on behavioral outcomes such as substance use behaviors.

Significantly, the longitudinal data from National Survey on Drug Use and Health, shows that adolescents in rural areas consume higher rates of alcohol than adolescents in urban areas (Lambert, Gale, & Hartley, 2008). Therefore, it is important to focus efforts on specific populations that might be at heightened risk. With the prevalence of rural adolescent drinking behaviors, interventions are needed to reduce adolescent alcohol use risk. The present study provides an initial step by providing basic research supporting the need for increased media literacy among early adolescents. These findings provide evidence that rural adolescents with higher levels of media literacy were less likely to drink alcohol in their lifetime. Therefore, more attention needs to be made to specifically target rural adolescents for effective media literacy intervention (Chang et al., 2016; Colby et al., 2013; Pettigrew, Miller-Day, Krieger, & Hecht, 2011; Rhew, Hawkins, & Oesterle, 2011; Shin, Miller-Day, Hecht, & Krieger, 2015).

This study also found that parent-adolescent communication about media portrayals of alcohol use protected adolescents from drinking alcohol. In other words, adolescents who reported higher levels of parental communication about media images were less likely to drink alcohol than others with lower levels of communication. This finding supports previous literature indicating the positive influence of parent-adolescent communication in general on substance use attitudes (Reimuller, Hussong, & Ennett, 2011; Shin et al., 2016), but extends it to highlight messages specific to media depictions of substance use. As found in previous studies, it is not just generally open communication about substances that is important, but specifically targeted communication about media portrayals that matters (Miller-Day, 2008; Miller-Day & Kam, 2010; Shin & Miller-Day, 2017).

Moreover, the specificity of parent-adolescent communication about depictions of alcohol in media needs further investigation with regard to different types of media. Considering the current study focused on general conversations about alcohol use on television and the Internet, future research should examine parental communication surrounding alcohol-related messaging on various channels of televised programs and social media (e.g., YouTube, Facebook, Twitter, Snapchat, Instagram). Other media such as film also need to be further investigated. One can argue that persuasion of media may differ, depending on different media channels. Different genres of media may have differential impacts on adolescents' substance use. Television dramas and movies are based on narrative storytelling, with the introduction, development, climax, and resolution, whereas postings on social media tend to be brief and include immediate feedback from others that might reinforce the message. Parents may need to use different strategies to communicate with adolescents about media messages depending on the media channel. It is plausible to assume that parental messages about television or advertisements might differ from parental messages about social media (e.g., Facebook posts, tweets).

There also is the question about whether the communication is concurrent or synchronous with media exposure (i.e., as it is being consumed or some immediately afterwards) or removed in time and place. Some media, like television (broadly defined to include digital manifestations) and Internet content lend themselves better to concurrent interactions and these effects may be more pronounced. Since youth are likely to be digital natives and their parents tend to be digital immigrants, special consideration of emerging social media and online gaming may be particularly difficult for parents. At present, this is all speculative. Future research may benefit from understanding media literacy-related parent-adolescent communication pertaining to various types of media and develop strategies to increase effectiveness of that communication.

The findings of this study suggest that family- and parent-based prevention interventions might consider including material that educates parents about how to add media depictions of substance use in their conversation with youth. While these interventions, like Strengthening the Family (Kumpfer & Alvarado, 2003), are powerful, the current findings suggest that effects can be enhanced and perhaps even more protective against influences by media if such content were added. For example, a session might be added to these programs with the objective of enhancing parental skill in discussing media content with youth. This session could address messaging strategies for when the content is being consumed concurrently with the youth (e.g., watching television together) and strategies for when the content is consumed separately or asynchronously (e.g., parent viewing the youth's Facebook page and past posts). This session could also consider strategies for setting family rules and norms regarding media consumption, including social media and online gaming.

Despite the significant findings of this study, it is not without limitations. First, it must be recognized that these findings do not assume causality. Future research should make an effort to collect the longitudinal survey data and examine the long-term effects of media literacy and parental communication on youth alcohol use. Second, the present study did not assess participants' exposure to media in the analysis model. Accounting for the frequency of media exposure and types of media would broaden our understanding of media and adolescent behavioral outcomes including attitudes, norms, intentions, and actual behavior. For instance, it would be interesting to investigate a comparison between the quantity of the media exposure and the quality of the media persuasion. As previously noted, different channels (e.g., television vs. Twitter) and genres of media (e.g., drama vs. entertainment show) may generate differential impacts on adolescent outcomes.

There is also the need to consider Internet content and online gaming, media that youth are likely to be far advanced of parents (e.g., digital natives). Are there separate literacies for Instagram and other social media content? Different ways these need to be discussed? What about the use of these social media in parent-child communication?

In conclusion, the present study provides evidence supporting the protective effects of adolescent media literacy and parent-adolescent communication about alcohol portrayals in the media. The findings suggest that interventions might be developed to enhance adolescent media literacy and to provide education for parents in ways to communicate with youth about media images promoting alcohol use. In this regard, we suggest more synergetic effects be developed in school and community-based programs to prevent adolescents from initiating substance use and continuous use.

Note

1 Rural was defined as any incorporated place, census designated place, or non-place territory and defined as rural by the United States Census Bureau (U.S. Department of Education, 2006).

References

Anderson, P., De Bruijin, A., Angus, K., Gordon, R., & Hasting, G. (2009). Impacts of alcohol advertising and media exposure on adolescent alcohol use: A systematic review of longitudinal studies. *Alcohol & Alcoholism*, 44(3), 229–243. doi: 10.1093/alcalc/agn115.

Austin, E. W., & Johnson, K. (1997a). Effects of general and alcohol-specific media literacy training on children's decision making about alcohol. *Journal of Health Communication*, 2(1), 17–42. doi: 10.1080/108107397127897.

Austin, E. W., & Johnson, K. K. (1997b). Immediate and delayed effects of media literacy training on third grader's decision making for alcohol. *Health Communication*, 9(4), 323–349. doi: 10.1080/108107397127897.

Banerjee, S. C., & Greene, K. (2007). Antismoking initiatives: Effects of analysis versus production media literacy interventions on smoking-related attitude, norm, and behavioral intention. *Health Communication*, 22(1), 37–48. doi: 10.1080/10410230701310281.

Center on Alcohol Marketing and Youth (CAMY). *Executive summary: Youth exposure to alcohol advertising on television, 2001–2009*. Retrieved January 15, 2016 from www.camy.org/research/Youth_Exposure_to_Alcohol_Ads_on_TV_Growing_Faster_Than_Adults/index.html.

Centers for Disease Control and Prevention (2012). *Alcohol-related disease impact*. Atlanta, GA: US Department of Health and Human Services, CDC; 2012. Retrieved January 29, 2016 from http://apps.nccd.cdc.gov/dach_ardi/default/default.aspx.

Centers for Disease Control and Prevention (2013). *Youth exposure to alcohol advertising on television—25 markets*, United States, 2010. Morbidity and Mortality Weekly Report. Retrieved January 20, 2016 from www.cdc.gov/mmwr/preview/mmwrhtml/mm6244a3.htm?s_cid=mm6244a3_w.

Chang, F. C., Miao, N. F., Lee, C. M., Chen, P. H., Chiu, C. H., & Lee, S. C. (2016). The association of media exposure and media literacy with adolescent alcohol and tobacco use. *Journal of Health Psychology*, *21*(4), 513–525. doi: 10.1177/1359105314530451.

Chen, Y. C. Y., & Austin, E. W. (2013). The role of parental mediation in the development of media literacy and the prevention of substance use. In A. N. Valdivia (Ed.) *The international encyclopedia of media studies* (pp.1–19). Hoboken, NJ: Blackwell Publishing.

Choi, H. J., Miller-Day, M., Shin, Y., Hecht, M. L., Pettigrew, J., Krieger, J., Lee, J. K., & Graham, J. W. (2017). Parent prevention communication profiles and adolescent substance use: A latent profile analysis and growth mixture model. *Journal of Family Communication*, *17*(1), 15–32. doi: 10.1080/15267431.2016.1251920.

Cin, S. D., Worth, K. A., Gerrard, M. G., Gibbons, F. X., Stoolmiller, M., Wills, T. A., & Sargent, J. D. (2009). Watching and drinking: Expectancies, proto-types, and friends' alcohol use mediate the effects of exposure to alcohol use in movies on adolescent drinking. *Health Psychology*, *28*(4), 473–483. doi: 10.1037/a0014777.

Colby, M., Hecht, M. L., Miller-Day, M., Krieger, J. L., Syvertsen, A. K., Graham, J. W., & Pettigrew, J. (2013). Adapting school-based substance use prevention curriculum through cultural grounding: A review and exemplar of adaptation processes for rural schools. *American Journal of Community Psychology*, *51*(1–2), 190–205. doi: 10.1007/s10464-012-9524-8.

Dalton, M. A., Adachi-Mejia, A. M., Longacre, M. R., Titus-Ernstoff, L. T., Gibson, J. J. Martin, S. K., Sargent, J. D., & Beach, M. L. (2006). Parental rules and monitoring of children's movie viewing associated with children's risk for smoking and drinking. *Pediatrics*, *118*(5), 1932–1942. doi: 10.1542/peds.2005-3082.

Draper, M., Appregilio, S., Kramer, A., Ketcherside, M., Campbell, S., Stewart, B., Rhodes, D., & Cox, C. (2015). Educational intervention/case study: Implementing an elementary-level, classroom-based media literacy education program for academically at-risk middle-school students in the non-classroom setting. *Journal of Alcohol and Drug Education*, *59*(2), 12–24.

Elek, E., Miller-Day, M., & Hecht, M. L. (2006). Influences of personal, injunc-tive, and descriptive norms on early adolescent substance use. *Journal of Drug Issues*, *36*(1), 147–172. doi: 10.1177/002204260603600107.

Fisher, D. A., Hill, D. L., Grube, J. W., Bersamin, M. M., Walker, S., & Gruber, E. L. (2009). Televised sexual content and parental mediation: Influences on adolescent sexuality. *Media Psychology*, *12*(2), 121–147. doi: 10.1080/15213260902849901.

Graham, J. W., Cumsille, P. E., & Elek-Fisk, E. (2003). Methods of handling missing data. In J. A. Schinka, & W. F. Velicer (Eds.), *Research methods in psychology* (pp. 87–114). New York, NY: John Wiley & Sons.

Greene, K., Elek, E., Catona, D., Magsamen-Conrad, K., Banerjee, S. C., & Hecht, M. L. (2015a). *Improving prevention curricula: Lesson learned through formative research on the Youth Message Development Curriculum.* Paper pre-sented at the National Communication Association, Las Vegas, NV.

Greene, K., Yanovitzky, I., Carpenter, A., Banerjee, S. C., Magsamen-Conrad, K., Hecht, M. L., & Elek, E. (2015b). A theory-grounded measure of adolescents' response to media literacy interventions. *Journal of Media Literacy Education*, 7(2), 35–49.

Griffin, K. W., Scheier, L. M., Botvin, G. J., & Diaz, T. (2000). Ethnic and gender differences in psychosocial risk, protection, and adolescent alcohol use. *Prevention Science*, 1(4), 199–212. doi: 10.1023/A:1026599112279.

Hansen W. B., & Graham, J. W. (1991). Preventing alcohol, marijuana, and cigarette use among adolescents: Peer pressure resistance training versus establishing conservative norms. *Preventive Medicine*, 20(3), 414–430. doi: 10.1016/0091-7435(91)90039-7.

Heatherton, T. F., & Sargent, J. D. (2009). Does watching smoking in movies promote teenage smoking? *Current Directions in Psychological Science*, 18(2), 63–67. doi: 10.1111/j.1467-8721.2009.01610.

Hindmarsh, C. S., Jones, S. C., & Kervin, L. (2015). Effectiveness of alcohol media literacy programmes: A systematic literature review. *Health Education Research*, 30(3), 449–465. doi: 10.1093/her/cyv015.

Hu, L., & Bentler, P. M. (1999). Cutoff criteria for fit indexes in covariance structure analysis: Conventional criteria versus new alternatives. *Structural Equation Modeling*, 6(1), 1–55. doi: 10.1080/10705519909540118.

Kam, J. A. & Middleton, A. V. (2013). The associations between parents' references to their own past substance use and youth's substance use beliefs and behaviors: A comparison of Latino and European American youth. *Human Communication Research*, 39(2), 208–229. doi: 10.1111/hcre.12001.

Kam, J. A., & Miller-Day, M. (2017). Introduction to special issue. *Journal of Family Communication*, 17(1), 1–14. doi: 10.1080/15267431.2016.1251922.

Kam, J. A., Potocki, B., & Hecht, M. L. (2014). Encouraging Mexican-heritage youth to intervene when friends drink: The role of targeted parent-child communication against alcohol. *Communication Research*, 41(5), 644–664. doi: 10.1177/0093650212446621

Kelly, K. J., Comello, M. L. G., & Hunn, L. C. P. (2002a). Parent-child communication, perceived sanctions against drug use, and youth drug involvement. *Adolescence*, 37(148), 775–783.

Kelly, K., Slater, M. D., & Karan, D. (2002b). Image advertisements' influence on adolescent perceptions of the desirability of beer and cigarettes. *Public Policy and Marketing*, 21, 295–304. doi: 10.1509/jppm.21.2.295.17585.

Kline, R. B. (2005). Principles and practice of structural equation modeling (2nd Ed.). New York: The Guilford Press.

Kumpfer, K. L., & Alvarado, R. (2003). Family-strengthening approaches for the prevention of youth problem behaviors. *American Psychologist*, 58(6–7), 457–465. doi: 10.1037/0003-066X.58.6-7.457.

Kupersmidt, J. B., Scull, T. M., & Austin, E. W. (2010). Media literacy education for elementary school substance use prevention: Study of media detective. *Pediatrics*, 126(3), 525–531. doi: 10.1542/peds.2010-0068.

Lambert, D., Gale, J. A., & Hartley, D. (2008). Substance abuse by youth and young adults in rural America. *The Journal of Rural Health*, 24(3), 221–228. doi: 10.1111/j.1748- 0361.2008.00162.

McClure, A. C., Tanski, S. E., Li, Z., Jackson, K., Morgenstern, M., Li, Z., & Sargent, J. D. (2016). Internet alcohol marketing and underage alcohol use. *Pediatrics*, *137*(2), 1–8. doi: 10.1542/peds.2015-2149.

Miller-Day, M. (2008). Talking to youth about drugs: What do late adolescents say about parental strategies? *Family Relations*, *57*(1), 1–12. doi: 10.1111/j.1741-3729.2007.00478.

Miller-Day, M., & Dodd, A. H. (2004). Toward a descriptive model of parent-offspring communication about alcohol and other drugs. *Journal of Social and Personal Relationships*, *21*(1), 69–91. doi: 10.1177/0265407504039846.

Miller-Day, M., & Kam, J. A. (2010). More than just openness: Developing and validating a measure of targeted parent-child communication about alcohol. *Health Communication*, *25*(4), 293–302. doi: 10.1080/10410231003698952.

Muthén, L. K., & Muthén, B. O. (1998–2012). *Mplus User's Guide* (7th Ed.). Los Angeles, CA: Muthén & Muthén.

Nathanson, A. I. (1999). Identifying and explaining the relationship between parental mediation and children's aggression. *Communication Research*, *26*(2), 124–143. doi: 10.1177/009365099026002002.

National Institute on Alcohol Abuse and Alcoholism (NIAAA). (2004/2005). *Alcohol and development in youth—Multidisciplinary overview* (Volume 28, Number 3). Bethesda, MD: NIAAA.

National Institute on Drug Abuse (NIDA) (2016). Monitoring the Future survey: High school and youth trends. Retrieved March 17, 2017, from www.drugabuse.gov/publications/drugfacts/monitoring-future-survey-high-school-youth-trends.

Oetting, E. R., & Donnermeyer, J. F. (1998). Primary socialization theory: The etiology of drug use and deviance: I. *Substance Use & Misuse*, *33*(4), 995–1026. doi: 10.3109/10826089809056252.

Peek, H. S., & Beresin, E. (2016). Reality check: How reality television can affect youth and how a media literacy curriculum can help. *Academic Psychiatry*, *40*(1), 177–181. doi: 10.1007/s40596-015-0382-1.

Pettigrew, J., Miller-Day, M., Krieger, J., & Hecht, M. L. (2011). Alcohol and other drug resistance strategies employed by rural adolescents. *Journal of Applied Communication Research*, *39*(2), 103–122. doi: 10.1080/00909882.2011.556139.

Pettigrew, J., Graham, J., Hecht, M. L., Miller-Day, M., Krieger, J., & Shin,. Y. (2015). Adherence and delivery: Implementation quality and program outcomes for the 7th grade keepin' it REAL program. *Prevention Science*, *16*(1), 90–99. doi: 10.1007/s11121-014-0459-1.

Pettigrew, J., Miller-Day, M., Shin, Y., Krieger, J., Hecht, M. L., & Graham, J. W. (2017a). Parental messages about substances in early adolescence: Extending a model of drug talk styles. *Health Communication.*, 1–10. doi: 10.1080/10410236.2017.1283565.

Pettigrew, J., Shin, Y., Stein, J. B., & Raalte, L. J. (2017b). Family communication and adolescent alcohol use in Nicaragua, Central America: A test of primary socialization theory. *Journal of Family Communication*, *17*(1), 33–48. doi: 10.1080/15267431.2016.1251921.

Phelps-Tschang, J. S., Miller, E., Rice, K. R., & Primack, B. A. (2016). Web-based media literacy to prevent tobacco use among high school students. *Journal of Media Literacy Education, 7*(3), 29–40.

Potter, W. J. (2013). *Media literacy.* Thousand Oaks, CA: SAGE Publications.

Primack, B. A., Douglas, E. L., Land, S. R., Miller, E., & Fine, M. J. (2014). Comparison of media literacy and usual education to prevent tobacco use: A cluster-randomized trial. *Journal of School Health, 84*(2), 106–115. doi: 10.1111/josh.12130.

Primack, B. A., & Hobbs, R. (2009). Association of various components of media literacy and adolescent smoking. *American Journal of Health Behavior,* 33(2), 192–201.

Primack, B. A., Kraemer, K. L., Fine, M. J., & Dalton, M. A. (2009). Media exposure and marijuana and alcohol use among adolescents. *Substance Use & Misuse, 44*(5), 722–739. doi: 10.1080/10826080802490097.

Reimuller, A., Hussong, A., & Ennett, S. T. (2011). The influence of alcohol-specific communication on adolescent alcohol use and alcohol-related consequences. *Prevention Science, 12*(4), 389–400. doi: 10.1007/s11121-011-0227-4.

Rhew, I. C., Hawkins, J. D., & Oesterle, S. (2011). Drug use and risk among youth in different rural contexts. *Health & Place, 17*(3), 775–783. doi: 10.1016/j.healthplace.2011.02.003.

Sargent, J. D., Wills, T. A., Stoolmiller, M., Gibson, J. J., & Gibbons, F. X. (2006). Alcohol use in motion pictures and its relation with early-onset teen drinking. *Journal of Studies on Alcohol, 67*(1), 54–65. doi: 10.15288/jsa.2006.67.54.

Scull, T. M., Kupersmidt, J. B., & Erausquin, J. T. (2014). The impact of media-related cognitions on children's substance use outcomes in the context of parental and peer substance use. *Journal of Youth and Adolescence, 43*(5), 717–728. doi: 10.1007/s10964-013-0012-8.

Shensa, A., Phelps-Tschang, J., Miller, E., & Primack, B. A. (2016). A randomized crossover study of web-based media literacy to prevent smoking. *Health Education Research, 31*(1), 48–59. doi: 10.1093/her/cyv062.

Shin, Y., & Miller-Day, M. (2017). A longitudinal study of parental anti substance-use socialization for early adolescents' substance use behaviors. *Communication Monographs, 84,* 277–297. doi: 10.1080/03637751.2017.1300821.

Shin, Y., Miller-Day, M., Hecht, M. L., & Krieger, J. (November 2015). *Effects of entertainment-education intervention for youth substance use prevention: Examining indirect effects of youth perception of narrative performance on alcohol use behavior via refusal efficacy.* Paper presented at the National Communication Association conference. Las Vegas, NV.

Shin, Y., Lee, J. K., Lu, Y., & Hecht, M. L. (2016). Exploring parental influence on the progression of alcohol use in Mexican-heritage youth: A latent transition analysis. *Prevention Science, 17*(2), 188–198. doi: 10.1007/s11121-015-0596-1.

Tanski, S E., Cin, S. D., Stoolmiller, M., & Sargent, J. D. (2010). Parental R-rated movie restriction and early-onset alcohol use. *Journal of Studies on Alcohol and Drugs, 71*(3), 452–459. www.jsad.com/doi/10.15288/jsad.2010.71.452.

U.S. Department of Education (2006). Documentation to the NCES Common Core of Data Public Elementary/Secondary School Locale Code File: School

Year 2003–04. U.S. Department of Education Institute of Education Sciences NCES 2006-332.

Van der Vorst, H., Engels, R. C. M. E., Meeus, W., Dekovic, M., & Van Leeuwe, J. (2005). The role of alcohol specific socialization in adolescents' drinking behaviour. *Addiction, 100*(10), 1464–1476. doi: 10.1111/j.1360-0443.2005.01193.

Wills, T., Sargent, J., Gibbons, F., Gerrard, M., & Stoolmiller, M. (2009). Movie exposure to alcohol cues and adolescent alcohol problems: A longitudinal analysis in a national sample. *Psychology of Addictive Behaviors, 23*(1), 23–35. doi: 10.1037/a0014137.

Wills, T., Sargent, J., Stoolmiller, M., Gibbons, F., & Gerrad, M. (2008). Movie smoking exposure and smoking onset: A longitudinal study of mediation processes in a representative sample of U.S. adolescents. *Psychology of Addictive Behaviors, 22*(2), 269–277. doi: 10.1037/0893-164X.22.2.269.

Wong, M. M., Nigg, J. T., Zucker, R. A., Puttler, L. I., Fitzgerald, H. E., & Jester, J. M. (2006). Behavioral control and resiliency in the onset of alcohol and illicit drug use. A prospective study from preschool to adolescence. *Child Development, 77*(4), 1016–1033. doi: 10.1111/j.1467-8624.2006.00916.

Yu, C. Y. (2002). Evaluating cutoff criteria of model fit indices for latent variable models with binary and continuous outcomes. Doctoral dissertation, University of California, Los Angeles.

3

COLLEGE STUDENTS AND LEGALIZED MARIJUANA

Knowledge Gaps and Belief Gaps Regarding the Law and Health Effects

Douglas Blanks Hindman

Communication research has shown a resurgence of interest in the impact of partisan identification in communication processes. For example, self-identification as a Democrat or Republican, or as a liberal or conservative, predicts perceptions of hostility and media bias against in-groups and in favor of out-groups (Gunther, 1992; Gunther, Miller, & Liebhart, 2009; Gunther, Edgerly, Akin, & Broesch, 2012). Partisan identification is associated with motivated reasoning in which conclusions complimentary toward one's in-group are favored over conclusions favored by nonpartisan experts (Kruglanski & Webster, 1996; Tabor & Lodge, 2012). Selective exposure to media that privileges one partisan group over all others is related to increased polarization between the groups (Dillipane, 2011; Iyengar & Hahn, 2009; Knoblock-Westerwick & Meng, 2011; Stroud, 2008).

The present study is informed by research in which group identity is shown to be a significant predictor of knowledge regarding heavily publicized topics. Drawing from the knowledge gap hypothesis (Tichenor, Donohue, & Olien, 1970) and its extension, the belief gap hypothesis (Hindman, 2009; 2012; Hindman & Yan, 2015), this study derives and tests hypotheses about changes in students' knowledge about long-term and short-term health effects associated with marijuana use by minors during the first three years following the legalization of recreational marijuana in Washington state.

An underlying question is whether student perceptions of the stigma of marijuana use have changed following the institutionalization of the

27

recreational marijuana industry in 2012. Student perceptions about stigma are addressed in questions about the individual's feelings about social media portrayals of their own marijuana use. In an evolving media environment, social identity, identity expression, and social media portrayals are increasingly intertwined. In an evolving political environment, truth claims associated with a variety of implied risks—climate change, health care affordability, and sexual health—are increasingly expressions of identity rather than expressions of knowledge (Hindman, 2009; 2012; Hindman & Yan, 2015).

Marijuana Legalization in Washington State

On Nov. 6, 2012, Washington state voters approved by a margin of 55.7 percent to 43.3 percent Initiative 502 legalizing possession of up to one ounce of marijuana for private recreational use by adults over age 21 (Washington Secretary of State, 2012, November 27). The voter-based initiative was the result of a petition drive that produced over 270,000 certified signatures in 2011 (Ammons, 2012, Jan. 27). The measure went directly on the November general election ballot after the legislature failed to put the issue to a vote.

The campaign for I-502 was supported by $6 million in donations, including $2 million from Progressive Insurance executive Peter B. Lewis (Martin, 2012, November 7). Proponents cited the potential windfall of tax revenues to the state that would result from ending ineffective and expensive law enforcement actions. Indeed, the state has collected over $400 million in excise tax and $137 million in sales tax since June of 2014; total sales topped $1 billion in 2016 (www.502data.com). In July of 2016, the formerly unregulated medical marijuana market was merged with the recreational marijuana regulatory system under the renamed Washington State Liquor and Cannabis Board (Preparations in place . . . n.d.).

Notably absent from the discussion leading to the vote to legalize recreational marijuana for adults was concern regarding health effects associated with marijuana use. Correlational evidence shows significant neuropsychological decline among those who initiated marijuana use in adolescence and who persisted through midlife (Meier et al., 2012). The highest percentage of US marijuana users in 2015 was among college-aged persons (19.8 percent of persons aged 18 to 25). This age group had significantly higher percentages of users in 2011 to 2015 as compared with the percentages from 2002 to 2010 (Center for Behavioral Health Statistics and Quality, 2016).

Literature Review

Knowledge Gaps

The main contribution of the knowledge gap hypothesis was acknowledging that the effects of mass media are constrained by social structural disparities, such as socioeconomic status, that are associated with the rate at which various groups acquire knowledge. Contrary to popular conceptions about the role of media in democracy, the authors showed that the mass media widened status differentials in knowledge. Because knowledge is tantamount to power, media ultimately serve to reinforce and exacerbate power disparities among the population (Tichenor, Donohue, & Olien, 1970).

The concept of mass media reinforcement of power differentials within society is a key component of the knowledge gap. That component takes on added explanatory power in an era in which facts and science are often disputed, disregarded, or denied when the facts conflict with political agendas. The current polarized political climate is markedly different from that in which the knowledge gap hypothesis was first proposed (Abramowitz & Sanders, 2008; Fiorina, Abrams, & Pope, 2008; Political polarization in the American public, 2015, June 12).

The original knowledge gap hypothesis included assumptions about knowledge that do not square with the polarized political climate. In the knowledge gap hypothesis, knowledge about science and public affairs was assumed to be unproblematic and universally accepted (Tichenor et al., 1970). The only requirement for knowledge to be diffused throughout the population was sufficient time. Knowledge, in this model, was cumulative, so that all groups gained knowledge, albeit at different rates (Tichenor, Donohue, & Olien, 1970). Media publicity was the primary means of diffusing knowledge about science and public affairs throughout social systems.

Missing from the extensive knowledge gap literature were studies about knowledge claims that were politically disputed (Hindman, 2009). Elected officials, political pundits, and spokespersons tend to dispute facts that negatively affect their goals or which pose the perceived risk of burdensome governmental regulations. Acknowledgement of a scientifically established connection between cigarette smoking and cancer, for example, was disputed by researchers representing the tobacco industry in order to forestall governmental regulation (Proctor, 1995). Similarly, the oil companies' own research first acknowledged the scientific consensus that the earth's atmosphere was warming and that the changes in the atmosphere were the result of human activity. In 1981, Exxon Mobil used knowledge of the connection between CO_2 and fossil fuels to make business decisions that would avoid future governmental regulation. The company funded 30 years of research designed to cast doubt on the connection between fossil fuels and global warming (Goldenberg, 2015, July 8).

Belief Gaps

The belief gap hypothesis is an extension of Tichenor, Donohue, and Olien's (1970) knowledge gap hypothesis. The belief gap hypothesis and the knowledge gap hypothesis both are based on issues for which there is a "correct" answer—an answer that can be easily verified or that has reached a level of consensus among nonpartisan experts who conduct evidence-based research. The belief gap hypothesis states that, in an era characterized by political polarization, indicators of partisanship will be better predictors than educational attainment of knowledge about heavily publicized and politically contested issues (Hindman, 2009).

Knowledge gap-era assumptions about the unproblematic and cumulative nature of knowledge are suspended when the knowledge consists of verifiable facts that are politically disputed. In the belief gap hypothesis, as the name implies, beliefs are privileged over knowledge. Whereas knowledge requires evidence to support the claim, beliefs are mere statements of personal opinion that are not burdened with the requirement to provide supporting evidence.

An individual, elected official, political pundit, or representative of a special interest group is free to believe or not believe anything that is contrary to the individual's self-interest, ideology, or values (Graham, Haidt, & Nosek, 2009). For example, spokespersons for tobacco industries, perceiving the risk of future governmental regulations that would affect company profits, learned that they could cast doubt on the scientific evidence linking smoking with cancer by stating, under oath, personal beliefs that were contrary to the facts (Proctor, 1995).

News reports of tobacco industry official's testimony at congressional hearings helped disseminate doubts about the risks of smoking. News media, relying on journalistic norms of balance, reported both scientific evidence of cancer risks and the tobacco industry's self-serving beliefs that cast doubt on the evidence. Industry officials knew that their doubts would be embraced by like-minded individuals throughout the country: individuals who were economically or physiologically dependent on tobacco (Proctor, 1995). This process, in which industry or political elites publicly express beliefs that are contrary to scientific evidence, is designed to exploit irrational impulses among individuals who are predisposed to accept the beliefs, regardless of the facts (Hindman, 2012).

Belief gaps are most obvious in polling about politically contested issues. This is because individuals filling out polls who don't know the correct answer to a question about facts will instead express their beliefs about the issue at hand. Hence, any statement that appears to favor their predispositions will be marked as true. Statements that subjects believe to be negative toward their predispositions will be scored as false (Zaller, 1992). When confronted with a factual question to which they do not know the correct answer, respondents will often use the opportunity for political expression (Bullock, Gerber, Hill, & Huber, 2013, May). Poll respondents would rather exhibit a political predisposition than ignorance—even though the two appear to be precisely the same when judged against the truth.

This paper applies the belief gap hypothesis to an analysis of knowledge among young adults. In the current study, the realms of knowledge that are of particular interest are a) knowledge about the Washington state law legalizing the recreational use of marijuana, and b) knowledge about the short-term and long-term health effects of marijuana use.

The first type of knowledge—knowledge about the contents of the marijuana legalization law—represents easily verified facts. A similar study compared the ability of Democratic and Republican partisans to identify which statements represented contents of the Affordable Care Act (Hindman, 2012). In that study, the belief gap was supported by evidence that Democrats knew more about the contents of the law over time. Republicans, however, appeared to know less. Contrary to the knowledge gap hypothesis, knowledge was cumulative only for groups that benefitted politically from the knowledge.

The second type of knowledge under consideration in this study requires the respondent to rely on the consensus of experts who conduct evidence-based research about the health risks of marijuana use. A study that employed this type of knowledge showed widening gaps between conservatives and liberals on acceptance of the value of abstinence-only sex education; a scientifically discredited teaching method that was shown to be ineffective in preventing unwanted pregnancies and sexually transmitted diseases (Hindman & Yan, 2015). Another study that relied on the knowledge claims of nonpartisan experts, in this case, climate scientists' consensus regarding the link between human activity and global warming, showed that ideology was a better predictor than educational attainment in accepting claims that there was solid evidence of global warming (Hindman, 2009). As with the knowledge gap, gaps in beliefs of liberals and conservatives widened over time.

In the knowledge gap hypothesis, both forms of knowledge—easily verified contents of heavily publicized laws and research about the health effects of marijuana use by minors—would be positively correlated with a measure of social status, operationalized as educational attainment. In the belief gap hypothesis, however, measures of social identity are expected to be better predictors than educational attainment of knowledge about marijuana laws and health effects.

Predictor Variables in Knowledge Gaps and Belief Gaps

Belief gaps are best conceptualized as special cases of the knowledge gap hypothesis. The knowledge gap hypothesizes a widening gap over time in knowledge between higher and lower status groups regarding heavily publicized scientific and public affairs issues (Tichenor, Donohue & Olien, 1970). On the other hand, the belief gap hypothesis is limited to cases in which the knowledge claim is politically disputed (Hindman, 2009). Knowledge as a criterion variable is replaced with beliefs, which accounts for cases in which individual beliefs are contrary to verifiable facts. In the case of facts that are not easy to verify, such as the cause of global warming or the effectiveness of abstinence-only sex education, a consensus of nonpartisan experts provide verification.

The main predictor variable in knowledge gaps is socioeconomic status, measured as educational attainment. Those with the highest levels of educational attainment are hypothesized to obtain knowledge at a faster rate than those with lower levels of education. The originators of the knowledge gap (Donohue, Tichenor, & Olien, 1975) provided an extension in the conceptualization of knowledge gaps. They argued that various indicators of social identity and social organization could serve as predictor of knowledge gaps. Community type and community economic structure were two indicators provided as examples of social organization affecting knowledge distribution among a social system. For example, studies showed knowledge gaps narrowing in communities in conflict. Similarly, communities engaged in conflict with outside groups showed considerable gaps in knowledge between local and non-local groups (Tichenor, Donohue, & Olien, 1980). More recent work has argued that indicators of identity are significant predictors of holding beliefs contrary to scientific consensus (Veenstra, Hossan, & Lyons, 2014).

The belief gap hypothesis also relies on indicators of social identity as predictors of beliefs about verifiable facts. Identification as a conservative or liberal, and political party identification, were both shown to be the best predictors of beliefs regarding politically contested but verifiable facts (Veenstra et al., 2014).

As Table 3.1 shows, knowledge gap and belief gap hypotheses share similarities and significant differences regarding the issues considered, the predictor and criterion variables measured, and the presumed impacts.

Social Identities and Risk Perceptions

Social identity is related to perceptual bias when the group is at risk for a negative health outcome. In a pioneering study, intravenous drug users and homosexuals significantly underestimated risk behaviors associated with contracting AIDS when compared with college students who were

Table 3.1 Assumptions in knowledge gap and belief gap hypotheses

	Knowledge gaps	Belief gaps
Issues	Verifiable truth claims about heavily publicized science or public affairs topics	Verifiable truth claims about heavily publicized and politically disputed topics
Criterion variables	Knowledge and beliefs	Knowledge and beliefs, risk perceptions
Predictor variables	Educational attainment, group affiliation (rural vs. urban community during conflict; occupational affiliation in environmental conflicts)	Partisan identification; self-identification on liberal-conservative scale; religious identification; social group identification.
Widening gaps		
Observations over time	Time x educational attainment or socioeconomic status	Time x partisan identification, political ideology, or group identification
Cross-sectional studies	Media use x educational attainment or socioeconomic status	Media use x partisan identification, political ideology, or group identification
Presumed impacts	Perpetuation/ exacerbation of status disparities	Perpetuation/ exacerbation of partisan, ideological, or group identification disparities
	Inability of social system to adjust to social change	Inability of social system to adjust to social change

not members of the at-risk groups (Campbell & Stewart, 1992). The minimization of known risk behaviors was consistent with the need to preserve one's positive identity as a member of a group (Campbell & Stewart).

A more contemporary study (McCright & Dunlap, 2013) demonstrated that even poorly defined social groups could have an impact on risk perceptions. It their study, conservative white males were significantly less concerned than the rest of the population about environmental risks such as the quality of the environment, pollution, and global warming. The researchers cited two cognitive mechanisms that help explain the rejection of environmental risks: identity-protective cognition and system justification (McCright & Dunlap, 2013, p. 212–214). Identity-protective cognition that appears as fearlessness among white males dismissing environmental risks is really defensiveness in protecting identity-central activities such as employment in energy-dependent industries (Kahan et al., 2007). Conservative white male group identification was enhanced through conservative media outlets promoting the system justification arguments of conservative white male elites occupying leadership roles in conservative politics and energy-dependent industries (McCright & Dunlap, 2013).

Social Identities Among College Students

The case of college student beliefs about the legalization of marijuana provides a number of potential extensions to the belief gap hypothesis. First, it offers an opportunity to observe belief gaps in the absence of media coverage of polarized debates among Republicans and Democrats. This is because legalization of recreational use of marijuana was not politically contested in the state. In the absence of Republican-Democrat polarization on the issue, citizens were not exposed to pundits and elected officials making public claims for or against the issue. Without news reports of elite contestation of evidence-supported claims, one would not expect citizens to associate issues surrounding marijuana legalization with their own political identities.

Another challenge and opportunity provided by the study is college students' indifference to partisan politics (Kiley & Dimock, 2014, September 25). Because college students' political identities are often not fully developed, partisan identity would not be expected to be a significant predictor of beliefs about the law or about the health risks of marijuana use by minors. Instead, other indicators of social group identity and self-interest in the norms of the group may come into play. The study provides the opportunity to consider aspects of social identity that might be relevant to legalization of recreational use of marijuana.

Religious Conservative Identities and Legalization of Marijuana

Although students may lack political identities, there is no shortage of opportunities for students to build an identity that they can share with others. Students can develop identities based on majors, living arrangements, and social group affiliations.

Of particular interest here is the degree of student identification as a conservative and religious person. Conservative groups in general tend to oppose legalization of recreational use of marijuana in favor of criminal approaches to control. Nationally, 47 percent of all Americans supported legalization of marijuana, up from 27 percent in 1979, and a larger percentage of Democrats than Republicans (51 percent vs. 27 percent) supported the legalization of marijuana in late 2012 (Backus & Condon, 2012, November 29). Federal law classifies marijuana as a Schedule 1 drug similar to heroin or cocaine because of its potential for abuse, threat to safety, and medical insignificance. However, the US Department of Justice has pledged to not interfere with states such as Colorado and Washington that have approved legalization of medicinal and recreational use of marijuana (Southhall & Healy, 2013, August 29).

Individuals affiliated with conservative community churches or with national conservative Christian organizations tend to publicly announce a formal set of beliefs, adhere to behavioral norms, and frequently attend social events and worship services with church members (Evangelical Protestants, 2015). Chemical dependency in general is anathema to conservative religious groups, which instead stress self-denial and dependence on the group's religious dogma (DeWall et al., 2014; Stewart, 2001).

Historically, religious groups have opposed marijuana use because of its tendency to intensify the user's focus on the present, as opposed to the spiritually transcendent, aspects of existence. The drug's effects are contrary to conservative religious emphases on self-denial, sacrifice, and the afterlife (Pollan, 2002). Religious identity would be expected to be a key predictor of differences with non-religious and non-conservatives in the perception of verifiable facts about the contents of the law and the health risks of marijuana use.

Frequency of Marijuana Use as a Social Identity

Another social group that would be relevant to questions about legalized marijuana would be the subculture surrounding marijuana use (Johnson, Bardhi, Sifaneck, & Dunlap, 2006). Status as a marijuana user would also likely become woven into a student's social identity. Students who frequently use marijuana would likely surround themselves with other users in order to share the experience of using and to participate in other social events while under the influence.

Students who are users of marijuana would be expected to view knowledge claims about health risks and the contents of the law through the perspective of self-interest and in support of the norms of the group. Among users, one might assume that statements about the contents of the law would be viewed positively, because of their group's support for the law, and statements about negative health effects of marijuana use would be viewed with skepticism or disbelief because the statements do not reflect well on the users' daily habits.

Acceptance of Social Media Portrayals of Marijuana
Use and Social Identity

Social media has become an important means of communicating individual and group social identities in an evolving media environment (Dominick, 1999; Livingstone, 2008; 2014; Taddicken, 2014). Among some individuals, the social media post about an activity is more important than the activity itself. If being a Christian conservative or marijuana user is a key part of one's identity, then attitudes toward social media portrayals of one's use would be closely tied to that identity. Hence, positive attitudes toward social media portrayal of one's own marijuana use would be related to rejection of knowledge claims regarding the negative health effects of marijuana use.

Hypotheses

In keeping with the belief gap hypothesis, measures of educational attainment would be less predictive of knowledge than would indicators of social identity. The issues chosen to test the hypotheses in this study are: easily verifiable facts about the contents of the law (H1a, H1b, H1c, RQ1) and statements representing evidence-based scientific research about the short-term and long-term health effects of marijuana use (H2a, H2b, H2c, RQ2).

Based on the previous discussion, the following hypotheses can be stated for testing:

> H1a: Measures of social identity will be better predictors than educational attainment of accurate beliefs about the contents of the law that legalized the recreational use of marijuana.

Individuals who tend to oppose an issue may express that opposition in polls. One way is to deny the truth of verifiable facts or expert knowledge claims that appear complimentary to the issue. Another way is to express belief in verifiable facts or knowledge claims that appear to put the issue in negative light. This is consistent with earlier findings by Jamieson and Cappella (2008, pp. 230–235) in which partisans were shown to agree with statements that portray their side favorably or portray opponents unfavorably, and to disagree with the converse: statements that portray their side unfavorably or that portray opponents favorably. It is also consistent with Bullock et al. (2013, May) who argue that partisans use knowledge questions in polls to express opinions consistent with their party's stance.

For example, Republicans appeared to know less over time about easily verifiable facts regarding the contents of Obamacare (Hindman, 2012).

This was likely because the Republican participants tended to deny the aspects of the Affordable Care Act that had widespread acceptance, such as allowing parents to keep dependents on their insurance until age 26 and requiring insurance companies to accept clients regardless of preexisting health conditions (Hindman, 2012).

In the current study, one would expect that various indicators of social identity will affect beliefs about the contents of the law, regardless of the truth. First, the expected negative predispositions toward the law legalizing recreational use of marijuana among conservatives, Republicans, and self-identified religious people would be reflected in their knowledge level about the easily verified facts regarding the contents of the law.

> H1b: Identification as a religious conservative will be negatively associated with accurate beliefs about the contents of the law legalizing recreational use of marijuana.

Second, frequent users of marijuana and those who embrace social media portrayals of their own use would show higher levels of knowledge about the law. This is because the respondents' self-interest is served by knowing the details of the law that legitimizes their own use of marijuana.

> H1c: Frequency of marijuana use, and approval of social media portrayals of one's own marijuana use, will be positively associated with accurate beliefs about the contents of the law.

The belief gap hypothesis predicts that social identity will grow over time in influence on individual beliefs. This is an extension of the knowledge gap hypothesis, which predicts a divergent interaction between educational status and time as predictors of knowledge. Previous studies have shown significant interactions between partisan and conservative social identities and with time. The current study provides an extension of the belief gap hypothesis into issues that are not politically contested, and among a population that is not overtly partisan. Hence, the relationships among social identity, time, and beliefs about the contents of the law that legalized marijuana will be stated as a research question.

> RQ1: Is there a relationship between the interaction of Time x Social Identity on the level of accurate beliefs about the contents of the law that legalized marijuana?

Whereas one would expect that opponents of the law would have lower levels of knowledge or beliefs about its contents than would proponents, the opposite would be expected for information that states facts about the negative health effects of marijuana use. Individuals who are opposed to marijuana use would be more likely to accept as true statements about negative health effects. Proponents of marijuana use would have the opposite reaction; they would express a disbelief in statements about negative health effects. In either case, indicators of social identity would be a better predictor of beliefs about the negative health effects of marijuana use than would educational attainment.

> H2a: Measures of social identity will be better predictors than educational attainment of beliefs about the negative health risks of marijuana use.

Those who are inclined to oppose marijuana use would tend to believe statements about the negative health risks of marijuana use. In the current study, beliefs about the negative health effects of marijuana use would be associated with identification as a religious conservative.

> H2b: Identification as a religious conservative will be positively associated with beliefs about the negative health effects of marijuana use.

Similarly, those who are predisposed to favor marijuana use because of their identities as frequent users, or as those who approve of social media portrayals of their use of marijuana, would not likely believe negative statements about the health effects of marijuana use.

> H2c: Frequency of marijuana use, and approval of social media portrayals of one's own marijuana use, will be negatively associated with beliefs about the negative health effects of marijuana use.

The traditional test of belief gaps over time is based on issues in which political elites contest verifiable facts based on partisan or ideological beliefs. Intense media coverage of the controversy widens over time the gaps between partisans in beliefs about the issue. As was stated above, the current issue of legalization of recreational use of marijuana was not politically contested in the state. Further, college students tend to be less politically polarized than older generations and elected officials. Hence, the nature of the relationships among social identity and beliefs about the health effects of marijuana use over time is best stated as a research question.

> RQ2: Is there a relationship between the interaction of time and social identity on beliefs about the negative health effects of marijuana use?

Methods

Overview

Data for testing the hypotheses came from three online surveys of students of 18 years of age or older in communication classes at a public university in Washington state. Each survey was reviewed by the university IRB and received exempt status. Students were recruited using an online subject pool management system, and received extra credit for their participation. Cases were deleted in which the respondent completed the survey in fewer than five minutes, left the majority of items blank, or showed evidence of straight-lining—giving the same response to a series of items.

The first survey was fielded following the November 2012 election and directly before the new Washington state marijuana law went into effect, Nov. 27–Dec. 7, 2012. The survey produced 312 usable cases. The second survey was fielded April 16–May 1, 2014, before legal retail sales began, and produced 402 useable cases. The third survey was fielded Sept. 22–Nov. 7, 2015, and produced 295 usable cases.

Predictor and Criterion Variables

Table 3.2 shows the means for each of the main predictor and criterion variables (operationally defined below) that were used in the study. The variable "month" was used to indicate the months between the first survey and the subsequent two. Hence, for the 2012 survey, "month" was zero; for 2014, "month" was 15; and for the 2015 survey, "month" was 34.

Measures

Female indicates the self-reported gender identity of the respondents with 0 representing male and 1 representing female. Table 3.2 also shows that 61percent of the respondents identified as female, which reflects the population of the classes from which the students were self-selected. The percentage of females was significantly lower in 2014 than in the other two years.

Educational achievement was operationalized as educational aspiration. If using traditional operationalizations of educational attainment, the entire sample for the present study would fit into the same category: "some college, no degree." Obviously, a sample of college students is relatively homogenous in terms of educational attainment. A more straightforward operationalization, "year in college," was not equally distributed across the years of the study. Instead, respondents were asked, "How far do you think you will go in school?" with options for "some

Table 3.2 Descriptive Statistics of Main Variables

		Mean	SD	Minimum	Maximum
Educational	2012	2.17[a]	0.43	1	3
aspiration	2014	2.27[b]	0.50	1	3
	2015	2.31[b]	0.50	1	3
	Total	2.25	0.48	1	3
Religious	2012	−0.10[a]	0.73	−1.40	1.94
conservative scale	2014	0.09[b]	0.71	−1.31	1.92
	2015	−0.02	0.76	−1.31	2.09
	Total	0.00	0.74	−1.40	2.09
Frequency of	2012	0.54	0.41	.00	1.00
marijuana use	2014	0.56	0.43	.00	1.00
scale	2015	0.53	0.44	.00	1.00
	Total	0.54	0.43	.00	1.00
Acceptance of social	2012	0.56[a]	0.39	0.00	1.00
media portrayals	2014	0.47[b]	0.42	0.00	1.00
of one's own	2015	0.45[b]	0.44	0.00	1.00
marijuana use	Total	0.49	0.42	0.00	1.00
Knowledge of law	2012	3.49[a]	1.92	.00	7.00
	2014	4.93[b]	1.50	.00	7.00
	2015	4.98[b]	1.31	.00	7.00
	Total	4.50	1.73	.00	7.00
Knowledge of	2012	2.32[a]	1.68	.00	5.00
short–term health	2014	3.40[b]	1.59	.00	5.00
effects	2015	3.48[b]	1.48	.00	5.00
	Total	3.09	1.67	.00	5.00
Knowledge of	2012	3.05[a]	2.81	.00	10.00
long-term health	2014	5.81[b]	3.34	.00	10.00
effects	2015	6.08[b]	3.06	.00	10.00
	Total	5.03	3.38	.00	10.00

Note: Means with different superscripts are significantly different ($p < .05$) (Scheffe) in tests with significant overall ANOVA ($p < .05$).

college, but less than four years," "graduate with my Bachelor's degree," "Graduate or professional school," and "I am not sure." The 12 cases in the final category were assigned to the variable mean of 2.2. This operationalization of educational attainment as educational aspiration was the best option, given the nature of the dataset.

Religious Conservative (Chronbach's α =.72) was formed as the mean of standardized measures of four items: self-placement on a liberal-conservative scale (very liberal, liberal, moderate or not political, conservative, very conservative); self-placement Democrat-Republican scale (1= strong Democrat or Democrat, 2 = Independent; 3 = Republican or Strong Republican; Religiosity (1 = not at all religious, 2 = not very religious, 3 = religious, 4 = somewhat religious, 5 = very religious); frequency of attending religious worship services (never, on major holidays only, several times a year, a couple of times a month, once a week, several times a week). Table 3.2 shows that the 2014 sample scored significantly higher on the religious conservative scale than did the respondents in the 2012 sample.

Frequency of marijuana use was computed first as the sum of four standardized indicators of frequency of marijuana use (Chronbach's α = .86). The first frequency indicator measured how much marijuana the respondents have used in their life (seven items ranging from 0 times to 100 or more times). The next item measured how much marijuana the respondents have used in past thirty days (I didn't use marijuana, 1 or 2 days, 3 to 5 days, 6 to 9 days, 10 to 19 days, 20 to 29 days and all 30 days). The third question measured typical marijuana use on one occasion (I don't use marijuana; 1–2 small hits on a marijuana cigarette, pipe, or bong, or 1–2 small bites of a marijuana food product; 3–5 hits on a marijuana cigarette, pipe, or bong, or 3–5 bites of a marijuana food product; smoke a whole joint, pipe, or bong, or eat an entire marijuana product; or smoke more than one joint, more than one pipe or bong, or consume a lot of marijuana product). Finally, the last question measured self-perception of marijuana use status with six items (non-user, very light user, light user, moderate user, heavy user, and very heavy user). The scale was positively skewed because 28 percent of respondents chose the non-user option for each item. The scale was recoded into a four-level measure with 0 representing non-users, .25 representing those respondents who identified as a user on one of the four indicators, .5 for those choosing two indicators of use, .75 for three indicators, and 1.0 for those who identified as a user on all four indicators. Table 3.2 shows that there were no significant differences across years on the frequency of marijuana use scale.

Approval of social media portrayals of one's own marijuana use (Chronbach's α .82) is a measure of five items, each preceded with, "How would you feel if friends or acquaintances of yours posted on social media pictures of you using marijuana?" The choices were "proud;" "angry" (reversed); "happy," "ashamed" (reversed); "embarrassed" (reversed). The five responses were "very (4), somewhat, a little, not at all (1)." The index was computed as the mean of the five measures. An examination of the distribution of the scale indicated a positive skew resulting from 35 percent of respondents selecting the lowest value on each scale item. To control for skew, the scale was trichotomized so that zero represented the 35 percent of respondents who chose the lowest value on each item in the scale, 1 represented the 30 percent of respondents that scored between 1 and 2 on the scale, and 2 represented the 35 percent who scored higher than 2 on the scale.

Beliefs about the contents of the law legalizing recreational use of marijuana was computed as the number of statements correctly identified as true about the Washington state marijuana law: *It will be legal for those over age 21 to possess up to two ounces of marijuana* (false); *all adults 21 and over will be allowed to have up to six marijuana plants in their homes* (false); *It will be legal to purchase marijuana only from state-licensed providers* (true); *it will be illegal to use marijuana in public* (true); *individuals under age 21 will be allowed to distribute marijuana* (false); *persons under age 21 will not be allowed on the premises of licensed marijuana retailers* (true); *driving under the influence of marijuana will be prohibited* (true); *advertising of marijuana sales will be restricted* (true); *taxes will be applied to the sale of marijuana by producers, processors, and retailers* (true). In 2012 respondents scored significantly lower on the index measuring knowledge of the state law legalizing recreational use of marijuana.

Beliefs about the short-term health effects was computed as the number of items correctly identified as true about the "immediate health consequences of using marijuana" including: *distorted perceptions* (true); *impaired coordination* (true); *problems with sleeping* (false); *difficulty with thinking or problem solving* (true); *sexual dysfunction* (false); *problems with learning and memory* (true); *numbness in the feet* (false); *increased heart related problems (palpitations, arrhythmias and heart attack)* (true); *ringing in the ears* (false); *there are no immediate health effects* (false) (Ammerman et al., 2015; Drug Facts, 2017, February; Meier et al., 2012).

Beliefs about the long term health effects was also computed as the number of items correctly identified as true about the long-term health effects of marijuana use: *compulsive drug seeking* (true); *tremors in hands* (false); *quitting withdrawal symptoms* (true); *anxiety* (true); *brain cancer* (false); *vision problems* (false); *depression* (true); *schizophrenia* (true); *sexual dysfunction* (false); *bone degeneration* (false); *increased respiratory problems* (true); *stomach cancer* (false); *irritable bowel syndrome* (false); *problems with short-term memory* (true); *decreased attention spans* (true); *learning impairments* (true); *lack of motivation* (true) (Ammerman et al., 2015; Drug Facts, 2017, February; Meier et al., 2012).

In 2012, respondents scored significantly lower on the index measuring both short-term and long-term health effects of marijuana use than in

2014 and 2015. This provides some evidence of higher levels of awareness of health effects over time.

Results

To test the hypotheses, the three dependent measures—knowledge of the contents of the law legalizing recreational use of marijuana, knowledge of short-term health effects of marijuana use, and knowledge of long-term health effects of marijuana use—were regressed on the predictor variables in a hierarchical multiple regression. Table 3.3 shows the results.

The first hypothesis was stated as:

H1a: Identification as a religious conservative will be a better predictor than educational aspiration of beliefs about the contents of the law that legalized recreational use of marijuana.

Table 3.3 Summary of Hierarchical Regression Analysis for Variables Predicting Knowledge of the Contents of the Law Legalizing Recreational Marijuana (N=1004)

	B	S.E.	β	Adj. R-square	F for change in R-square
(Constant)	3.92	0.27			
Sex (female)	−0.31	0.11	−0.09**		
				0.003	3.8
Educational aspiration	0.06	0.10	0.02		
				.005	3.100
Cannabis use	0.29	0.13	0.07*		
Religious conservative	−0.18	0.07	−0.08*		
Acceptance of social media images of cannabis use	−0.38	0.13	−0.09**		
				.021	6.4***
Time	0.04	0.00	0.34***		
				.130	125.9***
Time x religious conservative	0.14	0.07	0.06+		
Time x acceptance of social media images	0.12	0.06	0.07*		
Time x cannabis use	−0.05	0.06	−0.03		
				.134	2.6*

Notes: * $p < .05$, ** $p < .01$, *** $p < .001$

As shown in Table 3.3, both the coefficient for educational aspiration (β = .02, n.s.) and the F testing the change in R^2 were not statistically significant. In contrast, the three indicators of social identity, entered as a block in the Hierarchical Multiple Regression showed a significant F test of the change in R^2 (6.4, $p<.001$). All three coefficients representing social identity were statistically significant: frequency of marijuana use (β = .07), religious conservative (β = −.08), and acceptance of social media portrayals of one's own marijuana use (β = −.09). Together the findings support H1a.

The second hypothesis was stated as

> H1b: Identification as a religious conservative will be negatively associated with beliefs about the contents of the law.

The test for this hypothesis is shown in Table 3.3 as the statistically significant negative coefficients for religious conservative (β = −.08, $p < .05$). This indicates that those identifying as religious conservatives were less able than non-religious conservatives to identify true statements about the contents of the law legalizing recreational use of marijuana. The hypothesis was supported.

The third hypothesis was stated as:

> H1c: Frequency of marijuana use, and approval of social media portrayals of one's own marijuana use, will be positively associated with beliefs about the contents of the law.

The test for this hypothesis is shown in Table 3.3 as the statistically significant and positive coefficient for the frequency of marijuana use variable (β = .07, $p < .05$). This shows that those with higher frequencies of marijuana use were more successful at identifying true statements about the law. Contrary to the hypothesis, the other social identity indicator, approval of social media portrayals of one's own marijuana use, was negative and statistically significant (β = −.09, $p < .01$). In other words, those who approve of social media posts of their own marijuana use are less likely than those who don't post to know about the contents of the law legalizing marijuana use. Hence, the hypothesis was partially supported.

The first research question was stated as

> RQ1: Is there a relationship between the interaction of Time x Social Identity on beliefs about the contents of the law that legalized marijuana?

This research question is addressed by the interaction terms in Table 3.3. The F test measuring the change in R^2 was statistically significant (F 2.6, $p < .05$), which provides an indication of a relationship among the group of variables and knowledge about the contents of the marijuana legalization law. Two of the Time x Social Identity interaction measures were statistically significant, albeit one was only marginally significant (time x religious conservative, β = .06, $p < .1$) and was in the opposite direction as would be expected based on previous belief gap findings about declining knowledge among conservatives (Republicans) in knowledge about a disliked law (Hindman, 2012). The expectation would be that the more one knows about a disliked law, the more one disputes factual statements about its contents—particularly aspects that are widely viewed as favorable. The other significant coefficient, time x acceptance of social media images (β = .07, $p < .05$) was in the expected direction. The positive coefficient shows that, over time, acceptance of social media images of one's own marijuana use is positively associated with knowledge about the contents of the law. In other words, those who approve of social media portrayals of their own use tend to learn more about the law over time than those who don't want to see themselves using marijuana online. Overall, the research question shows a modest relationship between the interaction of Time x Social Identity on beliefs about the contents of the law that legalized marijuana.

To further test the extension of the belief gap hypothesis to questions surrounding student beliefs about the legalization of recreational marijuana, two measures of knowledge of the health effects of marijuana were used to test hypotheses relevant to the question of social identity as a predictor of beliefs. The general expectation is that those who are inclined to oppose marijuana use would tend to identify as true those statements that claim negative health effects resulting from marijuana use.

The first hypothesis about health effects was stated as:

H2a: Measures of social identity will be better predictors than educational attainment of negative health effects of marijuana use.

Tables 3.4 and 3.5 show results relevant to the hypothesis. The first indicator is a comparison of the F test of the change in R^2 for the Educational Aspiration block versus the F test of the change in R^2 for the Social Identity block (frequency of marijuana use, religious conservative, acceptance of social media portrayals of one's own marijuana use). In Table 3.4, the hypothesis was supported by a non-significant F (2.6, n.s.) test of the change in the R^2 in the Educational Aspiration block, and a significant F (22.1, $p < .01$) test of the change in the R^2 in the Social Identity block. Similarly, in Table 3.5, the hypothesis is supported by a non-significant F (3.7, n.s.) test of the change in the R^2 in the Educational Aspiration block, and a significant F (43.7, $p < .001$) test of the change in the R^2 in the Social Identity block. The hypothesis was supported.

Table 3.4 Summary of Hierarchical Regression Analysis for Variables Predicting Knowledge of the Short-Term Health Effects of Marijuana Use (N=1004)

	B	Std. Error	β	Adj. R-square	F for R-square change
(Constant)	2.91	0.27			
Sex (female)	0.16	0.10	0.05		
				0.01	11.9**
Educational aspiration	0.06	0.10	0.02		
				0.01	2.60
Frequency of marijuana use	−0.31	0.13	−0.08*		
Religious conservative	0.10	0.07	0.05		
Acceptance of social media images of marijuana use	−0.68	0.13	−0.17***		
				0.07	22.1***
Time	0.03	0.00	0.24**		
				0.13	65.9***
Time x religious conservative	−0.04	0.07	−0.02		
Time x acceptance of social media images	0.04	0.05	0.02		
Time x marijuana use	−.042	.054	−.025		
				.133	.360

Notes: * $p < .05$, ** $p < .01$, *** $p < .001$

The next hypothesis was stated as:

H2b: Identification as a religious conservative will be positively associated with beliefs about the negative health effects of marijuana.

Table 3.4 shows that the coefficient for religious conservative (β = .05, n.s.) was in the predicted direction, but was not statistically significant. Table 3.5 also shows that the coefficient for religious conservative (β = .05, n.s.) was in the predicted direction, but was not statistically significant. The hypothesis was not supported. Religious conservatives were

Table 3.5 Summary of Hierarchical Regression Analysis for Variables Predicting Knowledge of the Long-Term Health Effects of Marijuana Use (N=1004)

	B	Std. Error	β	Adj. R-square	F for change in R-square
(Constant)	4.99	0.51			
Sex (female)	0.07	0.20	0.01		
				0.01	8.68***
Educational aspiration	0.09	0.20	0.01		
				0.01	3.70
Frequency of marijuana use	−1.18	0.24	−0.15***		
Religious conservative	0.22	0.13	0.05		
Acceptance of social media images of marijuana use	−1.70	0.25	−0.21***		
				0.12	43.7***
Time	0.08	0.01	0.31***		
				0.22	123.80
Time x religious conservative	−0.04	0.13	−0.01		
Time x acceptance of social media images	−0.07	0.10	−0.02		
Time x marijuana use	−0.04	0.10	−0.01		
				0.22	.255

Notes: * $p < .05$, ** $p < .01$, *** $p < .001$

not more likely than anyone else to correctly identify truthful statements about short-term or long-term negative health effects of marijuana use.

The next hypothesis tests beliefs about negative health effects among those predisposed to support recreational use of marijuana. The hypothesis was stated as:

H2c: Frequency of marijuana use, and approval of social media portrayals of one's own marijuana use, will be negatively associated with beliefs about the negative health effects of marijuana use.

The test for this hypothesis is shown in the coefficients for the two pro-marijuana social identity variables. In Table 3.4, both frequency of marijuana use (β = -.08, p < .05) and acceptance of social media images (β = -.17, p < .001) were in the hypothesized direction and were statistically significant. In Table 3.5, both frequency of marijuana use (β = -.15, p < .001) and acceptance of social media images (β = -.21, p < .001) were also in the hypothesized direction and were statistically significant. The hypothesis was supported.

The second research question also attempts to determine whether indicators of social identity strengthen over time in predicting beliefs about the negative health effects of marijuana use. It was stated as:

RQ2: Will there be a relationship between the interaction of time and social identity on beliefs about the negative health effects of marijuana?

This research question is addressed by the interaction terms in Tables 3.4 and 3.5. In neither Table 3.4 or Table 3.5 was the F test measuring the change in R^2 statistically. This is strong evidence of a lack of a relationship. Similarly, none of the coefficients of the Time x Social Identity measures was statistically significant. No evidence was found of a relationship between social identity and time on beliefs about the negative health effects of marijuana use.

Summary and Conclusions

This paper applied the belief gap hypothesis to an analysis of young adults' knowledge about recreational marijuana laws and health effects. The knowledge indicators represented two types of knowledge: easily verified facts (about the contents of the law legalizing recreational marijuana use) and facts that require expert opinions (about the short-term and long-term health effects of marijuana use).

Findings showed that, in general, knowledge levels grew during the four years of the study. Knowledge of the law was significantly higher in 2014 and 2015 than in 2012. Similarly, knowledge of both short-term and long-term health effects was significantly higher in 2015 than in 2012. This supports the "cumulative knowledge" proposition of the knowledge gap hypothesis. Evidence from this study supports the proposition that *uncontested* scientific and public affairs knowledge tends to accumulate over time.

Contrary to the knowledge gap hypothesis, but consistent with the belief gap hypothesis, a measure of educational attainment (aspirational) was not a significant predictor of either types of knowledge: the easily verified contents of the law and the short-term and long-term health effects of marijuana use.

Consistent with the belief gap hypothesis, indicators of social identity were more significant predictors than was educational attainment (aspiration) of beliefs about the contents of the law and about the health effects of marijuana use. Further, hypothesized differences in social group identity were supported. Evidence showed contrasting beliefs about the law and about negative health effects between those with different social identities. The pattern that appears in the findings is consistent with the conclusion that individuals answer survey questions less to show knowledge than to express opinions consistent with their social identities (Bullock et al., 2013, May).

The present study advances the belief gap hypothesis in four ways. First, the study finds that belief gaps persist in the absence of political contestation of facts. The majority of belief gap studies concern factual issues that are politically contested. In contrast, the issue of legalization of recreational use of marijuana was not politically contested in the state. Hence, individuals could not rely on cues from political elites when answering questions about the law or health effects. Second, the study detected belief gaps among young adults—a demographic group that is less politically polarized than others (Kiley & Dimock, 2014, September 25). Whereas previous studies of adults show belief gaps developing between partisan groups, the present study showed that the belief gap hypothesis can be extended to include social identities. The study is notable for operationalizing three indicators of identities which were shown to predict knowledge, or, more formally, beliefs about knowledge, as was hypothesized. Finally, the study showed that the belief gap hypothesis can be extended to health risk perceptions. Individuals perceived the truth of negative short-term and long-term health effects in ways that were consistent with their behavior (frequency of use of marijuana) and online identities (accepting of online images associating them with marijuana use). This is consistent with previous studies showing group identification as significant predictors of risks relevant to group membership (Campbell & Stewart, 1992; McCright & Dunlap, 2013).

Three main indicators of social identity were chosen: religious conservatives, marijuana users, and individuals willing to be portrayed on social media as accepting of marijuana use.

Special attention was given to conservative religious groups because a) the significant presence of conservative religious groups on college campuses, b) the potential relevance of this identity to legalized recreational marijuana, and c) the intensity of the commitment required of members in those groups. As expected, religious conservatism was negatively associated with knowledge about the easily verified contents of the law that legalized recreational use of marijuana. This is in keeping with the belief gap hypothesis: respondents opposed to the law would claim to know less about its actual contents than would those predisposed in favor of the law. This effect was likely because religious conservatives disagree, on principle, with both the idea of the law but also with specific aspects of the law. In the absence of knowledge, beliefs take precedence.

Another identity expected to be relevant for the study was frequency of marijuana use. In college settings, the subculture of marijuana users would be expected to affect significantly beliefs about the health effects of marijuana use. As expected, frequency of use was a negative predictor of knowledge of the negative health effects of marijuana use. In the absence of knowledge, respondents use questions about negative health effects to express an opinion that serves their self-interest and group identity. Again, polls are used to represent beliefs about facts, not knowledge.

The third identity considered relevant to legalization of marijuana in this study was those who are proud, happy, and not at all angry, ashamed, or embarrassed when their friends post pictures of them using marijuana on social media. The central role of social media in creating and maintaining college students' social identities makes this variable of considerable interest. As expected, approval of social media portrayals of one's own marijuana use were negatively associated with knowledge of the negative health effects of marijuana use. Social identity was a better predictor than educational aspiration of knowledge about the negative health effects of marijuana use.

The findings of the study are relevant to the link between perceptions of risk and health. It is reasonable to expect that individuals who denied the truth of scientifically supported claims about health effects were, in effect, denying the health risk posed by marijuana use. Future work on beliefs about the health effects of marijuana use will include measures of the perceived degree of risk linking recreational use to specific effects, and expert assessments of the same risks. Measures of individual level of identification with various groups will be included with external indicators of group membership. The hypotheses would, however, be the same. Those individuals with identities predisposed to marijuana use will view risks as lower than those who oppose marijuana use. The "belief gap" in which social identities are more predictive than traditional predictors of knowledge, such as educational attainment, would be hypothesized to hold. Beliefs about facts, and beliefs about risk, are both expected to be supportive of social identities and existing behaviors. Perceptions of risk, particularly risks that are associated with meaningful social identities, are expected to be as prone to irrational and counter-factual interpretations as are political views.

In an evolving media environment, identities and media are more closely linked than ever. Audiences of traditional media expressed identity passively as taste publics. Audiences of social media use the platforms for self-presentation and identity creation. Through Facebook Likes researchers can accurately predict a wide range of personal attributes such as sexual orientation, ethnic origin, gender, and intelligence, as well as behaviors that social media users may not know they are revealing such as political views, religion, relationship status, and substance use (Kosinski, Stillwell, & Graepel, 2012).

Similarly, for many college students, online identities *are* social identities. How students present themselves, or how others present them through pictures taken at social events, is an indicator of how various forms of behavior evolve from stigmatized to accepted. In the present study, questions about how students would feel if images appeared online of themselves using marijuana or in settings in which marijuana was being used, became one of the strongest predictors of knowledge of the law or knowledge of associated health effects. Social identity, as mediated in social media, can be a key indicator in research on health and risk.

Limitations of the present study are numerous. First, the study relied on three self-selected samples of students seeking extra credit. The results cannot be generalized beyond the individuals participating in the study. The samples were too small and homogeneous to detect what might have been significant differences. The education measure, for example, was based on educational aspiration and not actual achievement. Clearly, results regarding that variable must be interpreted with caution.

Finally, the explained variance in the regression equations was small, particularly regarding knowledge of health effects. This suggests caution in drawing conclusions from the results described in this study. Clearly, there are other processes that drive college student knowledge and beliefs related to the legalization of marijuana.

References

Abramowitz, A. A., & Saunders, K. K. (2008). Is polarization a myth? *Journal of Politics*, 70, 542–555.

Ammerman, S., Ryan, S., Adelman, W., The Committee on Substance Abuse, & The Committee on Adolescence. (2015, March). The impact of marijuana policies on youth: Clinical, research, and legal update. *Pediatrics*, *135*(3). Available: http://pediatrics.aappublications.org/content/135/3/e769.

Ammons, D. (2012, Jan. 27). Marijuana Initiative 502 certified to Legislature/ ballot. Available: http://blogs.sos.wa.gov/FromOurCorner/index.php/2012/01/marijuana-initiative-502-certified-to-legislatureballot/.

Backus, F., & Condon, S. (2012, November 29). Nearly half support legalization of marijuana. CBS NewsNews Polls. www.cbsnews.com/8301-250_162-57556286/poll-nearly-half-support-legalization-of-marijuana/?pageNum=2#postComments.

Bullock, J., Gerber, A., Hill, S., & Huber, G. (2013, May). Partisan bias in factual beliefs about politics. NBER Working Paper Series, 19080. Available: www.nber.org/papers/w19080.

Campbell, L., & Stewart, A. (1992). Effects of group membership on perception of risk for AIDS. *Psychological Reports*, *70*(3, supplement), 1075–1092.

DeWall, C. N., Pond, R. S., Jr., Carter, E. C., McCullough, M. E., Lambert, N. M., Fincham, F. D., & Nezlek, J. B. (2014). Explaining the relationship between religiousness and substance use: Self-control matters. *Journal of Personality and Social Psychology*,*107*(2), 339–351. doi:http://dx.doi.org/10.1037/a0036853.

Dominick, J. R. (1999). Who do you think you are? Personal home pages and self-presentation on the world wide web. *Journalism & Mass Communication Quarterly*, 76(4), 646–658.

Donohue, G., Tichenor, P., & Olien, C. (1975). Mass media and the knowledge gap: A hypothesis reconsidered. *Communication Research*, 2(1), 3–23.

Drug Facts. (2017, February). National Institute on Drug Abuse: Marijuana. Available: www.drugabuse.gov/publications/drugfacts/marijuana.

Evangelical Protestants. (2015). *Religious landscape study*. Pew Research Center for Religion and Public Life. Available: www.pewforum.org/religious-landscape-study/religious-tradition/evangelical-protestant/.

Fiorina, M., Abrams, S., & Pope. (2008). Polarization in the American public: Misconceptions and misreadings. *The Journal of Politics*, 70, 556–560.

Goldenberg, S. (2015, July 8). Exxon knew of climate change in 1981, email says—but it funded deniers for 27 more years. *The Guardian*. Available: www.theguardian.com/environment/2015/jul/08/exxon-climate-change-1981-climate-denier-funding.

Graham, J., Haidt, J., & Nosek, B. (2009). Liberals and conservatives rely on different sets of moral foundations. *Journal of Personality and Social Psychology*, 96, 1029–1046.

Hindman, D. (2009). Mass media flow and the differential distribution of politically disputed beliefs: The belief gap hypothesis. *Journalism and Mass Communication Quarterly*, 86, 790–808.

Hindman, D. (2012). Knowledge gaps, belief gaps, and public opinion about health care reform. *Journalism and Mass Communication Quarterly*, 89, 585–605.

Hindman, D., & Yan, C. (2015). The knowledge gap vs. the belief gap and abstinence-only sex education. *Journal of Health Communication: International Perspectives*, 20(8), 949–957.

Iyengar, S., Sood, G., & Lelkes, Y. (2012). Affect, not ideology: A social identity perspective on polarization. *Public Opinion Quarterly*, 76, 405–431.

Jamieson, K. G. H., & Cappella, J. N. (2008). *Echo chamber: Rush Limbaugh and the conservative media establishment*. Oxford: Oxford University Press.

Johnson, G. (2015, July 4). Washington state has brought in $70 million in tax revenue from legal marijuana sales. *Business Insider*. Available: www.businessinsider.com/recreational-marijuana-washington-state-tax-revenue-2015-7.

Johnson, E., Bardhi, F., Sifaneck, N., & Dunlap, E. (2006). Marijuana argot as subculture threads: Social constructions by users in New York City. *The British Journal of Criminology*, 46(1), 46–77 Available: http://ssrn.com/abstract=905679 or http://dx.doi.org/10.1093/bjc/azi053.

Kahan, D., Braman, D., Gastil, J., Slovic, P., & Mertz, C. (2007). Culture and identity-protective cognition: Explaining the white-male effect in risk perception. *Journal of Empirical Legal Studies*, 4(3), 465–505.

Kiley, J., & Dimock, M. (2014, September 25). *The GOP's millennial problem runs deep*. Pew Reseach Center. Available: www.pewresearch.org/fact-tank/2014/09/25/the-gops-millennial-problem-runs-deep/.

Kosinski, M., Stillwell, D., & Graepel, T. (2013). Private traits and attributes are predictable from digital records of human behavior. *PNAS: Proceedings of the National Academy of Sciences of the United States of America*. Available: www.pnas.org/content/110/15/5802.full.pdf.

Livingstone, S. (2008). Taking risky opportunities in youthful content creation: Teenagers' use of social networking sites for intimacy, privacy and self-expression. *New Media & Society, 10*(3), 393–411.

Livingstone, S. (2014). Developing social media literacy: How children learn to interpret risky opportunities on social network sites. *Communications: The European Journal of Communication Research, 39*(3), 283–303. doi: 10.1515/commun-2014-0113.

Major, J. (2015, July 4). State presents new medical pot rules. *The Daily Record.* Avalable: www.dailyrecordnews.com/members/state-presents-new-medical-pot-rules/article_e8bd9c18-83e4-11e5-aa99-b737c89a0c35.html.

Martin, J. (2012, November 7). Voters approve I-502 legalizing marijuana. *The Seattle Times,* http://seattletimes.com/html/localnews/2019621894_elexmarijuana07m.html.

McCright, A. M., & Dunlap, R. E. (2013). Bringing ideology in: The conservative white male effect on worry about environmental problems in the USA. *Journal of Risk Research, 16*(2), 211–226. doi: 10.1080/13669877.2012.726242.

Meiera, M. Caspia, A., Ambler, A., Harrington, H., Houts, R., Keefe, R., McDonald, K. Ward, A., Poulton, R., & Moffitt, T. (2012). Persistent cannabis users show neuropsychological decline from childhood to midlife. *PNAS: Proceedings of the National Academy of Sciences of the United States of America.* Available: www.pnas.org/content/109/40/E2657.

Pollan, M. (2002). *Botany of desire: A plant's eye view of the world.* New York: Random House.

Political polarization in the American public. (2015, June 12). Pew Research Center. Available: www.people-press.org/2014/06/12/political-polarization-in-the-american-public/.

Proctor, R. (1995). *Cancer Wars: How politics shapes what we know & don't know about cancer.* New York: Basic Books.

Preparations in place for July 1 alignment of medical and recreational marijuana systems. (n.d.). Washington State Liquor and Cannabis Board: 2016 Press Releases. Available: http://lcb.wa.gov/pressreleases/alignment-med-and-rec-mj-systems.

Southhall, A. & Healy, J. (2013, August 29). U.S. won't sue to reverse states' legalization of marijuana. *The New York Times.* Available: www.nytimes.com/2013/08/30/us/politics/us-says-it-wont-sue-to-undo-state-marijuana-laws.html?_r=0.

Stewart, C. (2001). The influence of spirituality on substance use of college students. *Journal of Drug Education, 31,* 343–351.

Tichenor, P., Donohue, G., & Olien, C. (1970). Mass media flow and differential growth in knowledge. *Public Opinion Quarterly, 34,* 159–170.

Taddicken, M. (2014). The 'Privacy Paradox' in the social web: The impact of privacy concerns, individual characteristics, and the perceived social relevance on different forms of self-disclosure. *Journal of Computer-Mediated Communication, 19*(2), 248–273. doi: 10.1111/jcc4.12052.

Tichenor, P., Donohue, G., & Olien, C. (1980). *Community conflict and the press.* Beverly Hills, CA: SAGE.

Veenstra, A., Hossain, M., & Lyons, B. (2014). Partisan media and discussion as enhancers of the belief gap. *Mass Communication and Society, 17,* 874–897.

Washington Secretary of State. (2012, November 27). Nov. 6, 2012 election results: Initiative Measure No. 502 concerns marijuana. Available: http://vote. wa.gov/results/20121106/Initiative-Measure-No-502-Concerns-marijuana_ ByCounty.html.

Willis, H. H., & DeKay, M. L. (2007). The roles of group membership, beliefs, and norms in ecological risk perception. *Risk Analysis: An International Journal, 27*(5), 1365–1380. doi:10.1111/j.1539-6924.2007.00958.

Zaller, J. (1992). *The nature and origins of mass opinion.* New York: Cambridge University Press.

4

OUT OF SIGHT, OUT OF MIND?

Addressing Unconscious Brand Awareness in Healthcare Communication

Laura Crosswell, Lance Porter, and Meghan Sanders

On June 8, 2006, the FDA approved the world's first preventative vaccination for the human papilloma virus (HPV). Eager to initiate public discussion and perhaps activate consumer demand, Merck Pharmaceuticals quickly launched a national print, television, and online advertising campaign for the Gardasil(R) vaccination (Petersen, 2006). Prior to receiving FDA approval, however, Merck joined forces with nonprofits Cancer Research & Prevention Foundation and Step Up Women's Network to raise awareness for HPV through an unprecedented, three-tiered social marketing campaign.

While the HPV vaccination presented a hopeful defense against cervical cancer, Merck's early release of awareness messages sparked debate over corporate intentions. Reports characterized the social marketing campaign as "a commercial effort" that "primed the market" for Merck's new vaccine (Serono, n.d.). Critics also suggested Merck strategically engineered the awareness push to gain market lead, as GlaxoSmithKline was working on alternative inoculation developments (Herper, 2012). Though Merck insisted, "This campaign is part of a broad and longstanding public health commitment to encourage education about the disease" (Merck representative K. Dougherty in Schwartz, 2006), the pre-released messages prompted accusations of deceptive marketing agendas. Siers-Poisson (2007) further suggested that by "partnering with non-profits, especially non-profits that appear to have patients' health and women's issues as their primary concern, Merck reach[ed] audiences that may have rightly been suspicious of the motivations of a pharmaceutical company" (p. 32).

Current health communication research indicates the level of consumer trust in vaccination advertisements influences information seeking behaviors (Nan, 2012; Manika, Ball, & Stout, 2014). Therefore, it is important for researchers, medical practitioners, and marketing professionals to understand the relationship between pharmaceutical branding and consumer trust in public awareness health campaigns. Following the argument that "we should at least pause and think about what is happening when companies use social responsibility as an advertising strategy" (Pardun, 2009, p. 175), this work attends to the greater implications of corporate-driven healthcare messaging by framing the ways in which commercial interests threaten awareness efforts. In the following analysis, we focus on the disconnect between conscious and unconscious brand awareness as it relates to public trust in healthcare communication.

Commercializing Social Awareness

In 1969, Kotler and Levy coined the term "social marketing," arguing that macro-market scholarship did not adequately account for nonprofit fieldwork within business frameworks (Bolton, Cohen, & Bloom, 2006; Andreasen, 2012). Responding to the call for a broadening of industry terms, the American Marketing Association formally extended the term 'marketing' in 2007 to include "the activity, set of institutions, and process for creating, communicating, delivering, and exchanging offerings that have value for customers, clients, marketers, and society at large" (AMA, 2012). While AMA's new definition provides insight to changes occurring throughout the field of marketing, *social marketing* lacks such structured operationalization (Thackeray, 2012). Ambiguously interchangeable, the term is often applied to nonprofit activities, as well the overall social impact of marketing (Kotler & Zaltman, 1971; Lazer & Kelly, 1973). Further, social marketing is frequently misused as an appellation for social media/network marketing (Andreasen, 2012).

Today, most literature reflects variations of the notion that social marketing endorses "the design, implementation, and control of programs calculated to influence the acceptability of social ideas" (Andreasen, 2001, p. 71). Such definitions do not account for profit incentives or endorsement motives, limiting the term to philanthropic contexts. As a consequence of conventional standards and unclear definitions, researchers often overlook the canons of social marketing as a means for examining corporate campaigning. While the benefits of social marketing in the healthcare industry include an overall increase in consumer awareness, patient education, and medical discussion, questionable promotional efforts pose a threat to message reception and communication efficacy (Liang & Mackey, 2011). Davidson and Novelli (2001) support such a notion, explaining,

Society expects and accepts that business will promote its goods and services toward the end of making a profit. It is confusing and skeptical, however, when business ventures into the area of social marketing to promote the improvement of social good by changing behavior. This leads to an increase in the already worrisome level of cynicism about, and distrust of, business.

(p. 90)

The recent rise in media capabilities, combined with the extensive latitude of corporate liberties, make the commercial increasingly indistinguishable from the non-commercial (McChesney, 2000). These blurred boundaries bring into question our current understanding of public awareness campaigns, nonprofit messaging, and corporately sponsored cause-related marketing.

As a result of lax policies and regulatory oversight, corporate agencies often assume social marketing approaches to product promotion (Pardun, 2009). Such methods of consumer messaging increasingly surface throughout media airways, introducing an element of deception to the public health domain (Davidson & Novelli, 2001). As Jaramillo (2006) suggested, "The strategies that have defined such corporations as Nike and Disney have now been co-opted by the pharmaceutical industry. The actual pill is peripheral to the lifestyle that is being built and promised to consumers, not patients" (p. 271). Because people turn to various media sources when health concerns arise, it is necessary for stakeholders to recognize the internal, interpersonal, and mass mediated influences that shape healthcare decision-making.

Message Processing and Consumer Trust

Health awareness campaigns encourage message reception and behavior replication by relaying the information, knowledge, and skill necessary for goal attainment (Lundgren & McMakin, 2004; Lee-Wingate, 2006). In order for public health messages to have impact, however, receivers/audiences must process the information in some fashion. As D'Silva and Palmgreen (2007) note, "PSAs are created with the intention that the audience would at some point in the future respond positively to the information. Hence, apart from attention, encoding and recall become an integral part of developing appropriate messages" (p. 67). Health communication is more likely to be received if message senders are representative of targeted publics, modeled behaviors align with audience values, the information is constructed and relayed in a manner capable of being processed by the audience, and message design attracts viewer attention (Bandura, 1997).

Siefert, Gallent, Jacobs, Levine, Stipp, and Marci (2008) explain, "Cognitive-affective neuroscience clearly suggests that the brain processes information differently depending upon how information is presented and perceived" (p. 427). Tenets of social cognitive theory reflect such notions, emphasizing the importance of attention measures in information processing and decision-making. Though the effect may not be consciously recognized, the "mere association of a product with a positively evaluated stimulus such as an attractive picture. . .may be sufficient to alter attitude toward the product without any 'rational' belief change preceding the effect" (Rossiter & Percy, 1983, p. 112). Given that industry practices base message development and campaign implementation on the foundation of carefully orchestrated design, we can reason there lies a certain power in brand placement and sponsorship integration in public health messages.

Established research continually underscores consideration for message exposure, attention, comprehension, and retention in evaluating persuasive texts (Russell & Roskos-Ewoldsen, 2005; Bandura, 2001). Consumer scholarship indicates perceived trustworthiness heavily influences viewer identification with campaign communication and subsequent consumer behavior (Austin et al., 2002). Chatterjee and Chaudhuri (2005) found that trust significantly influences advertising efficacy through increased viewer attention, ad saliency, and brand recall. Studies also show that viewer skepticism negatively correlates with ad appeal, message reception, viewer attendance, and consumer responsiveness to the message (Obermiller, Spangenberg, & MacLachlan, 2005). Therefore, an ad's perceived trustworthiness largely determines message efficacy. In health communication, source credibility can also increase message efficacy by influencing beliefs, attitudes, and behavior (Pornpitakpan, 2004). Rhetorical scholarship suggests source credibility, a construct based on the believability of a communicator, derives from the perceived trustworthiness and expertise of the source (O'Keefe, 1990).

Value judgments regarding trust and credibility stem from "perceptions of knowledge and expertise; perceptions of openness and honesty; and perceptions of concern and care" (Peters, Covello, & McCallum, 1997, p. 2). We surmise that brand detectability may influence perceptions of openness and honesty, therefore influencing perceived trust and credibility. By deconstructing cases of commercialized health communication, scholars and practitioners can more effectively consider the means by which corporate agencies construct certain realities for healthcare consumers.

Semiological frameworks stress the power of corporate branding, promoting the notion that "the viewer is a knowledgeable, even masterful, decoder, moving skillfully from signifier to signified" (Bordwell, 2012, p. 44). Therefore, though it may not be a conscious thought process, corporate sponsorship in nonprofit health campaigns may influence viewer perception of campaign credibility and trustworthiness. As such, Merck's involvement in the HPV health awareness campaign, which eventually escorted audience members to a product promotion, may impact ways in which viewers perceive campaign credibility and trustworthiness. Our study compares implicit micro-level behaviors with explicit self-reported measurements to investigate the "hidden" effect of corporate sponsorship in health messaging.

While previous research has documented high recall for vaccination messages (Kobetz, Kornfeld, Vanderpool, Rutten, Parekh, O'Bryan, & Menard, 2010) and accounts of consumer apprehension toward the drug company advertisements (Shafter et al., 2011), there are few, if any, studies that investigate the potential influence of brand image in awareness campaigns. Given the lack of prior research in this area, we chose to conduct an inductive analysis. As such, we proposed the following research questions:

RQ1: Do consumers fixate on for-profit corporate sponsorship?

RQ2: Are participants able to recall for-profit corporate sponsorship?

In order to examine the ways in which different levels of brand awareness influence message reception, we first needed to determine brand discoverability. Physiological measures are often used as indicators of unconscious awareness and other responses that individuals may not think to or be able to articulate (Stern, Ray & Quigley, 2001; Potter & Bolls, 2012). Researchers can infer from physiological measures differences in individual's cognitive approach to media messages in regard to attention span and order in which information is seen and considered. Accordingly, the following research questions also guided this work:

RQ3: Do physiological measurements of corporate sponsorship fixation correlate with brand recall?

RQ4: Does physiological awareness of for-profit corporate sponsorship affect viewer perceptions of campaign credibility?

RQ5: Does physiological awareness of for-profit corporate sponsorship affect viewer trust in Merck Pharmaceuticals' social marketing campaign?

RQ6: In what ways does brand identification influence consumers' perceived effectiveness of the Gardasil vaccination?

Method

Consumer research heavily relies on specialized studies that dig into the psyche and behaviors of targeted audiences. Pre-conscious and unobtrusive data collection provides an advanced approach to modern advertising research (Briggs, 2006). Advanced measuring systems and calculations facilitate the evaluation of advertising effectiveness by revealing insight to the perceptual and cognitive processes that influence consumer decisions (Duchowski, 2007). Eye-tracking measures lend themselves to both qualitative and quantitative data analysis, offering researchers opportunities to interpret findings through illustrative mapped visualizations and/or statistical measurements of eye movement (Rosbergen, Pieters, & Wedel, 2004).

Maughan, Gutnikov, and Stevens (2007) argue eye-tracking techniques "put the study of consumer response to marketing and advertising materials on a firm scientific footing" (p. 342). Given the method's ability to obtain objective measures of attention and reliable indicators of consumer awareness, our eye-tracking analysis delivers a quantifiable assessment of brand influence in Merck's multi-phased campaign. By joining biometrics with survey responses, we offer a complex analysis of participant attitudes toward pharmaceutical branding in health communications.

Equipment and Materials

We monitored eye movement patterns using the Tobii T60, an eye-tracking device that resembles a regular computer monitor. Because tracking hardware is embedded in the monitor, head-mounting devices did not restrain participants. Therefore, subjects viewed Merck's social marketing campaign in a natural environment on what appeared to them to be a regular computer monitor.

Viewers watched a total of four broadcast messages aired in connection with Merck's roll-out campaign; including the two health awareness messages aired prior to FDA's approval of Gardasil ("Make the Connection" and "Tell Someone") and two post-FDA approved product commercials ("One Less" and "I Chose"). We used a 20-item pre-test questionnaire to measure previous awareness and knowledge of HPV and the Gardasil vaccination. We then used a 35-item post-test questionnaire to probe participant perceptions of each of the four commercial messages, their attitudes toward Gardasil, and any future vaccination intentions.

Procedures

We designed the pre-test questionnaire to gauge pre-exposure awareness and knowledge of HPV, cervical cancer, and the Gardasil vaccination. To prevent a priming effect, the survey addressed various other health issues (including influenza, the rotavirus, herpes simplex, colon cancer, lung cancer, skin cancer, heart disease, and alcoholism). Study guidelines also required the participants to complete the pre-test survey three to fourteen days prior to experiment participation.

During the second phase of the study, participants watched four of the HPV awareness campaign messages in the order in which they were released to the public ("Make the Connection," "Tell Someone," "One Less," "I Chose"). To avoid perceptual expectations and altered visual attention, participants were not given a specific viewing task, nor were they directly told that their eye movements were being tracked. Each participant viewed all four commercials without interruption and then completed a post-test questionnaire at a nearby computer station. The questions assessed participant demographics, as well as viewer recall, involvement, knowledge and exposure, and general attitudes toward the vaccine. We awarded students extra credit toward a mass communication course upon completing the second part of the study.

Participants

During the fall of 2013, we solicited participants through a subject pool at a midsized southern university. Though Merck's social marketing campaign largely focused on targeting women's healthcare behavior, men are often involved in medical decisions affecting female family members (i.e. daughters, wives, mothers). Beyond that, men are members of our consumer culture and actively participate in word of mouth marketing. Therefore, we did not issue gender-specific guidelines for participation. We collected information on sex, age, ethnicity, level of sexual activity, and vaccination status for categorical purposes after ensuring participant anonymity.

In total, 117 participants contributed to data collection. Three times as many females (65.8 percent) than males (21.4 percent) participated in the study. 12.8 percent of participants chose not to identify their gender. Ages ranged from 18–34, with a mean of 20.2 years. The majority of participants identified themselves as white, non-Hispanic (75.2 percent). Other races identified included African-American (11.1 percent), Hispanic (3.4 percent), Asia-Pacific Islander (1.7 percent), and Native-American (0.9 percent). 7.7 percent of participants did not report a race. Prior to the study, 70.9 percent of participants had heard of the Gardasil vaccination, 13.7 percent reported no prior awareness, and 2.6 percent were unsure. 12.8 percent of participants did not indicate their level of previous awareness.

Those who reported prior knowledge of the Gardasil vaccination most frequently identified commercial advertising as the source of initial awareness (58.1 percent), followed by physicians, (47.9 percent), friends/family (41 percent), and web sites (10.3 percent). 5.1 percent of participants reported "other," with sources including university health facilities, university faculty, and magazine advertisements.

Coding Procedure

For each of the four advertisements, we identified scenes in which Merck's branding appeared in the commercial spot. We then drew a rectangular area of interest (AOI) around any for-profit, nonprofit, or product branding that appeared in the defined scenes. Figures 4.1–4.4 illustrate the areas of interest (AOIs) for eye fixation data collection. The AOIs facilitated data analysis by tracking the number and length of participant fixations within each labeled area. In this study, a fixation was defined as directed gaze within an area of 35 pixels that lasted for at least 250 ms.

Although fixation data for these AOIs can be expressed in a number of ways, "the number of fixations and the cumulative dwell time of fixations recorded in each AOI have been reported as the most useful"

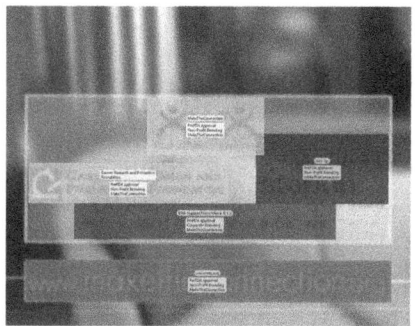

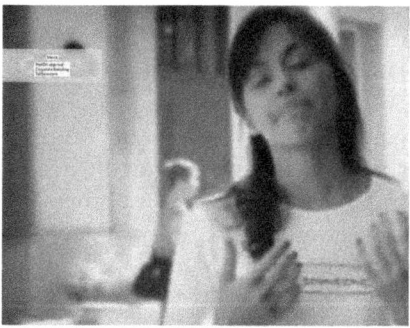

Figure 4.1 "Make the Connection"   *Figure 4.2* "Tell Someone"

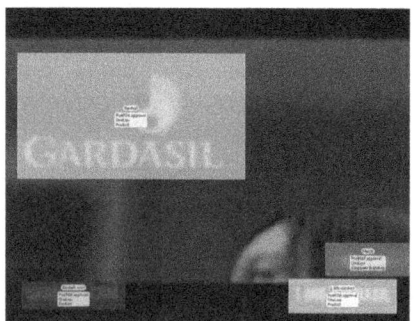

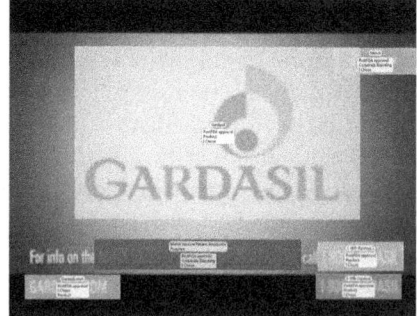

Figure 4.3 "One Less"   *Figure 4.4* "I Chose"

Figures 4.1–4.4 Scene Segments and AOIs. Figures illustrate the Areas of Interest (AOIs) for eye fixation data collection.

Table 4.1 Eye-Tracking Measurements: Metric Definitions

Visit Duration (VD)	"Defined as the interval of time between the first fixation on the AOI and the next fixation outside the AOI" (Tobii Studio, 2010)	Observation Length; Saccadic Movement
Time to First Fixation (TTFF)	Time in seconds from when the stimulus was first shown until the start of the first fixation within an AOI	Indicates discoverability (Bojko & Adamczyk, 2010)
Fixation Count (FC)	The number of fixations within an AOI	Believed to be indicators of both the depth and intensity of cognitive processing (Andreassi, 2007)
Fixation Duration (FD)	The length of the fixations in seconds within an AOI (inspireUX, 2010)	Generally provides best indication of the division of attention various elements on a page receive.

(Hallowell & Lansing, 2004, p. 23). As such, we collected the time it took for participants to first fixate on AOIs, fixation count, visit duration, fixation duration, and total fixation duration as our physiological awareness measurements. Table 4.1 provides an overview of the different tracking metrics used for statistical analysis.

Measurement Items

Fixation Metrics

We based our fixation data on the standardized Tobii gaze measurements defined in Table 4.1. Fixation count reflects the number of times participant gaze landed in a particular area of interest, whereas cumulative dwell time, or total fixation duration, reflects the sum of the gaze time devoted to all areas of interest (AOIs). To prepare for further analysis, we dichotomized fixation count measurements by separating participants that fixated on Merck branding at least once throughout the study from those who never established eye gaze within a Merck branding AOI. We also performed a mean split on the total fixation duration on corporate branding throughout the campaign (M=1.13 seconds, SD=1.11 seconds); therefore low durations represented fixations ranging from the lowest duration time to the mean viewing length (.00 –1.13), and high durations ranged from the mean time to the maximum total dwell time (1.131–6.53;

M=1.4, SD=.49). We followed the same procedure for branding fixations (M=1.4, SD=.50), with low fixation values ranging from .00 to 3.52 seconds and high fixation values ranging from 3.521 to 6.73 seconds.

While fixation times may seem low, the average is relatively large in comparison to branding airtime. Advertising regulations do require pharmaceutical companies to acknowledge message involvement through some degree of brand presence; however, industry research does not offer average fixation lengths for branding metrics in broadcast advertisements, nor does the FDA offer specific requirements for brand saliency in sponsored awareness campaigns (Code of Federal Regulations, Title 21). As such, we reference the average length of an eye blink to frame the subtleness of Merck's branding throughout the awareness campaign. Though reports vary, the average eye blink typically ranges from 0.1 to 0.4 seconds (Schiffman, 2001). In the pre-FDA messages, Merck's logo received roughly 2.406 seconds of airtime per message. Given the location, size, and limited air presence of the for-profit company branding, it is likely Merck managed to meet basic regulations and slip past viewer identification, in essentially, the blink of an eye.

Recall Metrics and Attitudinal Measurements

To examine the correlations between physiological fixation and self-reported awareness, we dichotomized self-reported awareness items and composite recall measurements. For each of the commercials, participants were asked to list any organizations/companies they recalled sponsoring the message. Unprompted recall indicators separated participants unable to identify Merck in any of the four prompted recall items from those who recalled "Merck" at least once. After completing all four of the unprompted awareness items, participants were asked to think back to specific messages and identify any of the listed sponsorships they recalled in specific advertisements. All aided awareness lists included the same items: Pfizer, GlaxoSmithKline, Merck & Co., Johnson & Johnson, Women's Step Up Network, American Cancer Society, Susan G. Komen Breast Cancer Foundation, and the Cervical Cancer Foundation. We then created an additive measurement score for total prompted awareness by adding together the amount of times "Merck" was correctly identified as a campaign sponsor. Our semantic differential scale stemmed from an adapted version of MacKenzie and Lutz (1989) and Priester and Petty's (2003) brand-related information processing measuring instruments. We used the five-point, six-item scale listed in Table 4.2 to survey participant perception of Merck's commercial messages. The survey questions provided a single sentence review of each commercial and asked participants to rate the specific message based on the dichotomous adjectives listed in Table 4.2. Participants rated their perceptions of each of the four commercials.

Certain items were reverse coded to prevent participant disengagement. Because we wanted an attitudinal index for the overall campaign, not per commercial, we conducted factor analysis for each item, collapsing the item across the four campaigns in order to construct our index.

Findings

RQ1: Do consumers fixate on for-profit corporate sponsorship?

Findings indicated most viewers did fixate on corporate sponsorship AOIs (M=.87, SD=.33). There were no significant differences between the ads.

RQ2: Do consumers consciously recall for-profit corporate sponsorship?

Findings showed 87 percent (n=101) of participants fixated on Merck's branding at least once, yet only 10.4 percent were able to identify or recall Merck as a corporate sponsor. Figures 4.5 and 4.6 illustrate areas in which participants fixated most, showing a moderate to heavy amount of traffic on Merck sponsorships. These examples highlight the dissonance between conscious awareness and physiological response.

Figure 4.5 illustrates the areas in which participants fixated most. Red coloring indicates areas that received longer and more frequent viewer fixations.

Figure 4.6 illustrates participant fixation counts.

RQ3: Do physiological measurements of corporate sponsorship fixation correlate with self-reported measurements of brand awareness?

As outlined earlier, physiological awareness is a measurement of viewer focus on corporate branding. Results indicated brand fixation and aided

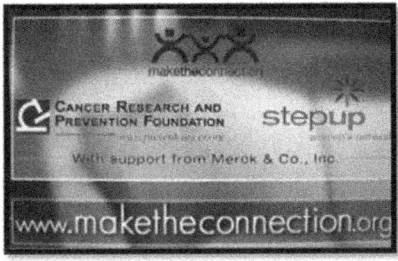 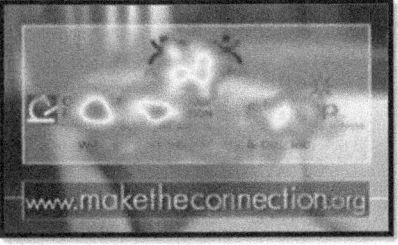

Figure 4.5 Heat Map Visualization for "Make the Connection."

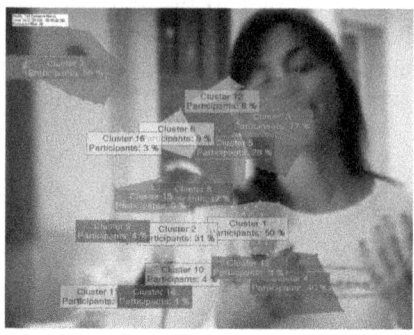

Figure 4.6 Cluster Visualization for "Tell Someone."

awareness are positively correlated, r(114)= .18, *p*< .01, suggesting the more often individuals fixate on Merck's logo (fixation count), the more likely they are to recall Merck's involvement in the awareness messages. The duration of fixations also demonstrated a positive correlation to corporate recall, r(114)= .29, p< .001. More simply, these numbers demonstrate that viewers became consciously aware of corporate sponsorship if they focused on Merck's branding long enough and/or frequently enough.

Table 4.2 Bivariate and Partial Correlations: Physiological Awareness and Recall Capacity

		Fixation Duration (FD)	Total Fixation Duration (TFD)	Fixation Count (FC)
Prompted Recall		273**	.291**	.183*
Sig. (1-tailed)		.003	.001	.025
N		101	116	116
Controlling for Prior Awareness			Total Visit Duration (TVD)	Total Fixation Duration (TFD)
Have you heard of the Gardasil vaccine?	Prompted Recall	Correlation	.313**	.326**
		Sig. (1-tailed)	.002	.001
		N	84	84
	Unprompted Recal	Correlation	.326**	.321**
		Sig. (1-tailed)	.001	.001
		N	84	84

As indicated earlier, our pre-test gauged prior awareness and knowledge of HPV, cervical cancer, and the Gardasil vaccination. A positive correlation remained between recall and fixation duration even after controlling for previous awareness, $r(82)= .326$, $p= .001$. Table 4.2 provides an overview of the significant correlations among brand fixations and recall measurements.

RQ4: Does physiological recognition of for-profit corporate sponsorship affect viewer perceptions of campaign credibility?

Those with low fixation counts (M=.22, SD=.98) rated the campaign as significantly more credible than those with high fixation counts (M=−.33, SD=.94), $F(1, 103)= 8.10$, $p<.01$. Findings also demonstrated that participants who spent less time fixating on for-profit sponsorship perceived Merck's campaign to be more credible (M=.15, SD=1.03) than viewers with longer corporate sponsorship fixation durations (M=−2.6, SD=.91), $F(1,103) = 4.32$, $p<.05$. In other words, as brand focus increases, perceived credibility decreases.

RQ5: Does physiological recognition of for-profit corporate sponsorship affect viewer trust in Merck Pharmaceuticals' social marketing campaign?

Brand discoverability (as measured by time to first fixation) and viewer trust in the campaign messages demonstrated a positive correlation, $r(99)= .30$, $p < .01$. This finding suggests that those who focused on corporate branding faster perceived the campaign to be less trustworthy than those who took longer to establish focus on corporate branding. Tests of variances showed neither brand fixation metrics nor recall measurement significantly influenced viewer trust in campaign messages. Table 4.3 outlines significant attitudinal and physiological correlations.

Table 4.3 Variable Correlations M(SD)

	Fixation Duration	Total Fixation Duration	Fixation Count	Time To First Fixation
	1.3(1.11)	1.13(1.11)	4.25(3.69)	4.07 (3.55)
Campaign Trust	−.025	.021	.024	.300**
Campaign Credibility	−.081	−.120	−2.70*	.153

**. Correlation is significant at the 0.01 level (1-tailed).
*. Correlation is significant at the 0.05 level (1-tailed).

RQ6: In what ways does brand identification influence the perceived effectiveness of the Gardasil vaccination?

An analysis of variance did not show any significant relationship between fixation duration $F(1,115)=1.296$, $p=.166$ and consumer perceptions of Gardasil vaccination efficacy, ($M=4.26$, $SD=.78$) or fixation count $F(1,115)= 1.335$, $p= .140$ and consumer perceptions of Gardasil vaccination efficacy.

In summary, while most individuals did see the branding at least once, only a very small percentage could report having seen it. The presence of sponsorship seemed to reach conscious awareness the more often and longer a person saw the branding. Given the brief duration of the sponsorship's presence in the message, it is very possible that for most people, awareness was not present enough to increase trust and credibility in the message.

Discussion

So what is the effect of corporate branding in social marketing campaigns? We found that most people focused their attention on corporate branding at some point while viewing this campaign. At the same time, however, participants largely did not identify the campaign with Merck. So where is the disconnect? What are the implications of audiences not comprehending the source of direct-to-consumer advertisements that are produced to resemble public service announcements? This difference in physiological fixation on branding and recall ability highlights the significance of Merck's off-label, promotional activities. While increased fixations can lead to more aided awareness, the awareness may not rise to the level of consciousness. Our findings present an opportunity to operationalize what we are calling unconscious awareness. We define unconscious awareness as one's sub-conscious, physiological response to visual indicators of corporate branding.

Other scholars have put forth similar accounts of what we describe as 'unconscious awareness,' coining terms such as "attentionless unconscious cognition" (Greenwald, 1992). However, as Jacoby, Lindsay, and Toth (1992) note, such notions "inherit the problem of ensuring that attention has been fully eliminated in supposed demonstrations of unconscious influences" (p. 806). More simply, the authors question the reliability of traditional measurements that claim to test 'automatic processing' through older, psychoanalytic methods (such as task dissociations, process dissociation procedures, and word-stem-completion tasks). Eye-tracking technology seemingly resolves prior limitations, offering a 'process-pure measurement' of unconscious awareness through physiological indicators.

In reviewing a series of studies in current psychology, Norman (2010) examined properties of 'the unconscious,' noting variations in operationalized indicators of the term. The author suggested theoretical assumptions stem from a wide range of experimental designs, specifically noting differences in subjective and objective measurements. Our study offers a new approach for measuring and defining 'unconscious awareness' by merging both qualitative and quantitative indicators. Norman's analysis also suggested empirical findings refuted traditionally dichotomized understandings of consciousness and unconsciousness, suggesting "the existence of intermediate states of conscious awareness" (Norman, 2010, p. 193). Our study supports modern interpretations, as we propose unconscious awareness occurs during a vulnerable stage of message processing—the interim between attention and retention.

Bandura suggested message processing involves attention, retention, production, and motivation. While attention requires the viewer to focus on, discern between, and extract information from relayed messages, retention entails rearranging the information into categories that the memory preserves. During the production phrase of message processing, the viewer relates the memory's impressions of communication efforts to specific actions, which results in behavior formation (Bandura, 1991). Our findings indicate unconscious awareness may result from incomplete message processing of stimuli stuck between stages of attention and retention.

We submit that brief brand fixations (physiological attendance) promote information recall at a subconscious level. Seemingly, the production phase of message processing incorporates biometric impressions that influence subsequent attitudes and behaviors. The physiological indices of viewer interaction with brand suggest that though viewers may not report any awareness of corporate involvement in a public awareness message, they oftentimes may still connect with the brand at a more implicit level—and perhaps at a lower degree of cognitive involvement.

Scholarship in visual persuasion confirms that unconscious considerations of ad elements (such as color patterns, ad copy, informative value, brand appeal, and exposure) motivate the nature of viewer response (Maddock & Fulton, 1996). Results from this study address the notable influences underlying branding strategies in health awareness campaigns. Our findings speak to source significance, indicating that the faster viewers noticed Merck branding, the less likely they were to perceive campaign messages as credible. Risk communication scholarship often highlights the power of information source when assessing message credibility. Regardless of communication presentation, consumer trust and source credibility heavily mediate successful communication (Ruth & Eubanks, 2005). Therefore, communication efficacy largely depends on how trustworthy the viewer perceives the source to be.

Studies suggest that "when people perceive themselves to be at risk, they understand and put into practice only those messages that come from sources they perceive as trustworthy and credible" (Lundgren & McMakin, 2004, p. 25). Therefore, citizen understanding of HPV, cervical cancer, and the Gardasil vaccination are inherently tied to Merck's ability to effectively communicate risk messages to target audiences. Assuming behavior is learned through observation, imitation, and identification, this analysis explored the means by which Merck Pharmaceuticals and partnering organizations shaped public awareness of HPV and cervical cancer.

While Merck's vaccination presents promising potential to reduce rates of cervical cancer, inoculation aptitude depends on pervasive acceptance and support for the HPV vaccination (Nan, 2012). The pioneering stages of Merck's awareness campaign indicate a concentrated corporate effort to mask pharmaceutical branding and conceal message involvement—and with good reason. The Edelman Trust Barometer surveys public trust in institutions, perceptions of source credibility, and specific issues influencing trust in business and politics. Rankings are based on the responses from 33,000 people in 28 different global markets. Findings from the 2016 index indicate trust in healthcare is relatively low, and in the US, the healthcare industry ties second to last with the automotive industry (White, 2016). American trust in pharmaceuticals and biotechnology also declined by two points since 2015. We expect that Merck strategically designed the subtle branding with an understanding that obvious corporate markings might prime viewers to connect the social awareness campaign to the company's eventual product release.

The suppression of presence is a particularly noteworthy phenomenon in advertising strategy (Perelman & Olbrects-Tyteca, 1971). Merck's strategic rotation and placement of required brand markings in the pre-FDA awareness broadcasts indicated conscious, active, and involved concern with the location and positioning of corporate markings. However, as our findings indicate, this may not have been the best strategy.

If we accept that "trusting consumers would take the stance that the advertiser designed the ad to be truthful and informative with the intent to lead the individual to an informed and beneficial choice," we can cautiously infer that skepticism rises when seemingly deceitful marketing tactics penetrate viewer cognitions (Ball & Stout, 2008, p. 4). Therefore, though brand presence often goes largely unnoticed in the realm of immediate consumer consciousness, the subtle corporate sponsorship may still impede communication effectiveness and future health behaviors through subconscious (or physiological) brand interaction. Indeed, our findings suggest commercialized social marketing campaigns threaten message efficacy, posing a potential breakdown in communication efforts and a collapse in public health advancement.

One of the largest gaps in consumer expectations and how they see healthcare lies in the area of transparency (White, 2016). Public health information becomes increasingly compromised by market motives as public awareness efforts evolve into direct-to-consumer advertisements through disguised social marketing. As indicated at the beginning of this chapter, our research stems from the premise that brand detectability may promote perceptions of openness and honesty, and therefore positively influence perceived trust in the message and source credibility. Accordingly, this research offers well-founded reasoning for regulating the size and visibility of corporate logos in commercialized healthcare messages.

While DTC guidelines required Merck to acknowledge message involvement through some degree of brand presence in the awareness effort, lax and ambiguous guidelines allow for creative (and deceptive) liberties. The early stages of Merck's campaign provide an excellent example of the pharmaceutical company's extensive effort to remain unidentifiable throughout the social awareness/product endorsement cycle. Current FDA regulations prohibit the visual presentation of commercial text that interferes with drug risk information. Given the influence of source credibility and transparency, it seems equally important to have regulations that prevent visual interference with corporate branding. Commercial design strategy also largely influences information retention, memory retrieval, and behavioral outcomes. Therefore, much like the guidelines that regulate risk information, the FDA should require full disclosure of any and all incentives related to sponsorships involvement, including corporate associations, compensations, partnerships, investments, and/or profitable opportunities linked to public awareness broadcasts.

America's aggressive marketing trends, combined with significant gaps in federal policies, reflect a contemporary need for regulation realignment in public healthcare communication. In order to honor citizen responsibility and informed decision making, healthcare consumers need a more accurate account of information realisms. Our proposed regulations level the playing field by providing opportunity for viewers to consciously process corporate involvement and potential message agendas. Such policies satisfy the demands of commercial speech rights and federal antitrust laws, while also protecting the sanctity of public health information.

Implications

As media changes, so do the ways in which individuals think, manage information, and relate to one another. Health communication operates in a new digital environment as our media industry is in a state of constant creative destruction and flux. Pharmaceutical influence, government policies, political agendas, media coverage, and now, Internet technology, increasingly host the changing nature of health information and communication reception (Kline, 2003). As more voices gain influence, stakeholders increasingly focus on and implement modern induction techniques to encourage target compliance among competing distractions. Advertising and editorial content, once as separate as church and state in traditional media, are now often indecipherable from each other in today's social media news feeds.

The American consumer, however, is not often equipped with the skills needed to tackle the foundational science, media framing, or political coloring that inform public health communication (Eysenbach, 2007; Lippman, 1922). Consequently, a steady flow of misinformation and disinformation plague healthcare decision-making and public well-being. The recent surge in social media and blogosphere activity and the rise of so called "fake news" further complicate dynamics driving public trust in healthcare information.

Changes in communication media denote a call for digital literacy. With an influx of messaging outlets and revolutionized notions of source credibility, consumers struggle to identify and navigate arenas of sound information. Studies already indicate information overload (even when useful) hinders audience message reception (Bawden & Robinson, 2009; Eppler & Mengis, 2004; Bawden, Holtham, & Courtney, 1999). However, it is still not clear how our evolving media environment influences notions of trust, credibility, and perceptions of reliable health information (Pearson & Raeke, 2000; Bradford et al., 2005). Mobile apps, social media trends, and digital innovations present complex challenges for healthcare professionals, and time-honored strategies are called into question as industry leaders navigate the evolving nuances of today's digital environment.

While experts confront the distractions that characterize our new media landscape, it is important for us to consider the social implications of industry tactics and shifts in communication practices. Though we may never know the true agenda driving Merck's involvement in the pre-released messages, in the long run, it may not matter. Sheila Rothman of Columbia University's Mailman School of Public Health, suggests, "If societies are just repeating the drug company's message, they are not really educating. They are blurring the line between educating and marketing" (Stein, 2009). Hybrid marketing strategies become increasingly dubious in light of the far-reaching and widespread messaging capabilities of today's informational age. Thus, it becomes ever more necessary for both researchers and practitioners in various fields and industries to better understand micro-dynamics of corporate influence on message processing.

Pharmaceutical interests in social awareness campaigns challenge the ethical and legal standards that regulate public health messaging. As Andreasen (2001) suggests, "If it is acceptable for societies to manage some behaviors, then the question to be considered should not be, 'Is social marketing ethical?' The proper questions should be 'What is the ethicality of marketing when compared to education and law as alternative tools of behavior management?' and 'Under what conditions will education, marketing and law be most appropriate and most ethical?'" (p. 17). This research promotes further exploration of such issues by introducing a quantifiable approach to examining unconscious awareness and conditioned tolerance of branded communication within the healthcare industry.

Limitations and Future Research

Merck's disguised endorsement demonstrates the degree to which corporations are silently setting the agenda within the healthcare industry. The burgeoning and increasingly invisible commercialized structuring of healthcare information presents alarming threats to public well-being. Our study offers preliminary insight to the influence of passive interaction with message sponsorship, and calls into question the dubious practices shaping public health communication. Data visualizations documented involuntary responses to awareness messages, offering opportunities to differentiate conscious brand recall from unconscious awareness of corporate influence. Essentially, participants' parasympathetic feedback facilitated the conceptualization of "unconscious awareness" as it relates to commercialized health communication. The dichotomy in physiological fixation and recall ability highlights the significance of strategic brand placement in off-label, promotional activities.

This research adds to health communication scholarship by documenting the influence of corporate branding in awareness messages and examining the impact of social marketing through "unconscious" viewer feedback. Because subjects viewed all commercial spots in one sitting, ecological validity was lessened in this experiment, making generalizability difficult. In addition, the effects were self-reported, and the experiment was conducted in a laboratory after the initial campaign was complete. While our work did control for prior awareness, we did not examine the differences in message processing between those who were vaccinated and those who were not. We also did not survey whether or not participants were aware that Merck was a for-profit pharmaceutical company, as we did not want to prime participants during pre-test or post-test surveys. Such limitations provide a strong platform for future research in this area. Further work in this area could serve to expand and confirm our findings.

Though our focus is case-specific, researchers can use similar methodological approaches to examine additional examples of branded health communication as it relates to consumer trust (for example, using biofeedback to gauge the influence of WebMD sponsorships). Additional examples and media platforms should be explored to paint a fuller picture of the phenomenon under investigation.

73

References

Alberts, H. (2008). Transcript: Trust as an economic driver. *Forbes*. Retrieved on December 19, 2014, from www.forbes.com/2008/06/16/covey-trust-transcript-oped-cx_hra_0616long.html.

American Marketing Association (2012). Definition of marketing. Retrieved on May 1, 2012, from www.marketingpower.com/AboutAMA/Pages/Defini tionofMarketing.aspx.

Andreasen, A R. (2001). *Ethics in social marketing*. Washington, DC: Georgetown University Press.

Andreasen, A. R. (2012). Rethinking the relationship between social/nonprofit marketing and commercial marketing. *Journal of Public Policy & Marketing*, *31*(1), 36–41.

Austin, E. W., Miller, A. C., Silva, J., Guerra, P., Geisler, N., Gamboa, L., Phakakayai, O., & Kuechle B. (2002). The effects of increased cognitive involvement on college students' interpretations of magazine advertisements for alcohol. *Communication Research*, *29*(2), 155–179.

Ball, J. G., & Stout, P. A. (2008, May). *Factors associated with consumers' trust of DTC advertising*. Paper presented at the annual meeting of the International Communication Association, TBA, Montreal, Quebec, Canada, Online. Abstract retrieved from http://citation.allacademic.com/meta/p232587_index. html.

Bandura, A. (1991). Human agency: The rhetoric and the reality. *American Psychologist*, *46*, 157–162.

Bandura, A. (1997). Self-efficacy and health behaviour. In A. Baum, S. Newman, J. Wienman, R. West, & C. McManus (Eds.), *Cambridge handbook of psychology, health and medicine* (pp. 160–162). Cambridge, UK: Cambridge University Press.

Bandura, A. (2001). Social cognitive theory: An agentic perspective. *Annual Review of Psychology*, *52*, 1–16.

Bawden, D., & Robinson, L. (2009). The dark side of information: Overload, anxiety and other paradoxes and pathologies. *Journal of Information Science*, *35*(2), 180–191.

Bolton, L. E., Cohen, J. B., & Bloom, P. N. (2006). Does marketing products as remedies create "Get Out of Jail Free Cards"?. *Journal of Consumer Research*, *33* (June) 71–81.

Bordwell, D. (May, 2012). The viewer's share: Models of mind in explaining film. Retrieved on April 30, 2013, from www.davidbordwell.net/essays/view ersshare.php.

Bradford, W., Hesse, B. W., Nelson, D. E., Kreps, G., Croyle, R. T., Arora, N. K., Rimmer, B. K. (2005). Trust and sources of health information: The impact of the Internet and its implications for health care providers: Findings from the first health information national trends survey. *Internal Medicine*, *165*(22), 2618–2624.

Briggs, R. (2006). Marketers who measure the wrong thing get faulty answers. *Journal of Advertising Research*, *46*(4), 462–468.

Chatterjee, S.C., & Chaudhuri, A. (2005). Are trusted brands important? *Marketing Management Journal*, *15*, 1–16.

Davidson, D. K., & Novelli, W. D. (2001). Social marketing as a business strategy: The ethical dimension. In Alan R. Andreasen (Ed.), *Ethics in social marketing* (pp. 70–88). Washington, DC: Georgetown University Press.

D'Silva, M. U., & Palmgreen P. (2007). Individual differences and context: Factors mediating recall of anti-drug public service announcements. *Health Communication, 21*, 65–71.

Duchowski, A. (2007). *Eye tracking methodology: Theory and practice* (2nd Ed). New York: Springer-Verlag.

Eppler, M. J., & Mengis, J. (2004). The concept of information overload: A review of literature from organizational science, accounting, marketing, MIS and related disciplines. *Information Society, 20*(5), 325–344.

Eysenbach, G. (2007). Health communication and mass media: An integrated approach to policy. *British Medical Journal, 324*(7337), 573–577.

Greenwald, A. G. (1992). New Look 3: Unconscious cognition reclaimed. *American Psychologist, 47*, 766–779.

Hallowell, B., & Lansing, C. (2004). Tracking eye movements to study cognition and communication. *ASHA Leader, 9*(21), 1, 4–5, 22–25.

Herper, M. (2012, April 4). The Gardasil problem: How the U.S. lost faith in a promising vaccine. *Forbes.* Retrieved March 20, 2015, from www.forbes.com/sites/matthewherper/2012/04/04/americas-gardasil-problem-how-politics-poisons-public-health/.

Jaramillo, D. L. (2006). Pills gone wild: Medium specificity and the regulation of prescription drug advertising on television. *Television New Media, 7*(3), 261–281.

Jacoby, L. L., Lindsay, D. S., & Toth, J. P. (1992). Unconscious influences revealed: Attention, awareness, and control. *American Psychologist, 47*(6), 802–809. doi: 10.1037/0003066X.47.6.802.

Kobetz, E., Kornfeld, J., Vanderpool, R. C., Rutten, L., Parekh, N., O'Bryan, G., & Menard, J. (2010). Knowledge of HPV amond United States Hispanic women: Opportunities and challenges for cancer prevention. *Journal of Health Communication, 15*, 22–29.

Kotler, P., & Levy, S. (1969). Broadening the concept of marketing. *Journal of Marketing, 33*, 10–15. doi:10.2307/1248740.

Kotler, P., & Zaltman, G. (1971). Social marketing: An approach to planned social change. *Journal of Marketing, 15*(4), 679–691.

Lazer, W., & Kelley, E. J. (1973). *Social marketing: Perspectives and viewpoints.* Homewood, IL: Richard D. Irwin.

Lee-Wingate, S. R. (2006). Alleviating mommy's guilt: Emotional expression and guilt appeals in advertising. *Advances in Consumer Research, 33*, 262–263.

Liang, B. A., & Mackey, T. (2011). Reforming direct-to-consumer advertising. *Nature Biotechnology, 29*(5), 397–400.

Lippmann, W. (1922). *Public opinion.* New York: Harcourt, Brace.

Lundgren, R., & McMakin, A. (2004). Approaches to communicating risk. In *Risk communication: A handbook for communicating environmental, safety, and health risks* (3rd ed.). Columbus, OH: Battelle.

MacKenzie, S. B., & Lutz, R. J. (1989). An empirical examination of the structural antecedents of attitude toward the ad in an advertising pretesting context. *Journal of Marketing, 53*, 48–65.

Maddock, R. C., & Fulton, R. L. (1996). *Marketing to the mind: Right brain strategies for advertising and marketing.* Westport, CT: Quorum Books.

Manika, D., Ball, J. G., & Stout, P. A. (2011). The influence of DTC advertising on college womens' decision to get vaccinated against HPV. American Academy of Advertising. Conference proceedings (Online): 46. Lubbock: American Academy of Advertising.

Manika, D. & Ball, J. G., & Stout, P. A. (2014). Factors associated with the persuasiveness of direct-to-consumer advertising on HPV vaccination among young women. *Journal of Health Communication, 19*(11), 1232–1247.

Maughan, L., Gutnikov, S., & Stevens, R. (2007). Like more, look more. Look more, like more: The evidence from eye-tracking. *Journal of Brand Management, 14*(4), 335–42.

McChesney, R. W. (2000). *Rich media, poor democracy: Communication politics in dubious times.* New York: The New Press.

Nan, X. (2012). Communicating to young adults about HPV vaccination: Consideration of message framing, motivation, and gender. *Health Communication, 27,* 10–18.

Norman, E. (2010). "The unconscious" in current psychology. *European Psychologist, 15*(3), 193–201. doi:10.1027/1016-9040/a000017.

Obermiller, C., Spangenberg, E. R., & MacLachlan, D. L. (2005). Ad skepticism: The consequences of disbelief. *Journal of Advertising, 34,* 7–17.

O'Keefe, D. J. (1990). *Persuasion: Theory and research.* Thousand Oaks, CA: SAGE Publications.

Pardun, C. (2009). *Advertising and society: Controversies and consequences.* Hoboken, NJ: Wiley-Blackwell.

Pearson, S., & Raeke, L. (2000) Patients' trust in physicians: Many theories, few measures, and little data. *Journal of General Internal Medicine, 15*(7), 509–513.

Perelman, C., & Olbrechts-Tyteca, L. (1971). *The new rhetoric: A treatise on argumentation* (J. Wilkinson & P. Weaver, Trans.) Notre Dame IN: University Press. (Original work published in 1958).

Peters, R. G., Covello, V. T., & McCallum, D. B. (1997). The determinants of trust and credibility in environmental risk communication: An empirical study. *Risk Analysis, 17*(1), 43–54.

Petersen, L. (2006). Merck to women: 'Get vaccinated,' be 'one less' cancer statistic. Retrieved June 10, 2007, from www.wcn.org/interior.cfm?featureid=7&id=1790.

Pieters, R. & Wedel, M. (2004). Attention capture and transfer in advertising: Brand, pictorial and text-size effects. *Journal of Marketing, 68,* 36–50.

Pornpitakpan, C. (2004). The persuasiveness of source credibility: A critical review of five decades' evidence. *Journal of Applied Social Psychology, 34*(2), 243–281.

Potter, R. F., & Bolls, P. D. (2012). *Psychophysiological measurement and meaning: Cognitive and emotional processing of media.* New York: Routledge.

Priester, J. R., & Petty, R. E. (2003). The influence of spokesperson trustworthiness on message elaboration, attitude strength, and advertising effectiveness. *Journal of Consumer Psychology, 13*(4), 408–421.

Rossiter, J., & Percy, L. (1983). Visual communication in advertising. In R. J. Harris (Ed.), *Information processing research in advertising* (pp. 83–125). Hillsdale, NJ: Lawrence Erlbaum.

Russell, F. H., & Roskos-Ewoldsen, D. R. (2005). Acting as we feel: When and how attitudes guide behavior. In T. C. Brock & M. C. Green, (Eds.), *Persuasion: Psychological insights and perspectives* (2nd ed.). Thousand Oaks, CA: SAGE.

Ruth, A., & Eubanks, E. (2005). Framing the mad cow media coverage. *Journal of Applied Communication*, 89(4), 39–54.

Schiffman, H. R. (2001). *Sensation and perception: An integrated approach*. New York: John Wiley and Sons, Inc.

Schwartz, J. (2006). More on Merck's "Tell Someone" HPV awareness program: Ethics of Vaccines. Penn Center for Bioethics. Retrieved on June 10, 2007, from http://vaccineethics.org/2006/05more-on-mercks-tell-someone-hpv.html.

Siefert, C., Gallent, J., Jacobs, D., Levine, B. Stipp, H., & Marci, C. (2008). Biometric and eye-tracking insights into the efficiency of information processing of television advertising during fast-forward viewing. *International Journal of Advertising*, 27(3).

Serono, M. (n.d.). A vaccine gives marketing lessons. Next Generation Pharmaceutical. Retrieved on April 2, 2013, from www.ngpharma.com/article/A-Vaccine-Gives-Marketing-Lessons/.

Siers-Poisson, J. (2007). Viral marketing (literally). COA News. Retrieved on August 10, 2007, from http://coanews.org/tiki-read_article.php?articleId=1980.

Stein, R. (2009, August 18). Medical groups promoted HPV vaccine using drug company money. *Washington Post*. Retrieved on May 1, 2017, from www.washingtonpost.com/wp-dyn/content/article/2009/08/18/AR2009081802499.html.

Stern, R. M., Ray, W. J., & Quigley, K. S. (2001). *Pyschophysiological recording* (2nd Ed.). New York: Oxford University Press.

Thackeray, R. (2012). Defining the product in social marketing: An analysis of published research. *Journal of Nonprofit & Public Sector Marketing*, 24(2), 83–100.

White, K. (2016, May 4). Warning signs for pharma. Edelman. Retrieved on December 30, 2016, from www.edelman.com/post/warning-signs-for-pharma/.

5

COMMUNICATING HEALTH-RELATED RISK AND CRISIS IN CHINA

State of the Field and Ways Forward

Zixue Tai, Zhian Zhang, and Lifeng Deng

Introduction: The Coming of Risk Society in China

Breakneck economic growth in the past three decades or so in China has ushered in an era of unprecedented prosperity in the country. Simultaneous developments on multiple fronts—including increasing technological advancement, further marketization, rapid urbanization, large-scale industrialization, and growing integration with the global society—have disentangled the milieu of forces turning contemporary Chinese society into one that bears resemblance to the risk society as conceptualized by Ulrich Beck (1992). It is no accident that the Chinese version of Beck's book was published in China in 2004, along with a few other works of his around the time (Beck, Deng, & Shen, 2010), when fears of an expansive assortment of risks became a nationwide plague in China. Beck's theory of risk society has become a steady inspiration for academic debates and scholarly contemplations in China since the late 1990s.

Historically, China has had its share of natural disasters and hazards such as floods, earthquakes, droughts, and tropical cyclones. This has been exacerbated by human-manufactured risks as a result of environmental deterioration ranging from "air pollution, biodiversity losses, cropland losses, depleted fisheries, desertification, disappearing wetlands, grassland degradation, and increasing frequency and scale of human-induced natural disasters, to invasive species, overgrazing, interrupted river flow, salinization, soil erosion, trash accumulation, and water pollution and shortages" (Liu & Diamond, 2005, p. 1179). The impact on everyday life is direct and far-reaching, often resulting in devastating loss of human lives and disruption of social order.

Against this backdrop, risk communication has garnered quite a bit of interest from researchers and practitioners alike in China lately. Our chapter aims to present a critical overview of the state of the field of risk communication in China and suggest a few key areas in which breakthroughs should and can be made to move the field forward. In the sections that follow, we first scrutinize the major issues and challenges in relation to a variety of health and medical risks, and then survey the current state of science communication as it relates to nuclear energy. We next highlight a few major areas of crisis and risk communication that are of special relevance to the community of researchers focusing on China and discuss how communication researchers may contribute to the improvement in the practices of risk assessment, risk management, and risk governance. We argue that the complexity of risk issues calls for an integrated and comprehensive approach embracing perspectives from—and collaboration with—natural sciences, government regulators, and the general public.

Public Health Issues and Medical Risks

Material prosperity has dramatically elevated the standard of life across China. Compared with the old days when food supply was scarce and dietary structure was highly limited for the vast populace, most people now enjoy an era of abundance and choice in the country. As a result, the average family pays an increasing amount of attention to what they have in the food basket and on the dining table. In response to this emergent popular demand, a specific genre of media content, led by TV programs, has garnered a large audience base in recent years. Focusing on various aspects of *yangsheng*, a foundational concept in Traditional Chinese Medicine (TCM) about the maintenance of good health, these programs promote lifestyles, diet, and therapeutic practices that are not found in standard Western medical prescriptions or treatments. For example, one deeply rooted doctrine of TCM emphasizes disease prevention through particular food ingredients in the daily diet. Feeding on that folklore belief, many cable channels have regular programs featuring proclaimed TCM masters preaching specific dietary recipes catering to people with different health issues and conditions.

Health-related programs on TV have become popular mainly for two reasons. First, rising public awareness about health issues and food safety in recent years has inflated popular demand for a variety of health-promoting information, and television, as the most popular medium of mass entertainment in China, naturally becomes the venue of choice for the general populace. Second, the typical format of *yangsheng* programs, which mostly feature a host plus a handful of special guests, often with limited interaction with a studio audience, makes this a low-cost endeavor in comparison with most other program genres. In one instance, Zhang Wuben, a self-branded TCM health expert who earned national fame through his appearance on a popular health diet program from Hunan Cable Channel, enjoyed ratings that were consistently ranked only second to CCTV News for primetime TV viewing. Using the slogan that "food diet can fight or feed the disease," what he preached on television reached such hype that the food ingredients he mentioned on the show would cause price hikes in grocery markets in many cities across the country. Of particular note is that the price of mung beans in many places nearly quadrupled for months in mid-2010 after Zhang claimed that mung bean soup could help cure diabetes, lung cancer, pneumonia, and cardiovascular disease, among others. Zhang's overnight fame on television made him the target of multiple investigative reports in late 2010 and early 2011, which revealed evidence of faked credentials and unsubstantiated qualifications. His clinic in Beijing was subsequently investigated for practicing TCM without proper licensing by the local government regulators. Zhang quickly fell into disgrace and oblivion.

This inglorious incident, however, has not diminished the public craze for health-related information, and *yangsheng* programs have continued their prominent presence on China's TV screen. The huge popularity of such programs has made them a prime target of state regulators. On August 26, 2016, the State Administration of Press, Publication, Radio, Film and Television (SAPPRFT) issued a directive regulating the production, format, and airing of television programs centered on food, diet, pharmaceuticals, and cosmetics (State Administration, 2016). Specifically, all such programs are required to be produced in-house by state television networks, hosts must be licensed and certified, and invited guests must show evidence of credentials in their field (e.g., official license for medicine, dietician, health professionals). For communication scholars interested in risk and crisis issues in China, some of the intriguing questions pertain to why certain audience members will almost unconditionally believe what they hear from a TV show, and what the main triggers are for mass behaviors such as the spread of misinformation, food hoarding, and crowd-based actions—a recurring theme during times of social disorder and mass panic in China.

Food has always been a defining element of Chinese culture, as testified by the oft-quoted age-old proverb in China: "To the commoners, food is heaven; To food, safety comes first." Unfortunately, food safety has been an area of looming risk in the life of ordinary Chinese citizens in recent years. Deterioration in the natural environment is greatly to blame. Yan (2012) notes three types of problems—namely, food hygiene (e.g., problems derived from food processing and sanitation), unsafe food (e.g., issues caused by excessive use of pesticides, chemical fertilizers, hormones, steroids, and preservatives), and poisonous food (e.g., deliberate contamination)—and points out that each of them constitutes a different type of risk that calls for different solutions from health officials, government regulators, and the general public. A high-profile case that is illustrative of the myriad problems China faces in health-related risks is the 2008 melamine adulteration scandal, a widespread industry practice in China, pointing to loopholes in the current inspection, surveillance, and regulatory process (Chan, Griffiths, & Chan, 2008).

A related topic that stirs up the popular pulse is genetically modified (GM) food. While the reasons behind the rise of this issue to prominence in public perceptions are manifold, television, as in the case of *yangsheng* controversies, has played an undeniable role. This is largely driven by Cui Yongyuan, an anchorperson from China Central Television (CCTV) who has achieved celebrity status for his outspokenness and prowess in picking on hot-button issues in his investigative reports. Cui has taken on GM food as his personal crusade through his primetime programs on China's only national TV in recent years, albeit with a clearly identifiable emphasis on skepticism, dread, and unknown risks of GM food. Parallel developments have been observed in many European nations in the 1990s with regard to the perceived risk of GM food, as Finucane and Holup (2005) note in their review of cross-national research literature.

As the most populous nation in the world, China naturally faces the daunting task of producing enough food to feed its people. This is exacerbated by the lack of enough arable land, loss of farming to rapid urbanization, and deterioration of soil conditions due to excessive use of chemical fertilizers. Genetically modified crops can offer distinct benefits, such as higher yields and lower agrochemical usage; but they may also bring harm to agriculture, the environment, and human health. In particular, the prospect of higher yield makes the cultivation of GM seeds a lucrative commercial endeavor, especially for developing countries with large populations and limited land resources.

Cui and his CCTV team repeatedly claim that China has been a testing ground for a variety of novel genetically engineered crop seeds over the years, and few efforts have been made to assess their possible hazards and risk factors. Limited media coverage of GM food in China has been overwhelmingly biased toward (often exaggerated) possible risks and potential hazards to public health, which bears similarity to press coverage of related issues in the UK and Spain (Vilella-Vila & Costa-Font, 2008). On the other hand, there has been a noticeable lapse of attention to the potential positive aspects of GM food to the farming industry and the people of China. It is imperative that a more balanced approach be promoted through the media and other public forums, because media coverage indeed plays a pivotal role in the shaping of public attitude toward GM food and animals (Marques, Critchley, & Walshe, 2015).

More importantly, an effective mechanism of government regulation and policymaking in China needs to be enforced. In that regard, experiences and lessons from other countries can enlighten debates and deliberations. As Finucane and Holup (2005, p. 1607) observe, "the reasons underlying objections to GM foods . . . often can be traced to important social-cultural beliefs, values, customs, and histories that orient and inform people making decisions in the face of uncertainty." A viable framework regulating the commercialization of GM food is hinged on both scientific and political considerations. This is the most obvious in risk regulation of Bt maize in the US and Europe, in which Levidow noted that "pressure by industry, NGOs, and the wider public influences regulators to focus on some risks and perhaps to downplay others [in different countries]" (1999, p. 21).

Diseases and epidemics have always loomed large in actual as well as perceived threats to public health in China. More than most other countries, outbreaks of epidemics often evolve into public crisis and wreak havoc in China due to the combination of high population density, large territorial span, and particular culinary preferences. On the one hand, economic prosperity in the reform era has allowed the government to invest more resources into state-led campaigns in combatting diseases and improving public health. One indicator of dramatic progress can be found in the increase of life expectancy from 65.5 in 1980 to 76 in 2004, as reported by the World Bank (World Bank, 2017). Due to increased official support in terms of grant money and state-of-the-art research facilities, medical research in various fields has made amazing strides. At the same time, modern hospitals with up-to-date equipment have been built mostly in major cities and urban areas.

On the other hand, it is rather recent that public communication has been acknowledged to have a role to play in gaining the upper hand over diseases and epidemics. A landmark development, ironically, was made possible by the outbreak of a rare virus that for months crippled the entire country—SARS in 2003. Based on the key finding that its old response mechanism to communicable diseases was both vulnerable and inefficient, the Chinese government totally revamped its disease surveillance system and enacted the Emergency Public Health Response Regulations "with a unified command, ready reaction, and coherent, ordered, and effective operation" (Yao, Chen, Chen & Gong, 2013, p. 290). Besides a consolidated nationally coordinated infrastructure, the newly implemented disease prevention and control system places considerable emphasis on the timely disclosure of disease information and global collaboration, and has demonstrated dramatic progress in the face of succeeding pandemics such as the H7N9 virus (Hvistendahl, 2013; Yao et al., 2013).

Improvement in communication and coordinated response has been a key area of focus in the new mechanism.

Although there is a growing realization of the importance of health-related communication as a research endeavor, academic research in various areas of health communication in its current state is still in its nascent stage in China, and is severely limited in both methodological approaches and theoretical perspectives (Tai, Zhang,Wang, & Lin, 2013). Therefore, much more needs to be done in order to make "communication" a critical component of the risk and crisis management process in China. Many problems affecting public health are medical as well as communicative. For example, rumors have been a vibrant part in the everyday practice of public health and popular medicine, particularly during epidemic outbreaks (Tai & Sun, 2011). In recent years, health-related rumors have maintained a noticeable presence on China's popular social media venues such as WeChat and Sina Weibo, which interconnect hundreds of millions of users and are important channels of public sentiments.

One hot-button issue that has haunted the health care field in China is deteriorating relations between patients and health care professionals such as doctors and nurses. De-coupling of health facilities such as hospitals from government funding in the current health care system means that delivery of health services is contingent upon financial vitality. Meanwhile, alleged over-treatment of common diseases often hits the headlines of conventional media and online postings. Common reasons cited as causes of patient-provider tensions include "defects in health policy and regulation, deficiency in humane quality, information asymmetry, poor doctor-patient communication, and physician's overloaded pressure" (Liu, Rohrer, Luo, Fang, He & Xie, 2015, p. 4). While patients with complaints and grievances in most Western countries typically use the weapon of litigation, their Chinese counterparts most often take matters into their own hands, frequently resulting in violence targeting doctors and nurses. This practice of blaming physicians—called *yinao* (or "medical riots")—is a common storyline across hospitals in China. As Liu et al. (ibid.) note, there has been intensified effort lately in improving doctor-patient communication skills in China, but much more is needed in terms of both evidence-based research and tailored assessment tools moving forward. Moreover, an effective solution to this problem will most likely require an integrated approach with participation from patients, their families, health care workers, and society at large, with communication of health risks as its core focus.

Public Understanding of Science and Environmental Risks

As we enter the second decade of the 21st century, science and technology has increasingly become an indispensable part of the overall quality of human life. Scientific literacy, which means the understanding by the general public of the nature, aims, and general limitations of science, has been recognized both as an important conceptual construct and a practical educational goal across the globe (Laugksch, 2000). China, which has benefited directly from its technology-centered approach in its national economic drives, is no exception. In the 2016 national convention on scientific and technological innovation, President Xi Jinping said improving scientific literacy among the general public, especially school-age youth, was just as important as achieving technological innovations, calling them the "two wings" of scientific development in the nation ("Cultivate," 2016).

There are monumental hurdles to surpass, however. Based on the three-dimensional construct (key terms and concepts; process of science; impact of science and technology) of scientific literacy as developed by Jon D. Miller (1983; 1992), the China Association for Science and Technology (CAST) has conducted multiple waves of national surveys to measure the level of scientific literacy among Chinese citizens. The CAST report published in September 2015 reveals significant differences along regional, occupational, educational, and most noticeably urban-rural lines; peasants, who make up the vast majority of the population, fall substantially behind city residents. It comes perhaps as no surprise that residents in the three metropolises of Beijing, Shanghai, and Tianjin are leading the nation (reaching proficiency levels of 18.71%, 17.56%, and 12% respectively), comparable to the percentage points scored by the US and Western Europe in 2000. China's national average of 6.2%, however, lags by a large margin behind the current measures in the US and Western European countries (News China, 2015).

Our purpose is, of course, not to discuss the niceties of the status of scientific literacy in China. Nonetheless, as a widely recognized measure for attitudes, attentiveness, and knowledge about science by the general public, these findings about scientific literacy in China set the appropriate background for us to assess the variety of challenges that lie ahead in our discussion of promoting understanding of risk factors in the context of an increasingly technologically dependent society in China. We confine our discussion to a number of environmental risks that have agitated the popular psyche in the past decade or so.

China's engine of economic growth begets more energy consumption, so electricity has figured prominently in state planning since the late 1970s. Explosive growth in electricity output is also necessitated by civilian use in China's sprawling urban areas. While coal-operated power plants supplemented by hydro-power were the norm in the 1980s, nuclear energy has been the primary target lately. At the start of 2016, the Chinese government announced that it will build a total of 30 nuclear reactor units in the next five years (2016–2020), equal to the number of units completed in the past 30 years (1985–2015) (China Business, 2016). Meanwhile, on January 27, 2016, the Information Office of the State Council issued a white paper titled "China's Nuclear Emergency Preparedness," which mapped out the country's nuclear policy including its overarching goals of utilizing nuclear energy and the national emergency response mechanism to ensure public safety.

This formation of a national nuclear policy stipulating the dual goal of promising security along with ambitious expansion takes place at a time when public anxiety about potential threat from nuclear energy is at a new high. In the early phase of China's nuclear power plant drive, around 1985, site selection was a competitive process among local governments, because being chosen for a new plant promised billions of dollars of investment from the state, new employment for local residents, and a guaranteed boost for electricity supplies in the area. All this, of course, eventually translates into an increase in the local GDP, an important benchmark for promotion and advancement in the Chinese official echelon. To a large extent, officials had also been quite successful in rallying support from the local residents in bidding for nuclear plant projects.

A turning point was the Fukushima Daiichi nuclear disaster that took place on March 11, 2011, in Japan. The tsunami triggered by a magnitude 9.0 earthquake caused nuclear meltdowns in the reactors, which led to radioactive material leakages the following day. This turned out to be the worst nuclear disaster since the 1986 Chernobyl incident, and the Chinese media went into full swing in covering this tragedy as it was unfolding. For months, gloomy images of fatalities, toppled buildings, and ensuing evacuations on China's television left a shocking and lasting impact on Chinese audiences about the catastrophic side of a nuclear power plant. Moreover, because this involves Japan, China's traditional foe, the media was relentless in subsequent coverage of a variety of short-term and long-term consequences for human life and the environment. All this produced the (very much unintended, probably) effect of changing public perceptions and inducing alarm in the general populace about nuclear energy.

This extensive coverage of nuclear technology, mostly focused on the disastrous fallouts, has been unprecedented in the Chinese media. What had happened in Japan, naturally, could happen in China. This prospect, no matter how remote the government alleges that may be, has triggered a series of discussions that had been lacking previously across multiple media platforms on the dark side of nuclear energy. As Xu (2008) observes, focal points of the debates from the 1980s to the 2000s had been largely centered on how to implement the government's nuclear expansion ambition; little challenge was raised to the government plan in expanding nuclear power use. In the new round of debates, a prominent voice of opposition has been Wang Yinan, senior researcher at the State Council Development Research Center. Wang was thrust into the center of national attention through an article she published on April 4, 2014, on *China Energy News*, China's national newspaper specializing in energy policy and technology (Wang, 2014). Wang made the case in the article against building nuclear power plants in inner areas in China due to technological and environmental constraints. Her affiliation with the main research arm of the national governing body, the State Council, probably garnered attenuated attention to her views, which had been widely circulated via conventional and online media forums. As a matter of fact, in the coastal province of Guangdong, news media were asked to remove coverage of her viewpoints and stay away from interviewing her for fear of invigorating public animosity toward nuclear power initiatives in their vicinity (Hu, 2014). Noticeably, dissenting voices that run against the state policy advocating more nuclear energy have been drastically diminished since 2015 when the government stepped up its effort of nuclear power plant construction.

The government plan, however, is increasingly becoming a hard sell to the general public. In recent years, public protests against local nuclear power plants have risen to an all-time high across the country. For example, days of public demonstrations halted the plan by the city officials of Lianyungang in Jiangsu Province to build a planned nuclear waste processing plant there (Meizhou Net, 2016); villagers in the suburbs of Lufeng in Guangdong Province confronted construction crews and obstructed on-site work for Lufeng Nuclear Power Plant, which is designated a National Key Project (NetEase, 2015). In one extreme case, about a year after the Fukushima Daiichi nuclear disaster, hundreds of local residents in the coastal city of Qingdao staged protests against the construction of a transformer substation within a kilometer of residential apartments for fear of health hazards due to radiation exposure (Phoenix Daily, 2016).

Environmental concerns that trigger mass protest and collective action go far beyond nuclear energy. Issues of increasing popular contention in the past decade have included grassroots efforts to halt p-Xylene plants and incinerators in multiple cities across China (Tai, 2015). Due to rising public awareness and shared concerns, major development projects that are lauded to bring in huge economic benefits by the government but are perceived to incur environmental risks are met with more and more resistance by local residents. As Steinhardt and Wu (2016) point out, this new repertoire of contention is becoming more widespread and often shapes government policymaking at the local and national levels. Within this context, it is imperative that all parties involved in environmental issues be properly informed in understanding and assessing potential risks before important decisions can be made and critical actions taken.

In actuality, various practices of information control and manipulation by invested individuals, advocacy groups, affected parties, and above all, government entities tangle up the communicative and deliberative processes for most undertakings that prioritize developmental opportunities over environmental concerns. In the case of nuclear energy, the survey of Chinese citizens after the Fukushima accident by He and colleagues (2014) shows that, despite a dramatic increase in public knowledge about the Fukushima disaster, most people still know little about nuclear power, nuclear technologies, and radiation risks in China; moreover, limited channels of information are available to the average citizen about nuclear energy in China, and government-supplied information—the dominant source of communication to the public—still sways public perceptions quite a bit. Sun and Zhu (2014) found evidence that more balanced information and transparency will decrease public perceptions of nuclear power risks and increase public support for state nuclear power policy.

We believe that now is the time to recognize the much-needed role that social sciences can play in the process of advancing public perceptions of risks in science and other fields in China. We call for an integrated approach incorporating insights of the natural, technical, and social sciences in risk assessment and risk management as mapped out by Renn (1998) to come to grips with dual aspects of risks in society as both a technical probability and as a social construction. Specifically, it is our contention that communication science has a vital part to fulfill with the tasks of the AEIOU (Awareness, Enjoyment, Interest, Opinion-forming, and Understanding of science) responses as suggested by Burns, O'Connor, and Stocklmayer (2003).

Moving the Field Forward in China: Bring Communication In

Although risk has always been an essential part of human existence, the systematic and scientific study of risk is only a post–World War II endeavor (Renn, 1998), and the identification of risk communication research as a distinct field of scholarly inquiry and professional pursuit has only occurred since the 1980s (Palenchar, 2009). By contrast, the history of risk research has a much shorter history in China, and risk communication as a subject matter is still in its nascent stage. But we must also acknowledge that we are witnessing a moment of juncture for the field in which exciting opportunities are emerging on the horizon amidst significant hurdles and variegated challenges.

Risk is often understood to be *"the possibility that human actions or events lead to consequences that affect aspects of what humans value"* (Renn, 1998, p. 51; emphasis original). Simultaneous developments in China in the past decades have led to the current era of proliferation of risks: rapid industrialization and technology-driven modernization in the country's economic expansion initiatives; massive urbanization in a relatively short span of time that disrupts conventional social structures and communal arrangements; widespread adoption of information technologies and changing media environment that heightens public attentiveness to and awareness of hazardous issues; increasing globalization and integration that bring more and more people up to speed with prevalent global practices of risk consciousness. These miscellaneous transformations in Chinese society naturally result in an elevated sense of uncertainty, and contribute to the physical (actual) presence and people's perceptions of risks, as aptly summarized by Lerbinger (2012, p. 22): "The incidence and severity of crises is rising with the complexity of technology and society." To exacerbate the situation, the crisis response mechanism, which tends to be largely government-centered, is still inefficient and inadequate under most circumstances.

Risk and crisis communication almost invariably assigns the media a central place in the process. Predictably, the role of the media has attracted considerable attention from communication scholars in the West. In the case of China, because journalism and media has dominated the history of communication research, perspectives on risk and crisis topics have displayed a lopsided focus on the media, with a heavy emphasis on media coverage of prominent events and key issues. Although media coverage is an important topic, as we have shown in our previous discussion of *yangsheng*-related TV programs, we need to move further by exploring the motivating factors influencing audience choice and perception of particular media sources, and more importantly, how mediated information shapes public behaviors.

The state's involvement in the media business is an important factor to consider, particularly in China. In general, the state media still plays a vital role in communicating risk-related information to the public, as He, Mol, Zhang, & Lu (2014) showed in their research on nuclear energy. Compared with the commercial media system in the West, state control of the media in China may create an advantage in the promotion of public interest that aligns well with state-designated goals, and the ability of the state to mobilize media in combination with other resources towards broad goals of informing the public, coordinating individual and collective efforts, and organizing mass actions. On the other hand, when there is a compelling state interest that conflicts with that of the public, the state power may be inclined to manipulate the media for its own gains, as we have seen in numerous cases in the past, especially under particular circumstances in which risks manifested into public crises (Tai & Sun, 2007). It may be beyond the capability of communication researchers to subvert the media system, but the media environment and related dynamics are important to keep in mind in evaluating the role and designing uses of the media in risk and crisis communication.

Meanwhile, social media and other new platforms of communication assume an undeniable place in the process. To a great extent, because new media is dominated by user-contributed content, new media communication affords new possibilities and often empowers the grassroots and the traditionally resource-poor constituents. This is a promising research stream for both academia and practitioners. Indeed, in an era of information abundance saturated by social media, smart phones, and personal devices, promising opportunities co-exist with emerging challenges. In that regard, staying current with the always-evolving new media environment is also an exciting way for researchers to develop fresh perspectives and make breakthroughs. A useful example is the research by Pei, Yu, Tian, and Donnelley (2017), which demonstrates techniques of forecasting mass concern about public health issues by monitoring news media on microblog (Weibo) sites. Research findings following similar lines have important practical implications, because early detection mechanisms, once proven reliable, may help crisis managers handle anticipated public reactions and social tensions in a timely, efficient, and proactive manner.

A hallmark of the science of crisis and risk communication has been its supra-disciplinary nature in perspectives and approaches. Because risk and crisis issues always intersect with people in a specific social setting, "we can only understand crisis and risk communication by first examining the nature of people and society they build" (Heath & O'Hair, 2009, p. 5). Cross-pollination involving sciences of different practices, therefore, is critically important in deciphering the puzzles of risk communication. Meeting the goals of science of communication, Baruch Fischhoff (2013, p. 14038) remarks, "requires collaboration between scientists with subject matter knowledge to communicate and scientists with expertise in communication processes – along with practitioners able to manage the process." Cecile Wendling (2012) astutely observes that when it comes to risk expertise in the Western nations, there is a noticeable gap between what social scientists do and what natural scientists and public policy makers actually expect from them; and natural scientists typically view the risk assessment and risk management processes as linear and instrumental, while social scientists assume the role of "mediator" or "communicator" between the natural scientists and the public. On the contrary, the participation of social scientists in the risk processes should lead to "a deeper debate" about offering alternative models to the linear approach, and moreover,

> They can help society rethink the process of risk assessment and risk management, which could become more iterative, more integrated, and more inclusive. Including social scientists in the expertise processes could be way to benefit from the extremely wide range of social science research available, and in so doing make better informed decisions and recommendations.
>
> (Wendling, 2012, p. 490)

This is a great guidebook for Chinese researchers to follow as well, especially with regard to the field of communication, which has not been aggressive in embracing inter-disciplinary approaches or collaborating with colleagues in other social sciences fields. Additionally, voices from social scientists are woefully needed considering that the current Chinese regulatory approach to environmental, health, technological, and other risks predominantly privileges the natural sciences perspectives, and social sciences are assigned the role of aiding what natural scientists have put on the table. In this regard, there is a noticeable parallel between the approach in China and what we have seen in the early years of risk regulation in the Western context (e.g., Jasanoff, 2009; Palenchar, 2009; Renn, 1998).

There is now a general consensus among scholars across national settings that risk is a multifaceted concept. The dichotomy between "objective risk" (based on scientific facts, technological data, or actuarial probability) and "subjective risk" (shaped by emotions and values) is often highlighted (Hermansson, 2012), and risk communication takes on both scientific (technical) as well as social-cultural dimensions (Heath & O'Hair, 2009). According to the risk rituals model, "the public perception of risk . . . is symbolic of social processes, dispositions, and deep cultural structures" (Moore & Burgess, 2011, p. 112). The Carnegie Mellon mental-model approach to risk communication, as elaborated by Morgan, Fischhoff, Bostrom and Atman (2002), argues that lay beliefs about risk are formed based on both specific facts and cognitive heuristics internalized through social and cultural learning; these perceptions are then reinforced or modified by the media and other communication processes. Of note is that communication is inherently built into these models. In the case of China, other important factors to take into account are special cultural values and social traditions that figure sizably into public perceptions of risk. These are the key areas that communication scholars can leave an imprint on risk research.

How risk is conceptualized affects how it is assessed, regulated, and managed. Because communication plays a pivotal role in all risk processes, it is imperative that communication experts share their insight over how risk is understood through evidence-based and theory-informed research (assessment), contribute to risk-informed policymaking by the government and public institutions (regulation), and have their say in suggesting pragmatic communication guidelines and preparedness in tackling important risk issues (management). Strategically, as an applied field of inquiry, risk researchers "need to maintain a balance between theoretical and practical significance" (Lindell, 2013, p. 812), and strive to link practical problems with appropriate broader theories and perspectives. More importantly, communication scholars should lead the charge in promoting dialogues with and participation from the general public in the risk communication process, and embrace the role of advocating for the vulnerable, the underprivileged, and the resource-poor groups that are easily impacted in the most negative way by risks in society. These are no easy tasks, especially in the political environment in China; but communication scholars have the moral and social obligation to bear the brunt of these responsibilities.

Concluding Remarks

Decades of economic expansion, industrialization, and urbanization in China have unleashed the risk genie from its bottle. As a result, the contemporary era of affluence has been concurrently plagued by the rise of uncertainty and risk in a wide range of areas spanning from environmental deterioration to food contamination to epidemics and natural disasters. Indeed, Ulrich Beck's risk society has found manifestations—with myriad parallels, unique twists, and drastic transformations—in its Chinese version. While the handling of potential and manifested risks in the form of public crises and emergencies has been high on the agenda of the Chinese government in recent years, the outcomes have been varied, showing significant accomplishments in some areas but leaving important improvement to be desired in other areas.

The SARS outbreak in 2003 has become a milestone event in risk and crisis communication in China because it has amplified attention to this area on an unprecedented scale from diverse constituents and stakeholders—scientists (both from the natural and social sciences), government agencies and regulators at the local and national level, media scholars and practitioners, and the general public. Vigorous research and debates among academics and practitioners have also produced encouraging outcomes, including a paradigm shift in the government response to public health crises and the elevation of the (both old and new) media to prominent roles in the process of communicating health risks to the public. Nonetheless, risk research in general and risk communication in particular is still in its nascent stage, monumental challenges still exist, and much is to be done in the field. At this juncture, we urge communication researchers in China to answer the call and rise to the challenge of the times. This coincides with a moment when communication as a discipline in China is searching for its identity and is seeking to make strides. Risk communication may be one of the subfields in which such breakthrough accomplishments are possible.

References

Beck, U. (1992). *Risk society: Toward a new modernity*. London: SAGE.
Beck, U., Deng, Z., & Shen, G. (2010). Risk society and China: A dialogue with Ulrich Beck. Published in Chinese. *Sociological Studies, 5*, 208–232.

Burns, T. W., O'Connor, D. J., & Stocklmayer, S. M. (2003). Science communication: A contemporary definition. *Public Understanding of Science*, 12(2), 183–202.

Chan, E. Y. Y., Griffiths, S. M., & Chan, C. W. (2008). Public-health risks of melamine in milk products. *The Lancet*, 372(9648), 1444–1445.

China Business News Online. The great leap forward in nuclear power plant construction. Retrieved from: http://finance.ifeng.com/a/20160304/14249005_0.shtml.

Finucane, M. L., & Holup, J. L. (2005). Psychosocial and cultural factors affecting the perceived risk of genetically modified food: An overview of the literature. *Social Science & Medicine*, 60(7), 1603–1612.

Fischhoff, B. (2013). The sciences of science communication. *Proceedings of the National Academy of Sciences*, 110(Supplement 3), 14033–14039.

He, G., Mol, A. P., Zhang, L., & Lu, Y. (2014). Nuclear power in China after Fukushima: Understanding public knowledge, attitudes, and trust. *Journal of Risk Research*, 17(4), 435–451.

Heath, R. L. & O'Hair, H. D. (2009). The significance of crisis and risk communication. In R. L. Heath & H. D. O'Hair (Eds.), *Handbook of risk and crisis communication* (pp. 5–30). New York: Routledge.

Hermansson, H. (2012). Defending the conception of "objective risk". *Risk Analysis*, 32(1), 16–24.

Hvistendahl, M. (2013). A decade after SARS, China's flu response wins cautious praise. *Science*, 340(6129), 130.

Hu Xuecui. (2014, August 6). Wang yinan: Shocked by responses to my nuclear power comments. *Phoenix Daily Business Report*. Retrieved from: http://finance.ifeng.com/a/20140806/12873200_0.shtml.

Jasanoff, S. (2009). *The fifth branch: Science advisors and policy makers*. Cambridge, MA: Harvard University Press.

Laugksch, R. C. (2000). Scientific literacy: A conceptual overview. *Science Education*, 84(1), 71–94.

Lerbinger, O. (2012). *Facing disasters, conflicts, and failures* (2nd Ed). New York: Routledge.

Levidow, L. (1999). Regulating Bt maize in the United States and Europe: A scientific-cultural comparison. *Environment: Science and Policy for Sustainable Development*, 41(10), 10–23.

Lindell, M. K. (2013). Disaster studies. *Current Sociology*, 61(5-6), 797–825.

Liu, J., & Diamond, J. (2005). China's environment in a globalizing world. *Nature*, 435(7046), 1179–1186.

Liu, X., Rohrer, W., Luo, A., Fang, Z., He, T., & Xie, W. (2015). Doctor-patient communication skills training in mainland China: A systematic review of the literature. *Patient Education and Counseling*, 98(1), 3–14.

Marques, M. D., Critchley, C. R., & Walshe, J. (2015). Attitudes to genetically modified food over time: How trust in organizations and the media cycle predict support. *Public Understanding of Science*, 24(5), 601–618.

Meizhou Net. (2016, August 9). Citizens of Liangyungang protest against construction of nuclear waste plant. Retrieved from: www.meizhou.cn/2016/0809/460894.shtml.

Miller, J. D. (1983). Scientific literacy: A conceptual and empirical review. *Daedalus, 112*(2), 29–48.

Miller, J. D. (1992). Toward a scientific understanding of the public understanding of science and technology. *Public Understanding of Science, 1*(1), 23–26.

Moore, S., & Burgess, A. (2011). Risk rituals. *Journal of Risk Research, 14*, 111–124.

Morgan, M. G., Fischhoff, B., Bostrom, A., & Atman, C. J. (2002). *Risk communication: A mental models approach.* New York: Cambridge University Press.

NetEase. (2015, September 14). Police arrest 19 protestors opposing nuclear power plant. Retrieved from: http://help.3g.163.com/15/0914/18/B3GC8OM900964K9G.html.

News China. (2015). China association for science and technology: Survey shows dramatic increase of scientific literacy in China. Retrieved from: http://news.china.com/domestic/945/20150921/20437563.html.

Palenchar, M. J. (2009). Historical trends of risk and crisis communication. In R. L. Heath & H. D. O'Hair (Eds.), *Handbook of risk and crisis communication* (pp. 31–52). New York: Routledge.

Pei, J., Yu, G., Tian, X., & Donnelley, M. R. (2017). A new method for early detection of mass concern about public health issues. *Journal of Risk Research, 20*(4), 516–532.

Phoenix Daily Business Report. (2016, February 29). Property owners in Qingdao protest against building of transformer substation close to their apartments. Retrieved from: http://news.ifeng.com/photo/hdnews/detail_2012_02/29/12869381_0.shtml.

Renn, O. (1998). Three decades of risk research: Accomplishments and new challenges. *Journal of Risk Research, 1*(1), 49–71.

State Administration of Press, Publication, Radio, Film and Television. (2016, August 26) Public notice on the regulation of medical, public health, diet programs and pharmaceutical commercials. Retrieved from: www.sarft.gov.cn/art/2016/8/26/art_113_31528.html.

Steinhardt, H. C., & Wu, F. (2016). In the name of the public: Environmental protest and the changing landscape of popular contention in China. *The China Journal, 75*(1), 61–82.

Sun, C., & Zhu, X. (2014). Evaluating the public perceptions of nuclear power in China: Evidence from a contingent valuation survey. *Energy Policy, 69*, 397–405.

Tai, Z. (2015). Finger power and smart mob politics: Social activism and mass dissent in China in the networked era. In P. Weibel (Ed.), *Global activism: Art and conflict in the 21st century* (pp. 396–407). Cambridge, MA: The MIT Press.

Tai, Z., & Sun, T. (2007). Media dependencies in a changing media environment: The case of the 2003 SARS epidemic in China. *New Media & Society, 9*(6), 987–1009.

Tai, Z., & Sun, T. (2011). The rumouring of SARS during the 2003 epidemic in China. *Sociology of Health & Illness, 33*(5), 677–693.

Tai, Z., Zhang, Y., Wang, D., & Lin, J. (2013). Researching health communication in China: Thematic orientations, methodological approaches, and topical enactments. *China Media Research, 9*(3), 84–95.

Vilella-Vila, M., & Costa-Font, J. (2008). Press media reporting effects on risk perceptions and attitudes towards genetically modified (GM) food. *The Journal of Socio-Economics, 37*(5), 2095–2106.

Wang Y. (2014, April 4). Nuclear power plant in hinterland areas is not an appropriate choice for China. *China Energy News*. Retrieved from: http://news.bjx.com.cn/html/20140414/503509.shtml.

Wendling, C. (2012). What role for social scientists in risk expertise? *Journal of Risk Research, 15*(5), 477–493.

World Bank. (2017). Life expectancy at birth, total (years). Retrieved from: http://data.worldbank.org/indicator/SP.DYN.LE00.IN.

Xin Jinping. Cultivate a vibrant management and operation mechanism in promoting science and technology. *People's Daily Online*. Retrieved from: http://scitech.people.com.cn/n1/2016/0603/c1007-28410557.html.

Xu, Y. C. (2008). Nuclear energy in China: Contested regimes. *Energy, 33*(8), 1197–1205.

Yan, Y. (2012). Food safety and social risk in contemporary China. *The Journal of Asian Studies, 71*(3), 705–729.

Yao, L., Chen, E., Chen, Z., & Gong, Z. (2013). From SARS to H7N9: The mechanism of responding to emerging communicable diseases has made great progress in China. *Bioscience Trends, 7*(6), 290–293.

Part II

COMMUNICATING AND EDUCATING THE PUBLIC AND MEDIA ABOUT RISK AND SCIENCE

6

RISK COMMUNICATION IN OCCUPATIONAL SAFETY AND HEALTH

Reaching Diverse Audiences in an Evolving Communication Environment

Juliann C. Scholl, Donna M. Van Bogaert, Christy L. Forrester, and Thomas R. Cunningham

The findings and conclusions in this report are those of the author(s) and do not necessarily represent the views of the National Institute for Occupational Safety and Health.

Introduction

As of 2015, the United States civilian workforce totaled over 157 million people (Bureau of Labor Statistics, 2015). Many American workers face threats to their safety and health in the form of exposures, injuries, illnesses, and even death, which cost over $250 billion in medical costs and productivity losses in 2007 (Leigh, 2011). However, such estimates are considered low because they do not include such costs as those associated with labor turnover, pain, and suffering. Another cost has to do with the lost impacts from "presenteeism" (or self-rated sickness presence), which is the tendency to go to work even while sick, often reducing productivity (Aronsson & Gustafsson, 2005; Guest & Conway, 2009; Hansen & Anderson, 2008). In an evolving workplace, this context shows there is significant need for information and interventions to address the risks posed by occupational exposures, such as illnesses attributed to chemical and other environmental hazards (Riegelman & Kirkwood, 2015) and fatal and non-fatal injuries (e.g., slips, trips, and falls) (Turnock, 2016). Fulfilling this need requires navigating several complex domains to reach workplace audiences:

- Occupational safety and health (OSH) research, to determine what constitutes a safe and healthy workplace
- Translation research, to understand the processes of transferring research findings into information that can be put to practice for meaningful impact
- Risk communication, to build awareness of risk and share information about best practices for eliminating injuries and fatalities and improving workplace safety and health
- New and emerging communication technologies, for effectively communicating OSH risk to workplace audiences.

This chapter first describes the field of occupational safety and health and the only US government agency specifically devoted to OSH research, the National Institute for Occupational Safety and Health (NIOSH). Next, the chapter discusses the role of risk and health communication in OSH and the changes in dissemination due to digital media. The chapter goes on to examine the challenges and opportunities created by new and emerging media technology and channels, and it concludes with recommendations for best practices and future research.

Background

Since the beginning of the Industrial Age, the domain of occupational safety and health has developed significantly on a global level. Alli, in *Fundamental Principles of Occupational Health and Safety* (2008), recognized the many facets of OSH in defining it as "the science of anticipation, recognition, evaluation and control of hazards arising in or from the workplace that could impair the health and well-being of workers, taking into account the possible impact on the surrounding communities and general environment" (p. vii). In other words, OSH is concerned with preserving the health and safety of workers and with reducing or preventing illness, injury, and death resulting from workplace exposures and hazards.

Many OSH standards and best practices have been endorsed by long-standing international leaders in the field, including the International Commissioner of Occupational Health (ICOH, founded 1906), International Labor Organization (ILO, founded 1919), World Health Organization (WHO, founded 1948), the Occupational Safety and Health Administration (OSHA, founded 1970), and the National Institute for Occupational Safety and Health (NIOSH, founded 1970). Several countries, including the United States and United Kingdom, established acts that mandate safe and healthy work environments for employees. In the United States, agencies were established for developing research to apprise hazards and enforce safety and health regulations. Federal agencies include NIOSH and OSHA, as well as the Mining Enforcement and Safety Administration (MESA) and the Mine Safety and Health Administration (MSHA), which were created in 1973 and 1977 respectively (MSHA, n.d.). There are currently 28 US states and territories that have OSHA-approved state plans, or federally funded safety and health programs (OSHA, n.d.).

National Institute for Occupational Safety and Health

Established by the Occupational Safety and Health Act of 1970, the NIOSH is the federal agency responsible for conducting research and making recommendations to ensure safe and healthy work conditions for all US workers. As reflected in its stated mission and values (NIOSH, 2016, January 11), NIOSH provides national and world leadership to prevent work-related illness, injury, disability, and death by gathering information, conducting research, and disseminating products, solutions, and services tailored to meet stakeholders' needs. As an institute within the Centers for Disease Control and Prevention (CDC) of the US Department of Health and Human Services (DHHS), NIOSH has more than 1,300 employees in eight research laboratories and offices across the United States. These represent a wide range of disciplines, including industrial hygiene, medicine, epidemiology, psychology, economics, statistics, communication, and engineering. NIOSH's mission is to generate new occupational safety and health knowledge and to translate or convert that knowledge into safe practices, procedures, and policies to protect workers (NIOSH, 2015, October). NIOSH is not a regulatory and enforcement agency; however, the institute often works with key federal regulatory partners, the Occupational Safety and Health Administration (OSHA) and the Mine Safety and Health Administration (MSHA) in the Department of Labor, to advance recommendations and best practices that reflect current research conducted by NIOSH and its partners (NIOSH, 2015, November 4).

Equally important to its research on occupational risk factors are the recommendations NIOSH provides for protecting the health and safety of the American worker. NIOSH must translate those findings into practical prevention information and communicate that information through guidance documents (which are non-binding or not enforceable), recommendations, educational materials, and interventions to improve working conditions. Communicating the information effectively is a challenge because of the continual changes in existing and emerging hazards and in the composition of the American workforce (for example, more part-time, temporary, aging, and small-business employees) (Bureau of Labor Statistics, 2013; Cummings & Kreiss, 2008).

Other significant challenges include cutting through Web information overload and competing for the attention of diverse audiences in the virtual environment; privacy mandates that prevent government agencies from fully engaging in customized content; and rapidly changing communication technology and norms. Amidst these challenges are opportunities for NIOSH to explore and use strategically in its OSH communications.

Communication Opportunities

One opportunity is better use of the advanced, interactive technologies now widely available. These technologies enable rapid dissemination of scientific knowledge. They also provide sophisticated networks that allow users to deliver content in multiple ways over numerous channels and modalities. Such technologies allow for consistent presentation of messages across several types of media.

Another opportunity is to better leverage the NIOSH identity, which is based on its long-established reputation for leadership and research excellence within the OSH community. NIOSH is recognized as an important and trusted source for information and resources that help advance worker health and well-being (NIOSH, 2016, January 11). Therefore, in meeting its mission to provide information that resonates with its diverse audiences, NIOSH works to uphold its reputation as a respected communicator through successful content creation and dissemination strategies.

NIOSH information products are grounded in research to identify risk factors and enable recommendations to prevent worker injury, illness, and death. The extent to which NIOSH information and resources are used, adapted, and adopted in the workplace, however, depends heavily on factors extending beyond risk factors and basic research findings. To that end, NIOSH relies on two initiatives—the NIOSH translation research program and the NIOSH Research to Practice (r2p) framework—to guide translation and transfer of NIOSH information, interventions, and technologies.

Translation Research

Translation research is the scientific investigation of how the products of research can be effectively translated or converted into practice and have an impact; it also encompasses the study of the barriers that prevent this process (Straus, Graham, & Mazmanian, 2006). In 2015, NIOSH established a translation research program, identifying translation research as one of four major research categories central to NIOSH. The program is built on four phases of exploration, which are based on the approach used by the National Institutes of Health (Khoury, Gwinn, & Ioannidis, 2010; Zerhouni, 2003).

The first phase studies the movement of basic risk research findings, such as pilot studies or case reports, into applications that have the potential to be turned into a global outreach effort or intervention. This involves generating solutions to workplace risks and engaging in limited testing. The second phase assesses internal validity by using observational and experimental testing of new interventions, processes, or training programs for their potential impact on an industry or workplace (such as a local construction site). Phase three focuses on external validity by moving evidence-based interventions and recommendations into well-accepted practice within the OSH field. This is done through diffusion research to identify barriers and facilitators to large-scale delivery and dissemination for adoption by broader audiences (such as the construction industry). Phase four studies the "real world" health outcomes or impact of newly developed interventions and recommendations. During this phase, research is conducted to examine the population-level outcomes of translation efforts, particularly their impact on injuries, illnesses, and fatalities.

Research to Practice (r2p)

The r2p framework drives the adaptation and adoption of NIOSH knowledge, interventions, and technologies into effective workplace practices and products. The framework does this by engaging six core elements: partnerships, intramural science, extramural science, technology transfer, communication, and impact evaluation. Each of these elements uniquely contributes to workplace safety and health; however, it is in their interactions and confluences that they fully align with NIOSH's mission and promote measurable impact (see Figure 6.1). The core element of communication is crucial to the way NIOSH science is translated into products

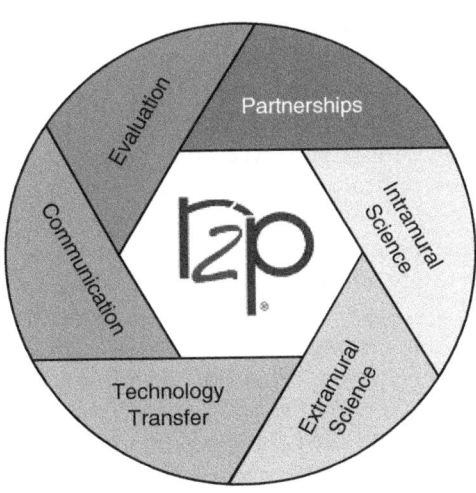

Figure 6.1 Elements of the Research to Practice (r2p) Approach

and then disseminated to intended audiences. Through communication, evidence-based strategies and tools are employed to deliver NIOSH information in ways that are understood and used by key stakeholders (NIOSH, 2015, December 4).

Communicating Risk

OSH Information

As in other areas of risk communication, the perception of risk is critical to motivating protective and preventive behaviors (Turner, Skubisz, & Rimal, 2011). Health-related risk is concerned with hazards or dangers to be identified, characterized, assessed, and managed for prevention of an adverse outcome (McComas, 2006; Parrott, 2004). In OSH, risk refers to the likelihood that harm will occur and is related to the hazards and exposures that exist in the workplace (Friend & Kohn, 2010). Risk communication involves directing information and persuasion toward diverse audiences to elicit behavioral changes (Olaniran & Scholl, 2016).

Risk communication requires understanding the nature of the target audience (Heath & O'Hair, 2010), particularly how they perceive the likelihood of a harm and its severity. Heath, Palenchar, and O'Hair (2010) argue, "There would be no discipline called risk communication if all of the people of any relevant society perceived the same risks, perceived them in the same way, and reacted to them as of one mind" (pp. 475–476). This claim underscores the importance of recognizing the diversity of the target audiences and how important it is to understand the variation with which they perceive and respond to risk. According to the risk perception attitude (RPA) framework (Rimal & Real, 2003), such variations can be seen when segmenting audiences according to their perceptions of a risk and their efficacy beliefs, particularly for the purpose of designing interventions that seek to change health-related behaviors (Rimal, Brown, Mkandawire, Folda, Böse, & Creel, 2009). The RPA framework suggests that individuals can be responsive (high perceived risk, high efficacy), avoidant (high risk perception, low efficacy beliefs), proactive (low risk, high efficacy), or indifferent (low risk, low efficacy). Real (2008) contends that "creating theoretically meaningful groups, communication researchers can make predictions about safety information-seeking and general safety behaviors" (pp. 342–343). Real's application of the framework to a study looking at manufacturing workers found that workers with greater efficacy beliefs displayed more positive safety behaviors. Moreover, the study found that responsive individuals reported safer outcomes than avoidants, while the proactive workers reporter safer outcomes than did indifferent workers.

Within the OSH field, perception of risk encompasses a wide range of concerns. Though the focus is on preserving the safety and health of

individuals in the workplace, by association, OSH includes loss prevention and the protection of natural and facility resources (Friend & Kohn,
2010). OSH research not only results in specific recommendations for
individual worker exposures but also has far-reaching implications. It
propels the development of policies and procedures that help employers
and workers reduce exposures to hazards or risk factors that contribute
to illness and injury. In the course of assessing risk and recommending
solutions, the OSH field also contributes to organizational efficiency and
quality. For example, finding better ways for warehouse employees to
move boxes from one place to another not only can help prevent back
pain but also can reduce time spent on the task, thus increasing productiv-
ity. Consequently, OSH audiences include multiple stakeholders beyond
safety professionals, including policy makers, efficiency experts, facility
designers, and employers.

Theories Underlying OSH and Risk Communication

Risk communication requires not only an understanding of how risk-related
messages are formed, sent, and received but also how individuals make
decisions given the perceived levels of risk they face. The risk communication process has traditionally meant identifying and verifying the evidence
(e.g., statistics, facts) associated with a particular risk, communicating and
explaining that evidence to a community at risk, and creating partnerships
with stakeholders to understand how to control the risks (Fischhoff, 1995;
Morgan, Fischhoff, Bostrom, & Atman, 2002). Partnership development
is argued to be an important component of this process, which promotes
two-way communication between the community and the entity informing
them about the risk (Chess, Salomone, Hance, & Saville, 1995).

Building relationships with stakeholders is exemplified through the
application of the CAUSE model (Rowan, 1991; Rowan, 1994; Rowan,
Botan, Kreps, Samoilenko, & Farnsworth, 2009; Rowan, Sparks,
Pecchioni, & Villagran, 2003), which suggests five communicative
goals: (a) Confidence—certainty felt by the audience in the message and
the source; (b) Awareness—attention to the warning signs of the risk
and being knowledgeable about the topic; (c) Understanding—ability
to visualize larger structures and complex processes related with the
risk; (d) Satisfaction—agreement with the proposed solution(s); and
(e) Enactment—moving an audience from agreement with the message to
action. These goals represent the ways risk messages can address the tensions experienced by audiences, such as skepticism about the message or
source, lack of awareness about the risk, and inadequate understanding
about the terms and complex processes associated with the risk (Rowan
et al., 2009).

The risk communication literature acknowledges that specific risk communication theory is limited in terms of application to diverse audiences (Lundgren & McMakin, 2013) and the uneven risk levels experienced by different populations. The most vulnerable populations have the most difficulty in accessing the information and resources they need to combat those very risks, despite the information they receive through health campaigns (Olaniran & Scholl, 2016). Moreover, not all cultures and populations view a risk the same way or with the same severity (Lachlan, Burke, Spence, & Griffin, 2009). Some racial and ethnic minorities use communication channels that are different from those used to disseminate crucial risk information, often leaving them without the information they need (Lachlan et al., 2009). The effective development of content and use of communication channels should take these population variances into consideration.

Other risk communication models have focused on individual-level audience information-seeking behaviors. For instance, PRISM, or the planned risk information seeking model (Kahlor, 2010), is an effort to link variables predicted by the theory of planned behavior (TPB; Ajzen, 1991) and the risk information seeking and processing model (RISP; Griffin, Dunwoody, & Neuwirth, 1999). PRISM conceptualizes an individual's efforts to seek information about the risks to their own personal health. Kahlor's test of this theory suggests that personal information-seeking has social-psychological complexities. Moreover, certain predictors, such as whether health issues are related to the environment or the difference between what an individual knows and what they need to know, can apply across specific health situations.

When considering risk communication at the level of organization or mass audience, scholars and practitioners can apply many different approaches to communicating risk (Breakwell, 2014; Morgan et al., 2002; Paek, Hilyard, Freimuth, Barge, & Mindlin, 2010). Most of these approaches are informed by health communication theory as well as theories in communication and other social sciences, such as psychology and anthropology. Table 6.1 provides some of the foundational theories used in teaching and practicing health communication.

Table 6.1 Published Theories on Health Communication

Theory	Researcher(s)	Description
Elaboration Likelihood Model	Petty & Cacioppo, 1986	A dual-process theory of persuasion that explains different ways of processing stimuli, why they are used, and how they influence attitude change

Social Learning Theory	Bandura, 1986	Identifies how individuals learn from each other through observed behaviors, attitudes, imitation, and modeling
Self-Efficacy	Bandura, 1993	A behavior model describing the extent or confidence an individual has in his/her ability to complete tasks and reach goals
Self-Determination	Ryan & Deci, 2000	A motivation and personality model that the degree to which an individual is capable is based on autonomy, relatedness, and competence
Theory of Reasoned Action	Azjen & Fishbein, 1980	Focuses on the combination of the individual's belief expectancies about outcomes related to health practices and evaluation of those outcomes; role of social norms in behavioral intention
Health Belief Model	Hochbaum, Rosenstock & Kegels, 1950	Likelihood that health-related action will lead to common health behaviors (contributed to self-efficacy theory)
Social Marketing	Kotlers & Roberto, 1989	Integrates marketing and behavior concepts to influence behaviors that benefit both individuals and communities for the greater good
Diffusion of Innovations	Rogers, 1983	Explains how, why, and the speed of how new ideas and technology travel through social systems
Transtheoretical Model of Health Behavior Change	Prochaska & Velicer, 1997	Health behavior changes involve six stages: precontemplation, contemplation, preparation, action, maintenance, and termination
Risk Perception Attitude Framework	Rimal & Real (2003)	Risk perceptions are considered along with efficacy beliefs, and audiences can respond in any of the following ways: responsive (high risk, high efficacy), avoidant (high risk, low efficacy), proactive (low risk, high efficacy), and indifferent (low risk, low efficacy)

There is room for expansion of digital and new media theories. New media refers to content that is available online and accessible through digital devices; such content enables user participation and feedback (Manovich, 2003). Theory development in digital and new media might address how risk and health information impacts on users and how they share and adopt recommendations and guidance. For example, Sublet, Spring, and Howard (2011) argue that Social Exchange Theory (Homans, 1958) can help explain the interactivity users might perceive with the channels they use, particularly blogs. Social exchange proposes that people assess the potential risks and benefits of their relationships and that most would abandon one when the risks become greater than the rewards. Based on this premise, Sublet, Spring, and Howard argue that blogs allow readers to go beyond consuming information by allowing them to connect with the people on the other end (that is, the blog writers and commenters), thereby creating the potential for connections that have their costs and rewards. Other scholars have identified ways new media have transformed intercultural communication (c.f., Shuter, 2012), and the ways new media support coordinated communication among individuals working together (i.e., media synchronicity theory, Dennis, Fuller, & Valacich, 2008; Dennis & Valacich, 1999).

Besides making information consumers feel a connection or relationship with the media they use, the ultimate goal of OSH risk communication is propelling behavior change that leads to prevention. To that end, and in addition to health communication theories, OSH risk communication must involve outreach efforts using ecological models of health behavior that "emphasize the environmental and policy contexts of behavior, while incorporating social and psychological influences. Ecological models lead to the explicit consideration of multiple levels of influence, thereby guiding the development of more comprehensive interventions" (Sallis, Owen, & Fisher, 2008, p. 503). In OSH, the levels of influence often include individual, community, organizational, and public policy (Sallis, Owen, & Fisher, 2008).

Communicating OSH Information in the Evolving Digital Media Environment

Communicating OSH information and workplace recommendations to the public has required OSH professionals to adapt to changes in the media landscape. The primary shift has been from paper-based to electronic documents, which has presented both challenges and opportunities in the way OSH organizations develop content, determine channel selection, and evaluate information dissemination. The Web and social media have also created an environment where anyone can publish—and do it quickly. The result is competition for audiences' attention in an environment where cognitive overload, navigation and search strategies, and information design are critically important. The great shift from traditional mass media (e.g., television, print magazines, radio) to a digital media environment has facilitated the emergence of new theory and best practices. Every organization is faced with figuring out to what level their target audiences have embraced the digital environment and how to effectively reach those audiences with new and traditional media channels. For most organizations, the new media environment has posed questions and required new decisions about where to place resources for communication efforts.

Like many longstanding OSH organizations, NIOSH historically relied on paper-based and hard media products such as journal articles, NIOSH documents, CD-ROMs, and videotapes to deliver OSH information. Just as they continue to do today through digital media, NIOSH has also relied on intermediaries to disseminate its research through print forms. Intermediaries are organizations or key individuals who have established connections to businesses and employers and can share NIOSH information (Cunningham & Sinclair, 2014). Such intermediaries have included health service providers, labor organizations, trade associations, insurance companies, and chambers of commerce. Evaluating the impact of these dissemination strategies largely rested on tracking publication distribution numbers, number of journal articles published, and citations of NIOSH journal articles. Though technical and educational documents continue to represent the most significant institute output, use of traditional printing and postal service for producing and disseminating document end products has been reduced significantly.

NIOSH and the World Wide Web

As with other government agencies, the availability of the World Wide Web has resulted in a significant shift in the generation and dissemination of NIOSH information. Since 1997, the NIOSH website (i.e., the NIOSH Web) has been the primary dissemination channel for NIOSH research, guidance, and information products. Primary audiences have included OSH professionals (NIOSH's primary intermediaries for reaching workers), workers, employers, decision-makers, and the general public. An early adopter of the Web, NIOSH originally offered plain-text information that was mostly accessed via file sharing by researchers and more savvy users of technology. In 2007, NIOSH added GovDelivery, a subscription service that enables users to set up automated delivery of regular NIOSH updates and newsletters via email. NIOSH expanded communication efforts to social media platforms including MySpace, Facebook, the NIOSH Science Blog, eNews (the NIOSH monthly electronic newsletter), and program-specific electronic newsletters. To reach hazard/industry-specific audiences, NIOSH has also added social media channels as their importance in key audiences emerged (www.cdc.gov/niosh/socmed.html). Impact measurement evolved to include the tracking of website views and visits as well as document downloads.

Many government agencies in the US and other countries find that Web and new media channels are an efficient and timely way to provide large amounts of information to the public (Wigand, 2010). In addition to functioning as a virtual library and archive, the Web allows agencies to improve the way they generate and disseminate information, as well as create products that intermediaries are more likely to share. These changes have also influenced how government researchers and communication specialists, and their stakeholders, approach the way they do their work. For example, through such channels as the NIOSH Science Blog, the NIOSH Web has become a virtual meeting place for NIOSH researchers, stakeholders, and the general public to obtain and share the latest information as well as leave comments.

Also, NIOSH has dedicated staff to write OSH-related content for Wikipedia, the second largest non-search engine driver to the NIOSH website. NIOSH became only the second federal agency and the first federal scientific agency to develop a formalized collaboration with Wikipedia (Temple-Wood, 2015). This partnership not only improves the availability of occupational safety and health information but also effectively extends the reach of NIOSH scientific findings and resources—to a far greater population than NIOSH could reach alone.

New Digital Communication Technology and Rich Media

Two significant aspects of new communication technology are media-rich products and evolving digital devices. Rich media are communication technologies that involve or combine audio, video, animation, and interactive features. Both audience attention and cognitive processing preferences are tied to rich media. The effect of rich media forms has been explained by media richness theory (Daft & Lengel, 1986), which ranks various communication media on the extent to which they allow for various social cues, such as gestures. Originally intended to refer to computer-mediated communication, media richness theory also finds relevance in more contemporary formats, such as text messaging.

Since the iPhone was introduced in 2007 (Reed, 2010), there has been a shift in ownership and use from personal computers to more media-rich mobile devices (Heggestuen, 2013). Mobile usage in the United States continues to increase, with people spending a majority of their time in digital media engagement on mobile apps (Marous, 2014). The demand for content delivery via mobile technologies is only expected to increase (Reed, 2014).

As media-rich digital products become increasingly prevalent in the communication environment, NIOSH and other government agencies continue to expand into other digital communication technology such as Web and mobile applications (apps). Apps are effective tools for taking knowledge gained from basic research and applying it to the field, as demonstrated by the NIOSH Ladder Safety App (www.cdc.gov/niosh/topics/falls/mobileapp.html) and NIOSH Pocket Guide to Chemical Hazards mobile web app (www.cdc.gov/niosh/npg/mobilepocketguide.html). These products often blend research, guidance, and training into a single tool. Such a tool creates the potential for more effective information and knowledge transfer, along with skill building.

Collaborative Content

Perhaps the most significant change in the digital environment is in how content is created and how information sources, such as government agencies, have to compete for audience attention when disseminating that information. While audiences are limited in the amount and kind of information they can retrieve from traditional media, users of new media have access to greater information storage, can demand quick delivery of content, and can give instant feedback on the content they consume (Wahl & Scholl, 2014). This interactivity with new media is characteristic of the "democratization" of the creation and consumption of media content (Manovich, 2003). Whereas users are consumers in traditional media, new media allow users to be producers, which implies more control over the information they can access.

Prior to the Web, the public relied on subject matter experts who were trained and credentialed in their fields and, as such, had access to authoritative printed references for their specialties. Subject matter experts included physicians and lawyers as well as industrial hygienists and other OSH professionals. By virtue of closed professional systems, such as peer-reviewed journals, they were information gatekeepers. As the World Wide Web became universally accessible, the gates opened and specialized information became easily available to everyone. Because the new media environment has encouraged users to be their own gatekeepers of information, audiences are far less beholden to more traditional gatekeepers and are even able to bypass gatekeepers altogether to retrieve the information they need and even redistribute it as they see fit.

The shift away from the more traditional notion of gatekeeping can be characterized as *gatewatching* (Bruns, 2008). Gatewatchers can take the form of sites that publish niche news or information that appeals to specialized audiences. Although gatewatchers cannot control what information passes through channels, they keep an eye at the "gates" for relevant information and choose what flows through those gates to pass on to others. According to Westerman, Spence, and Van Der Heide (2013), gatewatchers have a great deal of power in their promotion and diffusion of information. The emergence of gatewatching has created more demand for collaborative content, that is, content that can be written, edited, and managed by multiple users on a common platform. Online encyclopedias like Wikipedia are examples of formats with collaborative content because they can be edited by virtually anyone without the filter of peer review. The growing normalization of collaborative content has had a radical impact on traditional, centralized sources of information and opened wide the concept of citizen journalism. However, the prevalence of gatewatchers has made determining author expertise often difficult or impossible. Nevertheless, gatewatchers represent a new aspect of the digital media environment, which OSH communication science should seek to understand for more effective dissemination.

Despite the obvious challenges of collaborative content creation, communication norms have shifted. Users want to be involved in content, whether as contributors or as evaluators. To remain relevant to audiences, OSH organizations need to embrace and find appropriate ways to engage in this communication paradigm shift. NIOSH and other authoritative OSH resources are learning the importance of developing strategies to engage stakeholder and user collaboration in the creation and dissemination of health and safety information. For NIOSH, this has meant constructing Web content with the assumption that visitors to its website will likely reuse that content. This involves developing products and using Web content management systems that make it easy for users to retrieve information and repurpose it to meet their specific needs. Such an approach helps to ensure the integrity of highly technical research while allowing content to be translated into meaningful, impactful information products that fit the needs of audiences with diverse literacy levels, technical language, and demographic characteristics.

Opportunities and Challenges of New Media Channels

Technology is only part of the challenges and opportunities that face OSH organizations in developing risk communication strategies. For one thing, there is a lack of theory to guide strategy. Although there is a well-established theoretical foundation for the science of communication (as noted above), theory to guide newer types of digital, interactive communication modalities are not developing as rapidly as the technology. Moreover, the nature and systems of digital technology affect content and product development in ways that make it difficult for agencies to keep up with audience needs and demands. In addition, new media communication has created the need for alternative ways to measure impact (Barnes, 2015). Researchers and practitioners increasingly must document their work by faster measures (Priem, Piwowar, & Hemminger, 2012) and must consider a broader range of activities, such as online discussions and adoption in real-life settings, to show impact. Beyond these technology-driven challenges, OSH organizations must negotiate the additional complications of communicating to a diverse and changing workforce.

As the US workforce adapts to demographic shifts related to immigration and age diversity, OSH professionals must know more about how physical, mental, and cultural differences inform risk and prevention in the workplace. Some of the most significant changes in audience demographics are increasing numbers of temporary or contingent workers (Cummings & Kriess, 2008); workers employed by small businesses (Choi & Spletzer 2012; Cunningham, Sinclair, & Schulte, 2014); older workers (Hayutin, Beals, & Borges, 2013; Silverstein, 2008; Society for Human Resource Management, 2014; Toossi, 2012; Truxillo, Cadiz, & Hammer, 2015); female workers (Toossi, 2012); and vulnerable worker populations such as young immigrants (NIOSH, ASSE 2015) and Latinos (Diuguid, 2014).

Language is another dimension of variability among NIOSH audiences. Many immigrants to the United States are employed in jobs with high rates of injuries and fatalities, such as construction and agriculture (NIOSH, ASSE 2015). These workers are often unaware of their rights under US labor laws and lack critical English language skills that might otherwise make them less vulnerable to occupational hazards. Language barriers also can hinder the comprehension and usability of online and print resources designed to reduce illnesses, injuries, and fatalities, which occur more often among immigrant workers than workers born in the United States (NIOSH, ASSE 2015). While there remains a critical need for translating OSH information into languages other than English, OSH research has also demonstrated the need for culturally tailoring materials to meet the needs of specific audiences (Flynn, 2014).

Trends indicate that the digital communication environment will continue to evolve at a rapid rate (Holliman, 2017). OSH organizations will need to have more agile communication technology systems, which allow organizations to respond to new audience demands and regulatory changes faster, and to communicate with audiences across virtually any channel. Along with more agility, rich media content will need to include complex and interactive graphics, sound, video, and multiple data streams from digital device sources like GPS and photos. In addition, wearable technologies (e.g., smartwatches) and virtual reality products are expected to be commonly used and occupy more of the technology market by 2020 (Page, 2015). Creating such products requires new, high-level skills and problem-solving abilities such as identifying and removing program bugs and advanced graphic design (Robert Half Technology, 2015).

To be relevant in the digital communication environment, the OSH community will need to apply the same standards of evidence used in their research to measuring the performance and impact of new communication technologies, channels, and content types. To do this requires focused exploration in defining meaningful metrics. Web 2.0 interactivity has introduced new social tracking factors into communication and suggested new interpretations of impact. Use of new media has led OSH organizations to utilize "alternative metrics" or "altmetrics" to measure attention to research outputs (Priem, Taraborelli, Groth & Neylon, 2010). Altmetrics measure influence, reach, and engagement by tracking traffic to and conversations on NIOSH webpages, social media activity, and new media products such as the NIOSH Science Blog and Wikipedia. Used as qualitative attention indicators, altmetrics provide a broader picture of audience interaction with information. Although altmetrics do not measure the quality of information, they can provide a more comprehensive picture of how target audiences access and engage with information that fits their specific needs.

Digital communication is a system of complex subsystems influenced by a variety of audience factors. More than ever before, strategic planning is a paradox. The rapidly changing digital environment makes it difficult to plan very far into the future. However, organizations must still make decisions about a highly significant number of resource allocations. This requires a fundamental strategy and the ability to make effective choices in a media environment of endless opportunities. This is particularly true of many OSH organizations that are connected to governmental structures, often with modest resources. Strategic plans are essential, and in the digital environment they need to cover shorter periods of time and include subplans for complex subordinate components such as digital product strategies, Web plans, and mobile lifecycles.

Research supports continuing to use the Web as a platform for organizational communication (Klimchak, Sherman, MacKenzie, & Ward, 2013; Powell, Horvath, & Brandtner, 2016; Saffer, Somerfeldt, & Taylor, 2013). To this end, communication technology experts in government agencies like NIOSH need to maintain Web environments that are simple, flexible, and sustainable. For example, NIOSH has developed a Web and new media strategy that is informed by the history of the NIOSH Web that has incorporated significant changes in communication technology. The strategy identifies key Web challenges NIOSH and other government agencies will experience in the coming years, such as adapting Web content for mobile Web delivery, preparing for growth of current and new digital products, and assessing the sustainability of these products.

Recommendations for the Future in New Media and OSH Risk Communication

Communication strategies continue to undergo dramatic change as new technologies and channels emerge. To stay abreast of the changes and ensure optimal application of research, communicators can benefit from a number of key areas of research and best practice guidance. One area is the continued building of new media theory, which includes understanding the impact of new media on diverse audiences, particularly to promote behavioral change (Korda & Itani, 2013). While OSH research focuses on the environmental risks and nature of work, research cannot rely solely on traditional communication and health communication theory. New media has created the need for more interdisciplinary research and theory development in the areas of psychology, neurology, and technology-mediated communication and learning. One possible recommendation is to use case study methodology, which provides a look into the specific environments in which new media are used. Case studies allow for mixed methods and place more focus on risk communication geared toward applied environments (Urquhart & Vaast, 2012).

More specifically related to media theory is understanding how communication technologies influence and are used by different workforce audiences. This means extending knowledge beyond reach (that is, message exposure) to discerning the factors influencing audience engagement and understanding how to reach and engage audiences on specific issues (Hudson & Hall, 2013). OSH communication professionals must understand not only how information is shared but also how it is adopted and is influential in reducing worker illnesses, injuries, and fatalities. Specifically, there is still a lack of information on how social media can be used for health or risk communication, especially in determining the effectiveness of different types of social media (Moorhead, Hazlett, Harrison, Carroll, Irwin, & Hoving, 2013). More focused research into gatewatching (Bruns, 2008) could be beneficial. Understanding what kinds of content are more likely to be shared by users can shed light on what is relevant and useful to target audiences.

Another area is understanding the role of new media in translation research. One knowledge gap that still exists is the extent to which we understand how media can be used to increase the likelihood that products designed to reduce injuries and support safer work practices will be sought out, adopted, shared, and used in the workplace. This is especially the case where little information is available on the perceived value of downloadable apps in the field (Iris, Ellis, Yoder, & Keifer, 2016). More research is needed to discover how digital media can help move guidance, recommendations, and technology into practice in ways that maximize worker safety and health, well-being, and loss control in the most efficient and impactful ways possible (Desmarais & Lortie, 2011; NAS, 2009; Rantanen, 1999; Schulte, Okun, Stephenson, Colligan, Ahlers, Gjessing, Loos, Niemeier, & Sweeney, 2003).

Further investigation can help uncover the barriers that hinder certain translation efforts and approaches, such as passive methods that fail to reach those most affected in the workplace (Baker, Chang, Bunting, & Betit, 2015) and limited engagement of the audiences that are reached (Brace, Padilla, DeJoy, Wilson, Vandenberg, & Davis et al., 2015). To this end, the aforementioned NIOSH translation research program was established to broaden research in the areas of large-scale delivery, dissemination, and diffusion. As it relates to health communication and digital media, NIOSH is focusing translation research efforts on how audiences' awareness of NIOSH activities and outputs can be enhanced. To advance more audience-based research at NIOSH and to address the scarcity of this paradigm of research (Rantanen, 1999), health communication specialists are currently developing a database of survey items that can be used to collect audience data such as media preferences, health beliefs, and other communication and psychological characteristics that provides insight into the messages and dissemination strategies that resonate with certain audiences.

A third area of research and development is in best practice standards for creating new media content, particularly for diverse audiences that can be considered "moving targets" (Livingstone, 2004). Content about a particular topic or issue must be tailored to not only be relevant to the audience but also fit differences in literacy and languages (cultural and occupational). Content must also address communication barriers that contribute to health disparities across cultural and occupational audiences, because these disparities include access to worker protections (NIOSH, ASSE, 2015), disproportionate incidences of illness and injury (Pinkerton, Harbaugh, Han, Le Saux, Van Winkle, Martin, Kosgei, Carter, Sitkin, Smiley-Jewell, & George, 2015), and inadequate access to information or health promotion programs (Baron, Beard, Davis, Delp, Forst, Kidd-Taylor, Liebman, Linnan, Punnitt, & Welch, 2014).

Content development must also be informed by the format or delivery mechanism (such as a Web page or smartphone app). This requires creators to be more fluid in visualizing finished products. The digital device environment requires content to be more flexible, less static, and more dynamic. Dynamic content allows for the best user experience on any device. Standards are needed to guide the development of content versions for different devices. For instance, how should authorship be determined for versioned content (De Alfaro & Shavlovsky, 2013)?

These content versions, or scalable content packages, in some cases are edited differently, depending on who is using it and where it is being used. Versioned content allows users to either pull smaller bits of information from a larger content source and repackage it for their own purposes or pull shorter versions from different devices. More strategies may be needed to guide both development and management of versioned content as new channels of media continue to emerge.

A final area of continued research is in performance metrics, or tracking the use of OSH information for impact. Accurately measuring impact depends on knowing who is accessing and using OSH information. Continued focus can be placed on decision makers and intermediaries who are in the position to adopt and implement the guidance and recommendations in the workplace (Smith, 2008). Although intermediaries continue to be a prime audience for NIOSH, expanding internet use means that more audience-based research is needed to know who is accessing the information and how communication patterns have changed (Chou, Hunt, Hesse, Beckjord, & Moser, 2009).

Information seeking by target audiences is another important indicator of impact, which reflects the shift from the print-dominant paradigm to the current digital paradigm. Traditional ways of tracking the impact of research have included citation frequencies and journal impact factors. However, as previously discussed, alternative metrics (or altmetrics) are gaining more influence in discussions of impact and its definition. Future research must explore the weight carried by engagement and movement of information through social media networks in determining impact. Moorhead, Hazlett, Harrison, Carroll, Irwin, and Hoving (2013) recommend using a variety of research methodologies to determine the long- and short-term impacts of social media on best practices.

Conclusion

With the safety and health of 157 million US workers and 3 billion workers worldwide (Torres, 2013) at stake, effective communication of occupational risk is critical. Since 1970, NIOSH has been a world leader in risk communication. The Institute has demonstrated this through its theory-driven and evidence-based strategies and best practices in communicating research in occupational exposure, its progressive translation research program, and its track record for communication innovation.

The rapidly changing digital communication environment presents many opportunities and challenges. There will continue to be areas of risk communication in which NIOSH and other agencies need more foundational research on communication strategies and technology. These key areas include: (a) building new media theory; (b) identifying the role of new media in translational research; (c) developing best practice standards for new media content; (d) developing change and process management strategies; and (e) effectively evaluating impact through alternative and other communication performance metrics.

References

Ajzen, I. (1991). The theory of planned behavior. *Organizational Behavior and Human Decision Processes, 50,* 179–211.

Ajzen, I., & Fishbein, M. (1980). *Understanding attitudes and predicting social behaviour.* Upper Saddle River, NJ: Prentice-Hall, Inc.

Alli, B. (2008). *Fundamental principles of occupational health and safety* (2nd ed.). Geneva, Switzerland: International Labor Organization.

Aronsson, G., & Gustafsson, K. (2005). Sickness presenteeism: Prevalence, attendance-pressure factors, and an outline of a model for research. *Journal of Occupational and Environmental Medicine, 47*(9), 958.

Baker, R., Chang, C., Bunting, J., & Betit, E. (2015). Triage for action: Systematic assessment and dissemination of construction health and safety research. *American Journal of Industrial Medicine, 58*(8), 838–848. doi: 10.1002/ajim.22477.

Bandura, A. (1986). *Social foundations of thought and action: A social cognitive theory.* Upper Saddle River, NJ: Prentice-Hall, Inc.

Bandura, A. (1993). Perceived self-efficacy in cognitive development and functioning. *Educational Psychologist, 28*(2), 117–148.

Barnes, C. (2015). The use of altmetrics as a tool for measuring research impact. *Australian Academic & Research Libraries, 46*(2), 121–134. doi: 10.1080/00048623.2014.1003174.

Baron, S. L., Beard, S., Davis, L. K., Delp, L., Forst, L., Kidd-Taylor, A., Liebman, A. K., Linnan, L., Punnett, L., & Welch, L. S. (2014). Promoting integrated approaches to reducing health inequities among low-income workers: Applying a social ecological framework. *American Journal of Industrial Medicine, 57*(5), 539–556. doi: 10.1002/ajim.22174.

Brace, A. M., Padilla, H. M., DeJoy, D. M., Wilson, M. G., Vandenberg, R. J., & Davis, M. (2015). Applying RE-AIM to the evaluation of FUEL Your Life: A worksite translation of DPP. *Health Promotion Practices, 16*(1), 28–35. doi: 10.1177/1524839914539329.

Breakwell, G. M. (2014). *The psychology of risk.* Cambridge, UK: Cambridge University Press.

Bruns, A. (2008). The active audience: Transforming journalism from gatekeeping to gatewatching. In C. Paterson & D. Domingo (Eds.), *Making online news: The ethnography of new media production.* New York: Peter Lang.

Bureau of Labor Statistics. (2015). *Employment status of the civilian noninstitutional population, 1945 to date.* Washington, DC: U.S. Department of Labor. www.bls.gov/cps/cpsaat01.pdf.

Chess, C., Salomone, K. L., Hance, B. J., & Saville, A. (1995). Results of a National Symposium on Risk Communication: Next steps for government agencies. *Risk Analysis, 15,* 115–125.

Choi, E. J., & Spletzer, J. R. (2012). The declining average size of establishments: Evidence and explanations. *Monthly Labor Review*, 135(3), 50–65. www.bls. gov/opub/mlr/2012/03/art4full.pdf.

Chou, W. S., Hunt, Y. M., Hesse, B. W., Beckjord, E. B., & Moser, R. P. (2009). Social media use in the United States: Implications for health communication. *Journal of Medical Internet Research*, 11(4), 9. doi: 10.2196/jmir.1259.

Cummings, K. J., & Kreiss, K. (2008). Contingent workers and contingent health: Risks of a modern economy. *Journal of the American Medical Association*, 299(4), 448–50. doi: 10.1001/jama.299.4.448.

Cunningham, T. R., & Sinclair, R. (2014). Application of a model for delivering occupational safety and health to smaller businesses: Case studies from the US. *Safety Science*, 71(C), 213–225. doi: 10.1016/j.ssci.2014.06.011.

Cunningham, T. R., Sinclair, R., & Schulte, P. (2014). Better understanding the small business construct to advance research on delivering workplace safety and health. *Small Enterprise Research*, 21(2), 148–160. doi: 10.1080/13215906.2014.11082084.

Daft, R. L, & Lengel, R. H. (1986). Organizational information requirements, media richness and structural design. *Management Science*, 32(5), 554–571. doi: 10.1287/mnsc.32.5.554.

Dennis, A. R., Fuller, R. M., & Valacich, J. S. (2008). Media, tasks, and communication processes: A theory of media synchronicity. *MIS Quarterly*, 32(3), 575–600.

Dennis, A. R., & Valacich, J. S. (1999, January). Rethinking media richness: Towards a theory of media synchronicity. Proceedings of the Thirty-Second Annual Hawaii International Conference on System Sciences, 1, p. 1017.

Desmarais, L., & Lortie, M. (2011). La dynamique du transfert des connaissances: Une perspective centrée sur l'usager. [The dynamics of knowledge transfer: A user-centered perspective]. The workplace collection of chair in health and safety in the workplace management. Quebec, Canada: Presses de l'université Laval.

Diuguid, L. (2014). Latino family wealth projected to rise with the Hispanic population growth in U.S. *Kansas City Star*. Retrieved October 21, 2014, from www. kansascity.com/opinion/opn-columns-blogs/lewis-diuguid/article2357663.html.

Fischhoff, B. (1995). Risk perception and communication unplugged: Twenty years of process. *Risk Analysis*, 15, 137–145.

Flynn, M. A. (2014). Safety and today's diverse workforce: Lessons from NIOSH's work with Latino immigrants. *Professional Safety*, 59(6), 52–57.

Friend, M. A., & Kohn, J. P. (2010). *Fundamentals of occupational safety and health* (5th ed.). Lanham, MD: Government Institutes.

Griffin, R., Dunwoody, S., & Neuwirth, K. (1999). Proposed model of the relationship of risk information seeking and processing to the development of preventive behaviors. *Environmental Research*, 80, 230–245.

Guest, D., & Conway, N. (2009). Health and well-being: The role of the psychological contract. In G. L. Cooper, J. C. Quick, & M. Schabracq (Eds.), *International handbook of work and health psychology* (3rd ed.), pp. 9–23. Malden, MA: Wiley-Blackwell.

Hansen, C. D., & Andersen, J. H. (2008). Going ill to work—What personal circumstances, attitudes and work-related factors are associated with sickness presenteeism? *Social Science and Medicine*, 67, 956–964.

117

Hayutin, A., Beals, M., & Borges, E. (2013). The aging US workforce: A chartbook of demographic shifts. Stanford Center on Longevity. Retrieved November 3, 2014, from http://longevity3.stanford.edu/wp-content/uploads/2013/09/The_Aging_U.S.-Workforce.pdf.

Heath, R. L., & O'Hair, H. D. (2010). The significance of crisis and risk communication. In R. L. Heath & H. D. O'Hair (Eds.), *Handbook of risk and crisis communication* (pp. 5–30). New York: Routledge.

Heath, R. L., Palenchar, M. J., & O'Hair, H. D. (2010). Community building through risk communication infrastructures. In R. L. Heath & H. D. O'Hair (Eds.), *Handbook of risk and crisis communication* (pp. 471–487). New York: Routledge.

Heggestuen, J. (2013). One in every 5 people in the world own a smartphone, one in every 17 own a tablet. *Business Insider*. Retrieved October 21, 2014, from www.businessinsider.com/smartphone-and-tablet-penetration-2013-10.

Hochbaum, G., Rosenstock, I., & Kegels, S. (1952). *Health belief model*. United States Public Health Service.

Holliman, R. (2017). Telling science stories in an evolving digital media ecosystem: From communication to conversation and confrontation. *Connections, 10*(4), 1–4.

Homans, G. (1958). Social behavior as exchange. *American Journal of Sociology, 63*, 597–606.

Hudson, H., & Hall, J. (2013). Value of social media in reaching and engaging employers in Total Worker Health. *Journal of Occupational and Environmental Medicine, 55*(12), S78–S81. doi: 10.1097/JOM.0000000000000035.

Iris, R., Ellis, T., Yoder, A., & Keifer, M. C. (2016). An evaluation tool for agricultural health and safety mobile applications. *Journal of Agromedicine, 21*(4), 301–309. doi: 10.1080/1059924X.2016.1211054.

Kahlor, L. (2010). PRISM: A planned risk information seeking model. *Health Communication, 25*(4), 345–356. doi: 10.1080/10410231003775172.

Khoury, M. J., Gwinn, M., & Ioannidis, J. P. A. (2010). The emergence of translational epidemiology: From scientific discovery to population health impact. *American Journal of Epidemiology, 172*, 517–524.

Klimchak, M., Sherman, J. D., MacKenzie, W. I., & Ward, A. K. (2013). Effects of communication media, trust, accuracy and completeness on organizational commitment. Academy of Management Proceedings. doi: 10.5465/AMBPP.2013.17051.

Korda, H., & Itani, Z. (2013). Harnessing social media for health promotion and behavior change. *Health Promotion Practice, 14*(1), 15–23. doi: 10.1177/1524839911405850.

Kotler, P., & Roberto, E. L. (1989). *Social marketing: Strategies for changing public behavior*. New York: Free Press.

Lachlan, K. A., Burke, J., Spence, P. R., & Griffin, D. (2009). Risk perceptions, race, and Hurricane Katrina. *The Howard Journal of Communications, 20*, 295–309.

Leigh, J. P. (2011). Economic burden of occupational injury and illness in the United States. *The Milibank Quarterly, 89*(4), 728–772. doi: 10.1111/j.1468-0009.2011.00648.x.

Livingstone, S. (2004). The challenge of changing audiences or, what is the audience research to do in the age of the internet? *European Journal of Communication*, 19(1), 75–86. doi: 10.1177/0267323104040695.

Lundgren, R. E., & McMakin, A. H. (2013). *Risk communication: A handbook for communicating environmental, safety, and health risks* (5th ed.). New York, NY: Wiley IEEE Press.

Manovich, L. (2003). New media from Borges to HTML. In N. Wardrip-Fruin & N. Montfort (Eds.), *The new media reader* (pp. 13–25). Cambridge, MA: MIT Press.

Marous, J. (2014). Mobile banking not keeping pace with digital growth. *The Financial Brand*. Retrieved October 21, 2014, from http://thefinancialbrand. com/41827/banking-lacks-mobile-plan/.

McComas, K. A. (2006). Defining moments in risk communication research: 1996–2005. *Journal of Health Communication*, 11(1), 75–91. doi: 10.1080/10810730500461091.

Moorhead, S. A., Hazlett, D., Harrison, L., Carroll, J. K., Irwin, A., & Hoving, C. (2013). A new dimension of health care: Systematic review of the uses, benefits, and limitations of social media for health communication. *Journal of Medical Internet Research*, 15(4), e85. doi: 10.2196/jmir.1933.

Morgan, M. G., Fischhoff, B., Bostrom, A., & Atman, C. J. (2002). *Risk communication: A mental models approach*. Cambridge, UK: Cambridge University Press.

MSHA. (n.d.): History. Retrieved February 7, 2017, from: www.msha.gov/about/ history.

NAS. (2009). National Academy of Science. *Evaluating occupational health and safety research programs: Framework and next steps*. Washington, DC: National Academies Press.

NIOSH. (2015, October). National Institute for Occupational Safety and Health. Factsheet. Cincinnati, OH: U.S. Department of Health and Human Services, Centers for Disease Control and Prevention, National Institute for Occupational Safety and Health, DHHS (NIOSH) Publication No. 2013-140. www.cdc.gov/niosh/docs/2013-140/pdfs/2013-140.pdf.

NIOSH. (2015, November 4). NIOSH programs. National Institute for Occupational Safety and Health. www.cdc.gov/niosh/programs.html.

NIOSH. (2015, December 4). Research to practice (r2p). National Institute for Occupational Safety and Health. www.cdc.gov/niosh/r2p/.

NIOSH, ASSE. (2015). Overlapping vulnerabilities: The occupational safety and health of young workers in small construction firms. By Flynn, M. A., Cunningham, T. R., Guerin, R. J., Keller, B., Chapman, L. J., Hudson, D., & Salgado, C. Cincinnati, OH: U.S. Department of Health and Human Services, Centers for Disease Control and Prevention, National Institute for Occupational Safety and Health, DHHS (NIOSH) Publication No. 2015-178.

NIOSH. (2016, January 11). About NIOSH. National Institute for Occupational Safety and Health. Retrieved from www.cdc.gov/niosh/about/default.html.

NIOSH. (forthcoming). NIOSH translation research roadmap. Cincinnati, OH: U.S. Department of Health and Human Services, Centers for Disease Control and Prevention, National Institute for Occupational Safety and Health.

NIOSH. (forthcoming). NIOSH web 5-year plan, 2015–2019: A plan to meet NIOSH dissemination needs and new communication technology challenges. Cincinnati, OH: U.S. Department of Health and Human Services, Centers for Disease Control and Prevention, National Institute for Occupational Safety and Health.

Olaniran, B. A., & Scholl, J. C. (2016). *Handbook for the crisis communication center.* New York: Peter Lang.

OSHA. (n.d.) State Plans: Frequently asked questions. Retrieved February 7, 2017, from: www.osha.gov/dcsp/osp/.

Paek, H., Hilyard, K., Freimuth, V., Barge, K., & Mindlin, M. (2010). Theory-based approaches to understanding public emergency preparedness: Implications for effective health and risk communication. *Journal of Health Communication: International Perspectives, 15*(4), 428–444. doi: 10.1080/10810731003753083.

Page, T. (2015). A forecast of the adoption of wearable technology. *International Journal of Technology Diffusion, 6*(2). doi: 10.4018/IJTD.2015040102.

Parrott, R. (2004). Emphasizing "communication" in health communication. *Journal of Communication, 54*(4), 751–787. doi: 10.1111/j.1460-2466.2004. tb02653.x.

Petty, R. E., & Cacioppo, J. T. (1986). The elaboration likelihood model of persuasion. In R. E. Petty & J. Cacioppo, *Communication and persuasion* (pp. 1–24). New York: Springer.

Pinkerton, K. E., Harbaugh, M., Han, M. K., Le Saux, C. J., Van Winkle, L. S., Martin, W J., II, Kosgei, R. J., Carter, E. J., Sitkin, N., Smiley-Jewell, S. M., & George, M. (2015). Women and lung disease: Sex differences and global health disparities. *American Journal of Respiratory and Critical Care Medicine, 192*(1), 11–16.

Powell, W. W., Horvath, A., & Brandtner, C. (2016). Click and mortar: Organizations on the web. *Research in Organizational Behavior* [Online].

Priem, J., Piwowar, H. A., & Hemminger, B. M. (2012, March 20). Altmetrics in the wild: Using social media to explore scholarly impact. arXiv:1203.4745v1.

Priem, J., Taraborelli, D., Groth, P., & Neylon, C. (2010, October 26). Altmetrics: A manifesto. http://altmetrics.org/manifesto.

Prochaska, J. O., & Velicer, W. F. (1997). The transtheoretical model of health behavior change. *American Journal of Health Promotion, 12*(1), 38–48.

Rantanen, J. (1999). Research challenges arising from changes in work life. *Scandinavian Journal of Work and Environmental Health, 25,* 473–483.

Real, K. (2008). Information seeking and workplace safety: A field application of the risk perception attitude framework. *Journal of Applied Communication Research, 36,* 338–358. doi: 10.1080/00909880802101763.

Reed, B. (2010). A brief history of smartphones. *PCWorld.* Retrieved October 21, 2014, from www.techhive.com/article/199243/a_brief_history_of_smart phones.html.

Reed, M. (2014). Government indifference must not stand in the way of mobile health innovation. Retrieved October 21, 2014, from www.ihealthbeat.org/ perspectives/2014/government-indifference-must-not-stand-in-the-way-of-mobile-health-innovation.

Riegelman, R., & Kirkwood, B. (2015). *Public health 101: Healthy people—healthy populations* (2nd ed.). Burlington, MA: Jones & Bartlett Learning.

Rimal, R. N., Brown, J., Mkandawire, G., Folda, L., Böse, K., & Creel, A. H. (2009). Audience segmentation as a social-marketing tool in health promotion: Use of the risk perception attitude framework in HIV prevention in Malawi. *American Journal of Public Health*, 99, 2224–2229. doi: 10.2105/AJPH.2008.155234.

Rimal, R. N., & Real, K. (2003). Perceived risk and self-efficacy as motivators of change: Support for the risk perception attitude framework from two studies. *Human Communication Research*, 29, 370–399.

Robert Half Technology (2015, December 27). Must-have skills for mobile application development. Retrieved from www.roberthalf.com/technology/blog/must-have-skills-for-mobile-application-development.

Rogers, E. M. (1983). *Diffusion of innovations*. New York: Free Press.

Rowan, K. E. (1991). Goals, obstacles, and strategies in risk communication. *Journal of Applied Communication Research*, 19, 300–329.

Rowan, K. E. (1994). The technical and democratic approaches to risk situations: Their appeal, limitations, and rhetorical alternative. *Argumentation*, 8(4), 391–409. doi: 10.1007/BF00733482.

Rowan, K. E., Botan, C. H., Kreps, G. L., Samoilenko, S., & Farnsworth, K. (2009). Risk communication education for local emergency managers: Using the CAUSE model for research, education, and outreach. In R. L. Health & H. D. O'Hair (Eds.), *Handbook of risk and crisis communication* (pp. 168–191). New York: Routledge.

Rowan, K. E., Sparks, L., Pecchioni, L., & Villagran, M. (2003). The "CAUSE" model: A research-supported guide for physicians communicating cancer risk. *Health Communication*, 15, 239–252.

Ryan, R. M., & Deci, E. L. (2000). Self-determination theory and the facilitation of intrinsic motivation, social development, and well-being. *American Psychologist*, 55(1), 68–78.

Saffer, A. J., Sommerfeldt, E. J., & Taylor, M. (2013). The effects of organizational Twitter interactivity on organization-public relationships. *Public Relations Review*, 39(3), 213–215. doi: 10.1016/j.pubrev.2013.02.005.

Sallis, J. F., Owen, N., & Fisher, E. B. (2008). Ecological models of health behavior. In K. Glanz, B. K. Rimer, & K. Viswanath (Eds.), *Health behavior and health education: Theory, research, and practice*. San Francisco, CA: Jossey-Bass.

Schulte, P. A., Okun, A., Stephenson, C. M., Colligan, M., Ahlers, H., Gjessing, C., Loos, G., Niemeier, R. W., & Sweeney, M. H. (2003). Information dissemination and use: Critical components in occupational safety and health. *American Journal of Industrial Medicine*, 44(5), 515–531.

Shuter, R. (2012). Intercultural new media studies: The next frontier in intercultural communication. *Journal of Intercultural Communication Research*, 41(3), 219–327. doi: 10.1080/17475759.2012.728761.

Silverstein, M. (2008). Meeting the challenges of an aging workforce. *American Journal of Industrial Medicine*, 51, 269–280. doi: 10.1002/ajim.20569.

Smith, B. (2008). Can social marketing be everything to everyone? *Social Marketing Quarterly*, 14(1), 91–93.

Society for Human Resource Management (2014). Executive summary: Preparing for an aging workforce. Retrieved April 9, 2016, from www. shrm.org/Research/SurveyFindings/Documents/14-0765%20Executive%20 Briefing%20Aging%20Workforce%20v4.pdf.

Straus, S. E., Graham, I. D., & Mazmanian, P. E. (2006). Knowledge translation: Resolving the confusion. *Journal of Continuing Education in the Health Professions*, 26(1), 3–4.

Sublet, V., Spring, C., & Howard, J. (2011). Does social media improve communication? Evaluating the NIOSH Science Blog. *American Journal of Industrial Medicine*, 54, 384–394. doi: 10.1002/ajim.20921.

Temple-Wood, E. (2015, May 19). Collaboration with Wikipedia [Web log comment]. NIOSH Science Blog. http://blogs.cdc.gov/niosh-science-blog/2015/05/19/wikipedian/.

Toossi, M. (2012). Employment outlook: 2010–2020. Labor force projections to 2020: A more slowly growing workforce. *Monthly Labor Review*, 135(1), 43–64. Retrieved November 3, 2014, from www.bls.gov/opub/mlr/2012/01/art3full.pdf.

Torres, R. (ed.) (2013). *World of work report 2013: Repairing the economic and social fabric*. Geneva, Switzerland: International Labour Organisation, International Institute for Labour Studies.

Turner, M. M., Skubisz, C., & Rimal, R. N. (2011). Theory and practice in risk communication: A review of the literature and visions for the future. In T. L. Thompson, R. Parrott, & J. F. Nussbaum (Eds.), *The Routledge handbook of health communication* (2nd ed.). New York: Routledge.

Turnock, B. J. (2016). *Essentials of public health* (3rd ed.). Burlington, MA: Jones & Bartlett Learning.

Truxillo, D. M., Cadiz, D. E., & Hammer, L. B. (2015). Supporting the aging workforce: A review and recommendations for workplace intervention research. *Annual Review of Organizational Psychology and Organizational Behavior*, 2, 351–381.

Urquhart, C., & Vaast, E. (2012, October). *Building social media theory from case studies: A new frontier for research*. Thirty Third International Conference on Information Systems, Orlando, FL.

Wahl, S. T., & Scholl, J. C. (2014). *Communication and culture in your life*. Dubuque, IA: Kendall-Hunt.

Westerman, D., Spence, P. R., & Van Der Heide, B. (2013). Social media as information source: Recency of updates and credibility of information. *Journal of Computer-mediated Communication*, 19(2), 171–183. doi: 10.1111/jcc4.12041.

Wigand, F. D. L. (2010). *Adoption of Web 2.09 by Canadian and US governments*. New York: Springer.

Zerhouni, E. A. (2003). Medicine: The NIH roadmap. *Science*, 203, 63–72.

7

BEST PRACTICES OF "INNOVATOR" TV METEOROLOGISTS WHO ACT AS CLIMATE CHANGE EDUCATORS

Katherine E. Rowan, John Kotcher, Jenell Walsh-Thomas, Paula K. Baldwin, Janey Trowbridge, Jagadish T. Thaker, H. Joe Witte, Barry A. Klinger, Ligia Cohen, Candice Tresch, and Edward W. Maibach

THIS RESEARCH WAS SUPPORTED BY THE NATIONAL SCIENCE FOUNDATION (AWARDS DRL-0917566 AND DRL-1422431).

Introduction

The Challenge of Educating About Slow Onset Hazards

Social scientists studying natural disasters distinguish slow onset events such as drought, desertification, coastal erosion, and climate change from suddenly occurring harms such as hurricanes, wildfires, and landslides (e.g., Alexander, 1999; Gaile & Willmott, 2003). In health and risk communication, similar distinctions are made between acute health hazards such as heart attacks or strokes and slow onset harms such as increasing rates of Type II diabetes, sedentary behavior, and obesity associated with poor health outcomes (e.g., Slovic & Peters, 2006; Swain, 2007). In general, people are more able to become concerned about acute harms like wildfires and heart attacks—especially when such harms affect them—than they are about slow onset hazards. That is, as Sandman (1993) noted and numerous risk scholars have also shown (e.g., Slovic & Peters, 2006), the hazards that upset people are often not those most likely to kill or harm them and the hazards that kill or harm may not be especially upsetting. To illustrate this pattern further, possible transmission of the Ebola virus in the United States received widespread media coverage even though only two people were killed by it (Ashkenas et al. 2015). In contrast, excessive sedentary behavior such as watching television or sitting at a computer increases many sources of mortality risk (Matthews et al., 2012).

Given the challenge of galvanizing concern about slow onset hazards, research on the conditions under which people *do* learn about these harms is especially important. One line of work in which there are intriguing findings has to do with how people learn about the gradual hazard of climate change. Climate science says that the average global temperature is increasing because of the growing amount of heat-trapping gas emitted by human activities such as transportation, heating, and cooling. This rising global temperature causes a wide array of increasingly harmful effects including flooding, changes in patterns of insect-borne disease, increased risk of extreme weather, increased numbers of dangerously hot and humid days in warm, wet regions as well as increased risk of drought in drier regions (IPCC, 2007; National Research Council, 2011).

Unfortunately, many Americans' beliefs about climate change are currently out of step with the scientific consensus (e.g., IPCC, 2007). In one recent nationally representative survey, while 70% of Americans believed that global warming is occurring, 11% said that it is not happening, and 19% reported that they "don't know" whether global warming is occurring or not. Additionally, only 53% correctly indicated that it is caused mostly by human activity, while 34% said they believe it is caused mostly by natural forces in the environment (Leiserowitz, Maibach, Roser-Renouf, Feinberg, & Rosenthal, 2016). A growing body of research shows that there appear to be at least five key beliefs that are highly predictive of individuals' attitudes toward climate change and their support for taking societal action to address it: 1) belief certainty that climate change is real; 2) belief that climate change is caused mostly by human activity; 3) belief that climate change is harmful to people; 4) belief that climate change is a solvable problem; and 5) belief that most scientists agree that human-caused climate change is happening (Ding, Maibach, Zhao, Roser-Renouf, & Leiserowitz, 2011; Krosnick, Holbrook, Lowe, & Visser, 2006). From the standpoint of informal science education initiatives on climate change, these five key beliefs provide both a set of educational objectives for educators as well as a collection of important indicators for measuring the success of such efforts.

TV Meteorologists as Informal Climate Change Educators

In addition to systematically selecting important communication goals, research has long stressed the importance of strategically selecting a set of trusted messengers to communicate key messages to target audiences (Maibach & Covello, 2016). For a variety of reasons, local television meteorologists—a workforce of about 2,000 professionals nationwide—seem well positioned to act as important informal educators when it comes to the issue of climate change, and to help achieve better educational outcomes based on the key beliefs discussed above. The majority of American adults indicate that they learn about science primarily from television (Miller, Augenbraun, Schulhof, & Kimmel, 2006). Additionally, a majority of adults also regularly watch local television news and network television news (Miller et al., 2006). Since 2008, nationally representative surveys of the American public have found that most Americans trust television meteorologists as a source of information about climate change (Leiserowitz, Maibach, & Roser-Renouf, 2008). A September 2012 analysis found that television meteorologists are among the most trusted sources of information on the issue, with 60% of Americans saying they trust television meteorologists—a belief topped only by respondents' trust in climate scientists (76%) and other kinds of scientists (67%) (Leiserowitz et al., 2012).

Bases for TV meteorologists' credibility. But what exactly are TV meteorologists doing to be trusted? One source of their credibility is that they provide crucial information when people perceive they need it most: during storm and extreme weather coverage. As Daniels and Loggins (2007) explain, "Viewers of . . . commercial stations expect a weather forecaster to tell them when to take cover or other protective actions before it is too late. . . . Stations that ignore weather forecasters in favor of news talent may be ill-advised. Most stations in our sample chose to build wall-to-wall coverage of hurricanes around the forecaster" (p. 62). That is, local television stations are in competition for viewers. One way of winning viewers is to invest in TV meteorologists credentialed by the American Meteorological Society to provide evidence-based forecasts, computerized images of storms' locations, and useful, informed coverage during breaking weather news.

Another source of credibility for TV meteorologists—which may be more directly relevant to educating viewers about slow onset hazards, like climate change—are factors that have been identified more generally in research on source credibility and message reception: likability, knowledgeability, and attractiveness (O'Keefe, 2015). Positive evaluations of message sources generally lead to perceptions of increased credibility of the source, which lead to greater learning of message content (Petty,

Wegener, & Fabrigar, 1997). Indeed, in an experimental study, Anderson et al. (2013) found that viewers who liked a TV meteorologist learned more from an educational video about climate change presented by the meteorologist than those who did not view the meteorologist positively. As Anderson et al. (2013) noted, this finding is consistent with research on credibility of sources and message reception.

Best Practices for Informal Science Education

To guide our investigation, we drew from a consensus report by the National Research Council (Bell, Lewenstein, Shouse, & Feder, 2009) reviewing research on "best practices" for informal science education. Informal science learning environments are not school or work environments, but rather those where people choose to learn science, such as voluntarily selected television viewing, Internet exploration, visits to museums, science centers, or national parks, or play with computerized science games, and so forth. The report identified six "strands" or best practices that support science learning.

Best Practice 1: Educators engage audiences' emotions and interests. Research shows people learn science in informal settings when learning is exciting, interesting, and comfortable; that is, the learner feels physically comfortable and stimulated but not overwhelmed. For example, Sachatello-Sawyer et al. (2002) found museums usually design exhibits for families with children rather than adults and tend to over-use didactic methods such as lectures, which adults find dull. These authors report that adults want interactive experiences that let them build relationships with fellow enthusiasts.

Best Practice 2: Learners generate and use scientific facts, arguments, and models. For example, Randol (2005) found audiences were likely to learn when encouraged to discuss procedure and control variables (e.g., what happens when you turn this wheel or, perhaps, how might warming rivers affect fish like brook trout); that is, they learn when prompted to generate and use scientific observations and information.

Best Practice 3: People learn science when focused not just on content, but also on the scientific method. Specifically, people benefit from asking questions, exploring, experimenting, applying ideas, predicting, drawing conclusions from evidence, and thinking with others. For example, scientists and some TV meteorologists encourage involvement with the Community Collaborative Rain, Hail, and Snow Network or "CoCoRahs." Network members gather and report data on weather patterns. Taking and reporting careful measurements teaches aspects of scientific reasoning (Brossard, Lewenstein, & Bonney, 2005).

Best Practice 4: Learners benefit from understanding that science is not an established set of facts but rather involves ongoing knowledge construction. Some feel that helping audiences think about human, social, and historical processes affecting scientists confuses more than it helps. But informal science education scholars disagree. The Ontario Science Center has an exhibit, "A Question of Truth," exploring frames of reference (sun-centered vs. earth-centered) and bias as manifested in research on race and intelligence testing. Pedretti (2004) found through assessing comment cards on this exhibit by visitors that "84% of the comments were positive" (p. 146).

Best Practice 5: People learn science best in informal settings where they are active and participate, using scientific language and tools. Studies show interactive exhibits where visitors turn dials, make predictions, and compete with one another in "races" tend to attract more visitors and engage them for longer periods of time than do static exhibits (e.g., Allen, 2007; Borun, 2003). Goldowsky (2002) studied a penguin exhibit where visitors could move a light beam at the bottom of the penguin pool, and penguins would chase it. Those who used the light were more likely to reason about the penguins' motivations than those who did not (p. 141).

Best Practice 6: Informal science education should encourage people to like science and perhaps even enjoy contributing to it. For example, this best practice is instantiated in citizen science projects, which involve non-scientists in conducting research. A website, (www.citizenscience.org), identifies 50 articles published on citizen science projects such as reporting wildlife struck on highways or classifying galaxies. Citizen science networks support members in seeing themselves as individuals capable of science learning (Brossard, Lewenstein, & Bonney, 2005).

The NRC's (Bell et al., 2009) six strands or best practices may be critiqued for being interrelated. For example, finding ways to have audiences be active (Best Practice 5) seems to be encouraged as well in Best Practice 2, where learners are said to learn most when *they* generate observations and use scientific concepts to explain phenomena to one another as well as to educators. Overlaps among the best practices, however, may not be a limitation for this study. The purpose of this investigation was to learn the extent to which TV meteorologists' already established practices and outreach products were consistent with the National Academy's best practices for informal science communication and to generate new questions about the most effective ways to communicate about a slow onset hazard, climate change, in an informal science education outlet, television.

Thus, we had one research question:

RQ1: To what extent do TV meteorologists' practices, attitudes, and approaches to educating about weather and climate science align with the best practices delineated by the NRC (2009) report on best practices for informal science education?

Method

Participant Recruitment

To answer our research question, in 2009 we conducted in-depth interviews with 18 television meteorologists known to communicate climate change science. These "innovators" were identified using a snowball sampling approach, starting with several TV meteorologists known to the authors (including one of the authors, who himself was a TV meteorologist: JW), and proceeding with each person interviewed; additional suggestions were made by employees of an environmental science news service. Identification and recruitment continued until no additional "innovators" could be identified through this method. Each participant was offered $200 to participate in the study.

Of the 18 participants, 17 were from the United States and one was from Canada. Most (16) worked at local TV stations—in a range of geographic locations and media market sizes—although two worked at national channels or networks. All held a bachelor's degree, and seven also had master's degrees; 14 were men, and 4 were women.

Subsequent to the interviews being conducted, three specific criteria were specified for inclusion is this study. To qualify, weathercasters must have made clear in their interview that they: (a) educate audiences about climate science; (b) read peer-reviewed climate science; and (c) refrain from substituting peer-reviewed science with personal opinion. Of the 18 interviewed, 16 fit these criteria.

Interview Protocol

Interviews were conducted by phone, and were audio-recorded and transcribed. On average, interviews lasted approximately 75 minutes. Interviews explored motivations for explaining weather and climate science to television audiences, perceptions of what works well and what does not, and the extent to which interviewees enacted the best practices for informal science education described by NRC (Bell et al., 2009). A single experienced research interviewer—who is also an author of this study—conducted all interviews (PB). The interviewer was trained to use the interview protocol by conducting two practice interviews with a meteorologist and a climate scientist, receiving feedback from the first author.

Data Treatment and Qualitative Analysis

The transcripts were rendered "blind" so that coders were unable to determine the participant's name or geographic region. Three teams of coders (seven individuals) read and analyzed the data. Each team focused on differing aspects of the interviews and used different approaches to coding. This report is guided by both sets of findings of those coding teams, whose focus was on the extent to which TV meteorologists' practices matched the National Academy's evidence-based best practices for informal science education. That is, we used a theory-guided version of the constant comparison method for qualitative coding (Creswell & Clark, 2007). It involved reading and re-reading both the transcripts and the coding team's analyses to identify attitudes, approaches, or steps participants discussed when thinking about the best practices. The steps, attitudes, and message strategies reported are used by TV meteorologists in a wide range of media including community presentations, talks to school children, blogs, websites, and on-air reporting.

Results and Discussion

The 16 innovator TV meteorologists who educate their audiences about climate change do so in a variety of ways. Since they work on television, one might assume their outreach concerning climate change occurs mainly for their on-air audiences, but, consistent with Wilson's findings (2009), they are more likely to teach about climate change during invited presentations to schools and community groups and through websites and blogs. Here are their reported educational steps followed by analysis and further questions this analysis suggests.

Best Practice 1: Engaging Audiences' Emotions and Interests

Innovator meteorologists reported at least three ways they engage children and adults emotionally when sharing weather and climate science (Table 7.1). One approach involves *using visual aids and props to intrigue and entertain* audiences. Participant 1 brings a radiosonde, a set of weather instruments connected to a helium- or hydrogen-filled balloon, to his school presentations. Radiosondes are sent up to measure temperature, pressure, and humidity and send data back for analysis (NOAA, n.d.). As he notes, "Kids like balloons, and then they see this giant weather balloon. They get pretty excited about that. . . .There's that slim chance . . . a child could find one, [so he tells children] pay close attention because one of these might land in your front yard" (156–166).

Participant 11 uses props to engage adults emotionally as he explains the science of climate change: "For one of the talks I actually took out a loaf of bread and started eating a slice of bread. (Imitates having a mouth full of food) '. . . just eating this slice. Sorry, I know this is rude eating in front of you, but . . .'" (4116–4120). Poking fun at himself is also a tactic for explaining the greenhouse effect and climate change in a vivid, memorable way. That is, the Earth is like a greenhouse because radiation

129

Table 7.1 Best Practice 1 Summary Table: Engaging Audiences' Emotions and Interests

Approach	Example
Uses visual aids and props to intrigue audiences	Demonstrates using real scientific instruments (Participant 1)
Connects weather and climate to personal and professional ambitions	• Asks audience about interest in weather and climate • Encourages seeking peer-reviewed sources (Participant 13)
Avoids polarized statements	• Presents observations and collected data • Less focus on future projections and predictions (Participant 16)

from the sun passes through the atmosphere, heating the planet. This radiation bounces back from the Earth into space, but some of it is blocked by heat-trapping gasses, like carbon dioxide, which function like the glass roof of a greenhouse. This capturing of heat-trapping gasses helps the Earth to have an atmosphere. But *excess* carbon dioxide, somewhat like crust on bread or an extra blanket on a sleeper, captures *extra* heat, increasing Earth's temperature. As Participant 11 explained: "You can't just go up there and . . . give a lecture unless you're in [a] collegiate educational setting where that would be appropriate. . . . [I use] nonverbal cues [such as chomping on bread] to make sure that they're responding. I'm asking questions, seeing how [they are] getting what [I'm] saying" (4817–4859).

A second way several TV meteorologists engage audiences in weather and climate is by *connecting the study of weather and climate to personal and professional ambitions held by their audience*. For example, Participant 13, who often speaks to school groups, says:

At the beginning of the presentation I ask, "Does anybody want to be a scientist? Does anybody want to talk about the weather? Do you want to be in meteorology?" Maybe a few of the kids hold up their hands. [Then I say], "Does anybody want to be on TV?" And everybody raises their hand because everybody wants to be on TV for some reason. So I say, "What we're going to talk about today . . . [is] how to be a meteorologist and how to be on TV." And so those two things are very closely related because you have to know something to be on TV, you've got to have some information of some sort to share with people.

(4886–4899)

130

Participant 13 also said that "people are very eager to ask extreme questions that I maybe don't have the answers to, and I always encourage people, I say, 'Look up peer-reviewed science. Look up what kind of new studies are coming out.' Because if you can get your hands on the latest information that's coming out from the researchers, you'll be way ahead of even what they're talking about on television" (P13, 4945–4949). Her approach is an interesting way of both legitimizing an audience's engagement in asking "stump the expert" sorts of questions, but also using that tendency to *motivate* audiences to learn peer-reviewed science.

A third way innovators manage emotions is by *avoiding polarizing statements*. Often, they begin their discussions by focusing on *observable*, not future, phenomena or by reporting science, not politics. Other times they discuss environmental policy, but do so in a positive way rather than assigning blame. For example, Participant 16 describes his region's steps to reduce heat-trapping emissions as an approach to educating about climate change:

> I think talking about our air quality on a fairly regular basis and really showing people that air quality has improved on a regular basis simply because of regulation, which a lot of people don't want to hear, but showing that literally we have reduced the amount of emissions by more than half since the '80s, for example, just purely based on how we make our cars.
>
> (5956–5962)

As Wilson (2009) reported, some participants prefer to discuss climate science in community or school presentations; that is, in face-to-face settings rather than on air because face-to-face settings are contexts where they are invited to speak. In such a context, there is less likelihood of personal attacks or heightened emotions that could harm the chances of learning.

Further questions. The NRC (Bell et al., 2009) consensus report says learners need sufficient emotional engagement to want to learn science in informal settings but not so much stimulation that they feel overwhelmed. To engage their audiences, interviewees use visually intriguing props, appeals to audiences' interests and goals, and avoidance of polarizing statements. These tactics may have successfully assisted in providing sufficient, but not excessive, emotional engagement in why the climate is changing. Their use suggests that health and risk educators communicating slow onset hazards should explore:

What are the emotional conditions that encourage or discourage interest in slow onset health and risk hazards?

Best Practice 2: Explaining Key Science Concepts

NRC (Bell et al., 2009) does not offer a taxonomy of the types of scientific explanations learners generate in informal settings. To supplement that portion of NRC (Bell et al., 2009), we drew from Rowan's theory of explanatory discourse (1988, 1990, 1999, 2003), which identifies three classic sources of confusion in learning complex subjects and evidence-based steps for addressing each. Although we were unable to examine *audiences'* abilities to generate scientific concepts and information, we wondered whether TV meteorologists used steps similar to the approaches identified in research on explaining. Steps for addressing each difficulty are tailored to overcoming each type of confusion and are listed in Table 7.2's second row. Interestingly, as Table 7.2's third row illustrates, some innovator TV meteorologists discussed each confusion source but address

Table 7.2 Best Practice 2 Summary Table: Explaining Key Terms, Structures, Processes

Sources of Confusion	Confusing Key Terms	Hard-to-Envision Structures or Processes	Counterintuitive Ideas
Evidence-Based Explanatory Practices	Offers examples that do and do not illustrate phenomenon: e.g., compares what counts as weather (short term) with what counts as climate (long term)	Enhances visualization and links new information to established knowledge with diagrams, analogies, previews	First, acknowledges apparent reasonableness of erroneous lay view; then notes familiar experiences inconsistent with erroneous view. Then presents established science showing how it better explains experiences.
Examples of Innovator TV Meteorologists' Explanatory Approaches	Offers analogy for weather versus climate: single football play not the same as entire season performance (Participant 1)	Uses prop for illustrating high and low pressure (Participant 11)	Encourages audiences to document with photos changes they observe in animals' migrations (Participant 7)

these confusions with a range of tactics, sometimes tapping evidence-based approaches and sometimes using alternative approaches.

Distinguishing related concepts. Participants offered several tactics for helping audiences "break apart" related notions such as climate versus weather or event versus trend. Here is Participant 1's approach to teaching audiences the climate versus weather and trend versus event distinctions:

> P: [It's] actually not a difficult stretch to go from weather to cli-mate. Well, weather first being a short-term, fast-changing, then climate of course being much longer term. . . . I'll use [a football] analogy. . . . Weather is to climate as one play in a football game [is] to the entire season for all the teams. [You] can't decide that . . . this weather event means that we're having global warming, or it's because of global warming that this tornado occurred. That's absolutely not correct.
>
> (221–229)

Continuing his analogy, and reinforcing the distinction between a trend and a single event and the sorts of conclusions one can draw from single events as opposed to trends, Participant 1 says:

> P1: But . . . just because the greatest player in the league struck out doesn't mean, or threw an interception, doesn't mean they're not the greatest player in the league over the long term. And that's the way you kind of have to look at it, because it's too often that people would say, "Well how's it climate change, it was 10 below zero this morning, it can't be global warming."
>
> (231–234)

Using visualization to help audiences build simple mental models of complex structures or processes. Frequently, scientific accounts of complicated structures and processes are difficult to understand because their many parts or steps overwhelm the audience. If there are too many steps or processes, learners cannot find a simple way to visualize these phenomena, just as one might find a photograph of an anatomical part hard to understand and wish to locate instead a simplified diagram (Mayer, Bove, Bryman, Mars, & Tapangco, 1996; Rowan 1988, 2003). Several TV meteorologists recognized this challenge and described steps to assist visualization when they educate about climate change. For example, Participant 11 says:

> P11: So I developed this technique to use one of the props . . . which is a kids' squishy ball. . . . . I use [that] to represent the bulging ridges of high pressure.
>
> (4110–4112)

133

Participant 11 makes an unfamiliar phenomenon—bulging ridges of high pressure in the atmosphere—familiar by squeezing a child's toy ball and noting that the bulge created when the ball is squeezed is similar to what is occurring in the atmosphere with increasing levels of heat-trapping gasses.

Countering erroneous notions. Two techniques were used to counter erroneous notions. Some participants use visualization techniques to counter erroneous notions or unscientifically supported lay views. For example, Participant 5 discussed using a graphic to explain why, in spite of local weather variation (e.g., cool in some spots, hotter in others around the globe), there can still be an overall trend of global warming:

> P5, T22: On television . . . you have very limited time. And you can't go into detail on anything. But what we can do in a picture is worth a thousand words. So when, for instance, like last month, we at National Climate Data Center released the global temperature anomalies for the whole planet in June, July, and August. The oceans were the warmest on record. And they produced a great graphic that showed that with dots . . . the bigger the red dot on the map, the more the temperature was above normal.

> P5, T23: And most of the Midwest had a very cool summer this year, so even in [our state] I'd get [people saying], "We had a cool summer. What happened to global warming?" So I put that map up there on air and said, "Okay, now look at this. If you think it's been a cool summer, if you live in the Midwest in Denver or say North Dakota, it has been a cool summer, but look at the rest of the world. This is the temperatures for June, July, and August across the entire rest of the world, and it was way above average."

An important aspect of visualization techniques such as props, analogies, and graphics is that they function as "bridges" (Ausubel, 1978). That is, they link familiar, concrete, and tangible ideas to less familiar ones, rendering the newly introduced and less-familiar information more accessible and plausible. Photographs of glaciers shrinking over time (i.e., comparing glacier size near the beginning and the end of the 20th century) may function both as intellectual bridges and as compelling exemplars. Participant 5 reported his use of such photos:

> P5, T32: There are still a lot of people who don't even believe the planet is warming. I mean, I mean a lot of people. Of the people that are really skeptical on climate science, I'd say 60, 70% of them don't even think the planet's getting any warmer. And so what I have shown . . . is that USGS has an incredible array of

photos—based on before and after—taken from the same spot of glaciers around the planet. And I will throw those on at the end of a weathercast or put them up on my blog.

Participant 5 is also taking steps to render his explanations accessible by placing them in a variety of media. He discusses US Geological Survey before-and-after photos on the air, on his blog, in slides that are accessible through his website, and in presentations.

Several TV meteorologists reported countering erroneous notions by showcasing data from the past and emphasizing its status as *already occurring phenomena* rather than events predicted for the future. For example, Participant 6 said:

> P6, T50: [One] of the things that I talk about in the blog [is that] this [change in precipitation patterns from gentle rains that benefit crops to droughts and extreme downpours that do not] is not a computer projection. *This is based on observation* [italics inserted]. This was collected from the Global Precipitation Climatology Project. And it is covering a period of time from 1979 to 2007.

Similarly, Participant 7 encourages viewers to send her photos documenting environmental changes they have observed in their lifetimes, such as animals washing up on beaches in recent years that viewers do not recall seeing in their childhoods in the same locations, or photos of sea ice and glaciers that were considerably larger in their youth than in their adulthood. She incorporates these photos into slide shows that she shares at community presentations.

Further questions. Innovator TV meteorologists reported awareness of each difficulty noted in Rowan's (1999, 2003) taxonomy and offered intriguing steps for addressing them. For the most part, their steps were informed by intuition and experience rather than formal training. Some tactics such as analogies and visuals may be especially effective because they report using them frequently. It would be interesting to see if these innovators could be even more effective with exposure to brief educational materials alerting them to research on steps they already take and on other techniques backed by research but not used by the innovators. Further, the NRC best practices emphasize the value of learners *explaining science to one another*, not solely having experts handle all explaining. This peer-to-peer explaining occurs in museum settings, classrooms, and online interaction. Questions for further work are:

Would formal training in explanatory strategy assist health and risk educators in explaining the complexities of slow onset hazards to lay stakeholders?

135

What social conditions support learners in explaining com-
plexities of slow onset health and risk hazards to one another in
face-to-face interaction or online?

Best Practice 3: Encouraging Audiences to Learn
Scientific Methods and Reasoning

Best Practice 3 encourages informal educators to help audiences learn not just scientific results, but also the scientific *methods* that lead to results. In this study, innovator TV meteorologists were asked whether they helped audiences think about the scientific method, evidence, hypotheses, and how scientists test an idea in any context, but particularly in the context of climate change science.

Answers to this question were mixed (Table 7.3). Some said they do *not* cover the scientific method in presentations for schools or community and professional groups. For example, Participant 2 said, "When I talk about the climate models, I'll explain, for example, how the scientist tries to design these computer models that predict climate. I think that there are parts of the discussion that probably do discuss the scientific method, but I don't give the presentation with the goal of demonstrating the scientific method, if that makes sense" (49–54). Others said they do not help audiences to think about the scientific method, but were intrigued with the idea of doing so. Said Participant 7: "No, but I'm interested in being a better weathercaster, so maybe I should."

Those participants who said they *do* teach the scientific method take one of two approaches. Either they said that this step is essential, or they said

Table 7.3 Best Practice 3 Summary Table: Encouraging Audiences to Learn Scientific Methods and Reasoning

Approach	Example
Explains method and evidence that leads to the statement that humanly produced heat-trapping gasses are making the planet warmer	Shows audience climate models based on simulations and compares them with models based on observed data to illustrate that, but for humanly produced heat trapping gasses, the last 30 years would have been colder (Participant 15)
Describes scientific reasoning in a given case and provides ways for audiences to participate in asking questions about method and evidence	Explains certainty versus uncertainty (Participant 4) Encourages asking questions and researching answers (Participant 13)

that teaching aspects of the scientific method is not their principal goal, but likely an indirect effect of their presentations, discussions, or materials. Table 7.3 illustrates their approaches to teaching audiences about the scientific method. In the first group was Participant 5. Describing his websites for teachers and students, as well as his presentations, he said:

> I start with what science is, and what a theory is and what the definition of science is. I also run through things so they know . . . what isn't science, and what is science. And questions that science can answer. And I talk about, you know, religion is not a question that science can answer, because that's based on a belief system and science is based on *testable evidence* [italics added]. And I also point out to them that just because science can't answer it doesn't mean something's not true. It just means it's not science.
>
> (133–148)

Similarly, Participant 9 said: "That's one of the key things that I talk about. . . . If I talk about how scientists do their job, . . . I'll usually say, 'Okay, what's the first thing that you do? And we sort of guide them through things that they do that are basically showing that they're applying the scientific methods themselves, they just don't recognize it" (408–415).

In the second group were innovators who illustrated ways in which they demonstrate scientific reasoning that underlies weather forecasting or supports an anthropogenic explanation for climate change in the current era. Said Participant 4: "I definitely touched on it as well as the issue of certainty and uncertainty, which is what we call probability in our daily forecast. That what's happening has high certainty, but it doesn't have 100% certainty" (123–127). Another, Participant 13, illustrated her teaching technique, which involves prompting elementary school students to reason as scientists: "For example, [I ask students], 'What do you think happens with the sun? How does that work? Does it really heat the earth? Or does it heat the air?' I mean I try to give them an opportunity to come up with their own guess, and then I don't just give them the answer right away. I say, 'Here's some evidence, let's think about it. Now let's, let's say what do you think the answer's going to be?'" (469–473). Additionally, she explains the reasoning underlying her forecasts:

> We don't just come up with a conclusion of what it's going to be like by hitting the dart board, or stealing the forecast from NASA weather services. We come up with our own work every day. And the way we do that is, we sit down with a piece of paper, and we draw out what the week is going to be, what highs and low we think we're going to have, and we base this on the

computer models and the satellite and radar imagery. . . . So, I do go through some sort of . . . conceptualization of how that works without really saying, hey this is science, and here's the hypothesis, and here's the conclusion.

(488–498)

Participant 15 noted that when an audience member objected that, in prior decades, scientists have said there is evidence of global cooling, not warming, he showed slides comparing and contrasting simulated climate models with models based on observed data. He showed one audience that these models match well, until they remove increased carbon dioxide in the simulation. When that step is taken, one sees that the last 30 years should have been cooler than they have been, he said. Participant 15 emphasized that the models were not the work of a few individuals, but rather "a whole bunch of different simulations. It isn't one person's idea; I said this is an average of a whole bunch of models for differing simulations. They've all converged to this idea. . . . And they [the audience] got fairly quiet. I didn't have a lot of people saying, this is a bunch of hooey. . . . I think I convinced them. . . . I had stuff. I had pictures with me on my person to show them that I'd given this some thought" (560–596).

Perhaps this response is one of the clearest instances where an innovator reported a step-by-step argument, describing evidence for the claim that climate change is associated with increased heat-trapping gasses in the atmosphere. This participant reminded his audience that there were *not* just a few people making this argument, that instead there were multiple models converging on the same conclusion, and that conclusion led to the claim that increased levels of heat-trapping gasses being emitted by human activities is the best explanation for why global temperatures have risen at an alarming rate over the last century.

Further questions. Many of the innovators were either emotionally supportive of or already taking steps to involve their audiences in the reasoning and methods underlying scientific findings. Their apparent success with explaining scientific methods and connections between evidence and claims suggests these steps may be helpful in many contexts where audiences choose to learn science. Further questions for research raised by their responses are:

In what contexts are people most interested in learning scientific reasoning and methods?

How might experiences using scientific tools affect emotional engagement with and understanding of slow onset hazards such as climate change?

Best Practice 4: Helping Audiences See Scientists and Scientific Institutions as Fallible

According to NRC's (Bell et al., 2009) fourth best practice, informal contexts are most apt to encourage science learning if science is *not* presented as coming from an infallible source, but instead as a *human, fallible, and social process*. This means that presentation of scientists as people with flaws and strengths is helpful to science in the long run, and that lay audiences benefit from learning about processes for adjudication of claims in science, such as peer review.

Perhaps because of the challenges associated with communicating about a politicized science topic, innovators interviewed for this study responded in several ways to the question of whether they communicate the fallibility of science and the mechanisms for managing error. As summarized in Table 7.4, there were some who discussed how they encourage disagreement as people learn about any scientific topic. Others talked about their concerns regarding the scientific credentials of some of their fellow TV weathercasters. Still others discussed their approaches to climate change skeptics who are informed by advocacy groups, but not informed by peer-reviewed research.

Some participants explained that they explicitly teach audiences about peer review and its importance to scientific progress. Participant 5's website, designed for teachers and students in the English-speaking world, says, "Peer review is how scientists argue," (153) and this sentence is followed by a brief explanation of the essential role peer review plays in science. Similarly, Participant 1's endorsement of encouraging disagreement

Table 7.4 Best Practice 4 Summary Table: Portraying Scientists and Scientific Institutions as Fallible

Approach	*Example*
Explains peer review	Describes healthy discussion and disagreements among scientists that lead to deeper thinking and more detailed findings and conclusions (Participant 1)
Discusses internal professional debate related to credentials needed for meteorology	Explains that not all TV meteorologists have scientific degrees but have other qualifications (Participant 8)
Illustrates an approach for addressing advocacy groups who deny global warming is occurring	Draws comparisons to similar issues such as the ways in which uncertainty was exaggerated in early days of controversy over risks associated with smoking (Participant 2)

is emphatic and consistent with ethical theories of communication such as that of Habermas (Burleson & Kline, 1979). Habermas argues that ethical communication occurs when social conditions allow only the "force of the better argument" to be a consideration in deciding the merits of a claim, not concerns about power or consequences. Asked, "But do you address the fact that even within the field that there can be discussion and differing opinions, and that that's a healthy part of the process," Participant 1 said, " Oh, yeah, absolutely. It's very healthy. There's nothing wrong with people being skeptical about things because hopefully that makes you think deeper and not be so convinced, oh, I'm absolutely right, I don't need do anything anymore" (14–18).

Participant 5 also comments on the usefulness of peer review in settling scientific disputes. He says, "In science . . . one of the good aspects of peer review, is once something is settled, then you just can't keep bringing that question up over and over. If you want to get your paper published, you need to provide something new. If you just say, 'No, I still am right,' your paper is not going to get published" (143–153).

Still others commented on the joy of science being the process of disagreeing and discovery. Participant 6 said: "Science is not just a monolithic thing, it's very dynamic. That's one of the things that I think that scientists enjoy. It's like detective work. They enjoy exploring and finding the truth, and they will debate you to the nth degree if they think they're right. But it always comes back to the facts. What is debated is not the facts, but the interpretation of those facts" (164–169).

A few respondents discussed an internal professional debate on credentials for TV weathercasters. There are science-based programs throughout the world where students study meteorology and can be certified as meteorologists. However, television companies will also hire some individuals who obtain a bachelor of arts or an associate of arts, rather than someone with a grounding in science. Participant 8 commented on this situation saying: "[These individuals] don't have the true degree in science. It's not a bachelor in science. It's a bachelor in arts. Or it's an AA or it's simply a certificate that allows them to communicate weather information, and the AMS [American Meteorological Society] decided years ago to recognize this group, that doesn't have the physics- and calculus-based true bachelor in science degree" (312–315). He continued: "I understand if the morning weather anchor in [city] is going to be a pretty girl who wears tight sweaters, because it's the reality of what TV is, okay?" (348–350).

This debate over who should be a TV meteorologist is an important part of the conditions outlined in Best Practice 4. This best practice says that audiences should learn about the flaws and strengths of the people who do science as well as the flaws and strengths of social institutions like the AMS. Encouraging public discussion of a professional debate of this sort is not easy, but in the long run, according to NRC (Bell et al., 2009),

140

airing of such matters is apt to enhance stakeholders' abilities to learn from science and to trust scientists because it casts scientists as people with both strengths and limitations.

A third way interviewees responded to this question about discussing the fallibility of scientists and scientific institutions was to illustrate ways they manage advocacy groups who insist that global warming is not occurring or is occurring but is not caused by humans increasing the amount of heat-trapping gas pumped into the atmosphere. Participant 2 said:

> There are some very prominent [groups] in expressing those opinions and putting their opinion out to the public. They are very well-funded. That's why there's still some confusion among the public. . . . If you go back fifty years or so when the very first medical studies came out that cigarette smoking made you predisposed to a number of health risks and conditions, when those first studies came out, there were doctors that said "No, that can't be."
> (45–53)

Further on, Participant 2 said:

> So in the same way that there was a social aspect of the smoking issue with society, it's kind of the same thing with this issue, in that people talk about if you're going to do something about global warming there's going to be ramifications. Now I don't get into so much of the policy ramifications [in my community talks and talks with professional groups], I only talk about the science of global warming, but inevitably someone will ask a question, and you know I'll have to talk about it, but I don't go with the goal of talking about policy, so maybe there is a social [and] economic component to this, but the analogy is to the cigarette smoking issue (70–75). . . . I don't always agree with the policy recommendations, but I don't get into that in my talks.
> (98–99)

Participant 2's view was that some of the skepticism about climate change is a function of funded efforts to generate such skepticism. This sort of skepticism may differ from the questions and disagreements scientists and others thinking about the science of climate change might express when trying to make sense of the extent to which studies support scientific claims.

Participant 2's comments on advocacy groups that promote skepticism about climate change science are consistent with the comments of other innovators interviewed for this study. They discussed the importance of helping audiences reflect on the differences between facts and opinions as well as between science and policy, and on reasons to take the science of climate change seriously, while still acknowledging uncertainty in its findings. For example, Participant 10 said:

> The interesting thing is that, some of the preeminent scientists who were first looking at this . . . pronounced [that this] warming would take place at higher latitudes. And indeed, that's what's being observed. So the, even with the uncertainty, the observations of what appears to be taking place with the climate system, which is not just the air, it's the land, it's soil moisture, it's the oceans, . . . [are consistent with the predictions].
>
> (5415–5420)

Further questions. The notion of explaining the fallibility of science was daunting to some of the innovators. Some felt it best to stay focused on facts and not discuss ways the science of climate change might be wrong or its proponents might be individuals with human frailties. But others clearly accepted and even relished this task, saying that laypersons needed to understand that scientific argument among scientists is a healthy thing, an inherent part of good science. They also thought laypersons needed to understand the essential role peer review plays in adjudicating disagreements among scientists. Further questions suggested by the innovators' responses are:

> *Is learning about specific climate scientists as individuals, their life stories, failures, and triumphs, associated with deeper understanding of climate science?*
>
> *How does learning about scientific failures in the study of slow onset hazards such as sedentary lifestyles, nutrition, obesity, and climate science affect understanding of these hazards? How does it affect attitudes and behaviors associated with them?*

Best Practice 5: Support Audiences in Being Active as They Learn Science

Participants reported two ways in which they created conditions for audiences to be active, not solely listeners or readers, when learning weather and climate science. As illustrated in Table 7.5, the first approach involved welcoming and encouraging communication about weather and climate from audiences. Several participants said that the simplest of steps, beginning a talk with students or an adult group with a question about the day's weather, typically yielded response. For example, Participant 3 said, "When I walk in, especially with kids, I'll say, 'What's the weather like outside?'" (75–76). Participant 6 encourages comments and questions

Table 7.5 Best Practice 5 Summary Table: Inviting Audiences to Be Active as They Learn Science

Approach	Example
Welcomes and encourages communication about weather and climate from audience	Asks audience to comment on weather and weather forecasts based on their observations (Participant 6)
Creates or shares resources for activities involving data collecting and reporting	Encourage audience to join groups that collect and report data (i.e., CoCoRahs) (Participant 5)

about items he posts on his website. He said: "Look. Don't worry about whether you're wrong or not. Go ahead and respond. Because it's the only way I know what you perceive to be the truth, and I can't correct that thinking if I don't know what it is. So I'm encouraging people to comment [on materials posted to his site], and they do think that they know a lot about the science" (218–222).

The second approach involves creating activities for data gathering and reporting. Several interviewees noted the popular program, "CoCoRahs," [Community Cooperative Rain, Hail, and Snow Network], where volunteer weather observers measure rain and hail near their homes, sending their data to scientific organizations and local television stations. Participant 5 said, "Any time an adult or a kid or a teacher says, 'What can I do to get my kids interested,' . . . I say, 'I can get you a great project for twenty-nine bucks. Go get a CoCoRahs gauge, put it out there . . . and it's real science because that data is really helpful. It'll be collected for a hundred years, and we've got several students using it now, and several classes using it" (137–141).

Participant 9 noted that his station has dozens of schools participating in weather watching activities: "We started out in [year], with 10 different school-based weather observation sites. And I think we're up to probably close to 160 right now" (292–293). Participant 18 focuses on collecting weather emergency information: "I'm a great advocate of Sky Warn. . . . We will encourage students and parents and families to become Sky Warn trained and to provide weather" (485–487). Participant 13 discusses a weather watching program and activities he created:

We have a Weather Watcher program which they can email us . . . pictures. They can email us their storm report. . . . I created on [name].com a series of experiments for kids, basically making a thermometer from recycled materials, making a wind gauge, you know that kind of stuff. . . . I've also designed two weather activity books for kids. One's a basic weather activity book and the other is how science and baseball are related.

(379–380)

These participants seem aware of the way hands-on learning engages audiences in science, and in the case of Participant 18 especially, makes them more alert to weather emergencies. They also see the marketing potential for television stations: involving dozens of schools in reporting weather data to a station is one way to enhance station visibility.

Some use activities to teach aspects of climatic change, such as documenting the times when flowers bud or birds arrive, and whether those times are changing. Participant 9 says: "Oh, what they call phenology, and that sort of thing. . . . And very often I'll make that part of a . . . Weather Minds question because it's just one of those nice teachable moments" (317–323). By "Weather Minds" he means an opening segment for his on-air weather report where he fields viewer-sent questions about, for example, why avalanches are occurring, whether trees are budding earlier, or other topics that teach viewers about regional weather and climate conditions, especially conditions relevant to outdoor recreation.

Further questions. Innovators were almost uniform in their support for finding ways for learners to be active by asking questions, using instruments, or becoming citizen scientists. Their intuitions and experience supported the benefits of having audiences be active, rather than solely listening, as they learn about a slow onset hazard. Their responses lead to the following questions:

Are some forms of active involvement in learning about a slow onset hazard more emotionally engaging and more likely to deepen scientific understanding than others? That is, do people gain more from asking questions, using scientific tools, observing phenomena in the field, or coding data?

When active involvement involves asking questions, drawing inferences, and peer-to-peer explanations of science—rather than using scientific tools or coding data along with scientists—to what extent do such experiences deepen understanding and affect attitudes about slow onset hazards?

Best Practice 6: Encourage Audiences to See Themselves as Scientists

Best Practice 6 involves encouraging audiences to see themselves as people who like and can contribute to science. As illustrated in Table 7.6, several participants encourage such identification and feel gratified when audience members report feeling that they identify with the TV meteorologist or take pride in their (the audience member's) ability to learn science.

Consider, for example, Participant 13's response when asked, "Do you think it [your action] encourages them, those individuals to see themselves as scientists?"

> I hope so. I mean sometimes when the kids write back, you know they'll say, I know what a front is. I think that that once kids have . . . a direct connection to somebody in some field, they think they feel a lot more a part of it. Definitely adults talk about it, if they've met you and . . . they have had an intimate time with you to talk about something. All of a sudden they know exactly what you know.
>
> (560–570)

Similarly, Participant 4 and Participant 16 report that they believe everyone is a bit of a scientist.

> [P4]: I get a lot of people who say that they always had some sort of interest in science, but either the math got in the way, or life got in the way, or something happened where they just didn't pursue it, so I'm thinking there's a little scientist in everybody.
>
> (126–129)

Table 7.6 Best Practice 6 Summary Table: Encouraging Audiences to See Themselves as Scientists

Approach	*Example*
Encourages audiences to identify as people who like science and who can contribute to science	• Connects face-to-face with people through community outreach activities involving science (Participant 13) • Notes high number of citizen scientists contributing to astronomy and meteorology (Participant 5)
Celebrates or recognizes audience contributions to science	Recognizes individuals who send in observations, data, comments, and questions on air (Participant 5)
Helps audience learn how to be a scientist or do science	• Encourages citizen science and sharing resources in website or blog posts (Participant 5) • Encourages studying math so one can succeed in a scientific career (Participant 1)

[P16]: Oh sure. Especially when we talk about the need to have a thermometer, rain gauge of your own. That's exactly what I'm trying to send across the message that anyone can be—and is—a scientist. And if you're ever curious about anything, then you're already asking the right questions, and you're already going in trying to prove [your] own thoughts and theories.

(643–652)

Being scientific is generally viewed as a sophisticated state, a role in which one can take pride. Research shows that people value friends for their provision of ego and emotional support (Burleson, 2003), and if a TV meteorologist such as those interviewed in this study encourages an audience to take pride in their inherent curiosity and enjoyment of learning science, and treats them as friends, worthy of one-on-one, respectful interaction, that experience may lead to the audience feeling proud of themselves and motivated to learn science.

A second way in which innovators encourage identification with science, weather observation, and sometimes climate science is by celebrating or recognizing scientific contributions and accomplishments by audience members. For example, several interviewees discussed programs that involve schools, sometimes hundreds of schools, in sending observational data (measurements of temperature, rainfall at the schools' locations) to the television station. Those contributing data to the television station are recognized on the air. Their school names may be listed in the crawl text that runs during weather reports. Another innovator gives school science fair winners recognition from the American Meteorological Association and rewards high school valedictorians with gifts of sophisticated calculators. A third recognizes and respects viewers by engaging them in what he terms "intelligent conversation" through a blog that reports peer-reviewed science with regional implications. He said:

[P5]: They love the fact that I will engage them in the conversation [when they comment on his blog and he responds]. Now, part of it may be the fact that I'm on TV. But if you look at the comments closely, you're going to see that the sense I get from the comments is, they're hungry for a conversation. They're hungry for an intelligent conversation. They're not hungry for a lot of the positioning that's taking place.

(215–219)

A third way in which TV meteorologists encourage identification with science is to help audience members learn steps for becoming a scientist or doing science. This tactic, known as enhancing a person's sense of efficacy, or perceived ability to do a task, is important because when people feel efficacious, they are more apt to address problems (e.g., Bandura, 1986; Witte, 1992). Some TV meteorologists explicitly encourage viewers to believe in their ability to do science. Says Participant 5:

> You can do science yourself. You don't have to be in a lab coat and have a PhD to do science. I did a blog awhile about how astronomy and meteorology are the two greatest sciences with the highest number of citizen scientists involved.
>
> (153–158)

Participant 1 tells school children:

> If you want to be the type of meteorologist that would fly into the eye of a hurricane or chase tornados or go to the South Pole . . . it's really important that you have to be studying your science and your math. And even at the second grade level, they get this. If you're not very good at it, work with your teachers to get better.
>
> (11–14)

In summary, a number of TV meteorologist innovators who share climate science sense that their audiences like science and like learning, but feel somewhat intimidated by science. They address these feelings by providing emotional support and advice, with some explicitly encouraging audiences to recognize their inherent curiosity as a scientific trait and to get involved in scientific activities such as measuring rain fall and reading blogs that summarize peer-reviewed climate science. They also encourage audience members to study math in school and get involved in citizen science activities outside of school or work.

Further questions. The innovators generally like the idea of encouraging audiences to notice that they (the audiences) enjoy learning scientific information and processes and may think like scientists in some contexts. Several use this approach in their educational efforts to encourage mathematical skills and love of learning, assets important for professional success in science and other fields. Their responses suggest these questions for further research:

> *Under what social and educational conditions do people come to view themselves as individuals who enjoy science and would enjoy contributing to science?*

> *Does enjoyment of science and viewing oneself as someone who likes science, across their lifetime, lead to understanding of slow onset hazards reported in traditional media?*

147

Summary: What Did We Learn From Innovator TV Meteorologists?

From in-depth, theory-guided interviews with TV meteorologists already educating audiences about climate change in 2009, we learned—to a greater or lesser degree—these innovators are embracing the NRC best practices, or are open to embracing them, although few are currently using all of them. This offers some face validity to the findings of the NRC report, and it suggests that these innovators' climate education efforts are likely having a positive impact (though their efforts are almost certainly informed more by their intuition, their willingness to take risks, and trial and error, than through any formal training).

Beyond the questions generated by responses to specific best practices, the NRC (Bell et al., 2009) framework as a whole may be helpful for addressing slow onset hazards. That is, risk perception and risk communication research indicates that adults feel ambivalent about being educated on health and environmental risks. On the one hand, as Douglas and Wildavsky (1983) argue, society itself is organized to protect people from dangers such as wild animals, enemy combatants, starvation, and so forth. On the other hand, research in interpersonal communication shows that adults do not like unsolicited advice (e.g., MacGeorge, Feng, & Thompson, 2008). Therefore, those who educate about slow onset hazards, even when there are compelling reasons to do so, need to communicate carefully.

The best practice framework places considerable emphasis on getting audiences to *think with* an educator, not simply listen and accept. Interviewees' responses to questions about whether they discuss the scientific method and whether they discuss the fallibility of science were particularly illuminating. A number of interviewees embrace these ideas. That is, several reported that they do teach the scientific method to their audiences (i.e., Best Practice 3) by encouraging observation of changes in animals' migration patterns or shrinking glaciers and by encouraging audiences to make observations or use scientific instruments like rain gauges.

Not all participants are comfortable inviting audiences to think about the fallibility of science, particularly when educating about a politicized topic like climate change, but several embrace this ethic. Recall Participant 5, whose website, designed for teachers and students in the English-speaking world, says, "Peer review is how scientists argue," (153), and several other participants who said disagreement is healthy and essential in science. Why might such a stance contribute to the effectiveness of a slow onset hazard communicator? Although it makes that educator's job difficult in some ways, it also invites the audience to see scientists as people like them, not infallible entities to be resented, but professionals worried about problems and trying to find ways to address them. Clearly, there are contexts when debating climate science with climate science deniers is a futile exercise, but recall that 70% of Americans say global warming is occurring, but many are unsure about why (Leiserowitz et al., 2012, 2016). This suggests that most audience members are not deniers, but are also not especially informed or emotionally engaged with this topic. These conditions indicate that education about the fallibility of science and about methods for adjudicating claims in science may, over time, be a way of educating and engaging audiences in how climate change matters in their region.

Finding ways for audiences to be active makes learning enjoyable. The new media environment increasingly shows that people enjoy being message senders as well as receivers, and they like environments where they are active in some way, whether the activity involves blogging, functioning as a citizen scientist, or taking a nature hike to study coastal plants and erosion. Best Practice 6, which encourages people to see themselves as individuals who like science, is a welcoming and flattering message strategy. Rather than setting up an "us versus them" context for learning about a hazard or insisting that only scientists know what counts as a danger, it invites audiences to learn more because they are scientist-like themselves. As Participant 5, says, "You can do science yourself. You don't have to be in a lab coat and have a PhD to do science." Interestingly, Kahan (2015) maintains that an adversarial context can be created simply by uttering words such as "climate change" or "vaccination." For some, these words signal that people with an interest in such topics have little interest in *their* group's needs and values. Encouraging people to become involved in community-relevant scientific concerns and the joy of scientific activities may help to de-politicize controversial science topics.

Linking This Study of the Innovators With Current Findings

In the few years since these interviews were conducted, there has been a significant shift in the views of TV meteorologists about climate change (Maibach et al., in press) and a marked increase in the number of TV weathercasters who are embracing the role of local climate educator (Maibach et al., 2016). This has occurred in part by building on the insights offered by these innovators, in part by leveraging their positive role modeling, and in part through systematic efforts of universities, government agencies (i.e., NASA and NOAA), AMS, and nonprofit organization Climate Central to make it easier for weathercasters to embrace this role through the provision of timely, localized information and broadcast-ready graphics (Placky et al., 2016). Climate Central develops content for TV meteorologists to use in their broadcasts, social media, and community presentations. For example, its team of meteorologists, research scientists, data analysts, journalists, and graphic designers is able to localize climate change stories and develop graphics effective on television and in social media for sharing this information. Climate Central analyzes data from NOAA and NASA and distributes it widely. These data show warming trends throughout the United States have accelerated since 1970 (Samenow, 2012). Articles like Samenow's that highlight relevant information for readers of his publication (*Washington Post*) are apt to get attention because of their emphasis on hazards with local impact.

Implications of best practices for evolving media. There can be a tendency to adopt new technologies because they are new, rather than tapping a clear conceptual framework for *why* one might use new tools such as blogs, interactive graphics, animations, or compelling video as opposed to more traditional efforts such as news stories or nature hikes. The NRC (2009) best practices provide guidance for considering why one might want to use, for example, a cartoon one can share online versus creating an instructional activity, as well as *what* one wants to communicate about a slow onset hazard. TV meteorologists have frequently noted that constraints on the length of on-air segments hamper efforts to explain complexities (e.g., Wilson, 2009). The NRC (2009) best practices alert users to several key conditions that help audiences enjoy scientific material, learn complexities, and feel motivated to learn more, even when material is presented in short on-air formats. For instance, this framework says segments that encourage audiences to be active by participating in the methods of science, not just hearing about results, intrigue viewers. It also says casting audiences as people who like science encourages engagement with scientific material. Future work should explore the effectiveness of teaching the NRC (Bell et al., 2009) best practices to interdisciplinary teams comprised of natural scientists, social scientists, science educators, and communication professionals. Evidence of the effectiveness of interdisciplinary science communication teams is available in Zhao et al. (2014). These scholars showed that a series of explanatory videos developed by Climate Central and presented by chief TV meteorologist Jim Gandy (CBS affiliate, WLTX, Columbus, SC) increased understanding of the regional effects of climate change among CBS viewers over a one-year period. CBS viewers were more knowledgeable about the harmful effects of climate change (e.g., more high heat, high humidity days; more illness-inducing pollen in the air) than were viewers of the other major networks, the comparison groups.

Limitations

This study explored ways that innovator TV meteorologists approach the task of communicating about a complicated, slow onset, politically contested societal risk—climate change—in 2009, a time when relatively few TV meteorologists were educating audiences about climate change's impacts. One limitation is that its theory-guided qualitative methods allow generation of further questions, not findings. Another is that the sample size (16) is small.

Conclusion

Studying best practices for educating about slow onset hazards in this evolving media environment is one of the more important goals applied communication research can pursue. Communicating the ethics and methods of science by inviting audiences to be active and scientist-like may be an effective approach to gaining stakeholders' interest in slow onset hazards. We show through interviews with 16 innovator TV meteorologists, studied in 2009, that they, in general, either agreed with or already used many evidence-based best practices for effectiveness in informal science education contexts, such as television. However, they may benefit from formal training in these best practices.

Current approaches to informal science education may unduly emphasize insistence on scientific conclusions without sufficient opportunities for stakeholders to consider scientific methods, failings, systems for fixing error, and contexts where stakeholders can actively reason with and even conduct research with scientists. TV meteorologists, like many other science communicators such as resource managers, extension agents, park rangers, physicians, health communicators, docents, journalists, commentators, and bloggers, as well as scientists in other fields, may be able to draw from the National Research Council's (Bell et al., 2009) best practices for guidance on involving audiences in learning science. Such steps may engage audiences emotionally and encourage them to learn more about slow onset hazards that are seemingly distant but often harm or kill more so than do acute harms to which people more easily give attention.

References

Alexander, D. E. (1999). *Natural disasters*. Dordecht, Netherlands: Kluwer.

Allen, S. (2007). *Secrets of circles summative evaluation report*. Report prepared for the Children's Discovery Museum of San Jose. Available: www.informal science.org/evaluation/sow/115 [accessed October 2008].

Anderson, A. A., Myers, T. A., Maibach, E. W., Cullen, H., Gandy, J., Witte, J., Stenhouse, N., & Leiserowitz, A. (2013). If they like you, they learn from you: How a brief weathercaster-delivered climate education segment is moderated by viewer evaluations of the weathercaster. *Weather, Climate, and Society*, 5(4), 367–377.

Ashkenas, J., Buchanan, L., Burgess, J., Fairfield, H., Grady, D., Keller, J., Lai, K. K. R., Lyons, P. J., Murphy, H., Park, H., Peçanha, S., Tse, A., & Yourish, K. (2015, Jan. 26). How many Ebola patients have been treated outside of Africa?

New York Times. Available: www.nytimes.com/interactive/2014/07/31/world/africa/ebola-virus-outbreak-qa.html?_r=0 [accessed May 31, 2016].

Ausubel, D. P. (1978). In defense of advance organizers. *Review of Educational Research, 48,* 251–257.

Bandura, A. (1986). *Social foundations of thought and action: A social cognitive theory.* Englewood Cliffs, NJ: Prentice-Hall.

Bell, P., Lewenstein, B., Shouse, A. W., & Feder, M. A. (Eds.). (2009). *Learning science in informal environments: People, places, and pursuits.* National Research Council, Committee on Learning Science in Informal Environments. Washington, DC: The National Academies Press.

Borun, M. (2003). *Space command summative evaluation.* Philadelphia: Franklin Institute Science Museum. Available: www.informalscience.org/evaluations/report_24.pdf [accessed October 2008].

Brossard, D., Lewenstein, B., & Bonney, R. (2005). Scientific knowledge and attitude change: The impact of a citizen science project. *International Journal of Science Education, 27*(9), 1099–1121.

Burleson, B. R. (2003). The experience and effects of emotional support: What the study of cultural and gender differences can tell us about close relationships, emotion, and interpersonal communication. *Personal Relationships, 10*(1), 1–23.

Burleson, B. R., & Kline, S. L. (1979). Habermas' theory of communication: A critical explication. *Quarterly Journal of Speech, 65*(4), 412–428.

Creswell, J. W., & Clark, V. L. P. (2007). *Designing and conducting mixed methods research.* Thousand Oaks, CA: SAGE.

Daniels, G. L., & Loggins, G. M. (2007). Conceptualizing continuous coverage: A strategic model for wall-to-wall local television weather. *Journal of Applied Communication Research, 35*(1), 48–66.

Ding, D., Maibach, E. W., Zhao, X., Roser-Renouf, C., & Leiserowitz, A. (2011). Support for climate policy and societal action are linked to perceptions about scientific agreement. *Nature Climate Change, 1*(9), 462–466. doi: 10.1038/nclimate1295.

Douglas, M., & Wildavsky, A. (1983). *Risk and culture: An essay on the selection of technological and environmental dangers.* Berkeley, CA: University of California Press.

Gaile, G. L., & Willmott, C. J. (Eds.). (2003). *Geography in America at the dawn of the 21st century.* New York: Oxford University Press.

Goldowsky, N. (2002). *Lessons from life: Learning from exhibits, animals, and interaction in a museum.* UMI #3055856. Unpublished doctoral dissertation, Harvard University.

IPCC. (2007). *Climate change 2007: Synthesis report.* Contribution of working groups I, II and III to the Fourth Assessment Report of the Intergovernmental Panel on Climate Change. (R. K. Pachauri & A. Risinger, Eds.). Geneva, Switzerland: IPCC.

Kahan, D. M. (2015). Climate-science communication and the measurement problem. *Advances in Political Psychology, 36*(S1), 1–43.

Krosnick, J., Holbrook, A., Lowe, L., & Visser, P. (2006). The origins and consequences of democratic citizens' policy agendas: A study of popular concern about global warming. *Climatic Change, 77*(1), 7–43. doi: 10.1007/s10584-006-9068-8.

Leiserowitz, A., Maibach, E., & Roser-Renouf, C. (2008). Climate change in the American mind: Americans' global warming beliefs and attitudes in November 2008. New Haven, CT: Yale Project on Climate Change Communication, Yale University and George Mason University. Available: http://environment.yale. edu/climate/files/Climate-Beliefs-September-2012.pdf.

Leiserowitz, A., Maibach, E., Roser-Renouf, C., Feinberg, G., & Howe, P. (2012). Climate change in the American mind: Americans' global warming beliefs and attitudes in September 2012. Yale University and George Mason University. New Haven, CT: Yale Project on Climate Change Communication. Available: http://climatecommunication.yale.edu/wp-content/uploads/2016/02/2012_10_Americans%E2%80%99-Global-Warming-Beliefs-and-Attitudes-in-September-2012.pdf.

Leiserowitz, A., Maibach, E., Roser-Renouf, C., Feinberg, G., & Rosenthal, S. (2016). Climate change in the American mind: March 2016. Yale University and George Mason University. New Haven, CT: Yale Program on Climate Change Communication. Available: http://climatechangecommunication.org/wp-content/uploads/2016/06/Climate-Change-American-Mind-March-2016-FINAL.compressed.pdf.

MacGeorge, E. L., Feng, B., & Thompson, E. R. (2008). "Good" and "bad" advice: How to advise more effectively. In M. Motley (Ed.), *Applied interpersonal communication: Behaviors that affect outcomes*, pp. 145–164. Thousand Oaks, CA: SAGE.

Maibach, E., & Covello, V. (2016). Communicating environmental health. In H. Frumkin (Ed.) *Environmental health: From global to local* (3rd ed.), pp. 759–780. San Francisco, CA: Jossey-Bass.

Maibach, E., Cullen, H., Placky, B., Witte, J., Seitter, K., Gardiner, N., Myers, T., & Sublette, S. (2016). TV meteorologists as local climate educators. In M. Nisbet (Ed.) *Oxford Research Encyclopedia of Climate Science*. New York: Oxford University Press. doi: 10.1093/acrefore/9780190228620.013.505.

Maibach, E. W., Leiserowitz, A., Roser-Renouf, C., & Mertz, C. K. (2011). Identifying like-minded audiences for global warming public engagement campaigns: An audience segmentation analysis and tool development. *PLoS ONE*, 6(3), e17571. doi: 10.1371/journal.pone.0017571.

Maibach, E., Mazzone, R., Myers, T., Seitter, K., Hayhoe, K., Ryan, B., Witte, J., Gardiner, N., Hassol, S., Lazo, J., Placky, B., Sublette, S., & Cullen, H. (in press). TV weathercasters' views of climate change appear to be rapidly evolving. *Bulletin of the American Meteorological Society*.

Maibach, E. W., Roser-Renouf, C., & Leiserowitz, A. (2008). Communication and marketing as climate change–intervention assets: A public health perspective. *American Journal of Preventive Medicine*, 35(5), 488–500. doi: 10.1016/j.amepre.2008.08.016.

Matthews, C. E., George, S. M., Moore, S. C., Bowles, H. R., Blair, A., Park, Y., Troiano, R. P., Hollenbeck, A., & Schatzkin, A. (2012). Amount of time spent in sedentary behaviors and cause-specific mortality in US adults. *The American Journal of Clinical Nutrition*, 95(2), 437–445.

Mayer, R. E., Bove, W., Bryman, A., Mars, R., & Tapangco, L. (1996). When less is more: Meaningful learning from visual and verbal summaries of science textbook lessons. *Journal of Educational Psychology*, 88(1), 64.

Miller, J. D., Augenbraun, E., Schulhof, J., & Kimmel, L. G. (2006). Adult science learning from local television newscasts. *Science Communication, 28*(2), 216–242. doi: 10.1177/1075547006294461.

National Research Council. (2011). *America's climate choices*. Washington, DC: The National Academies Press.

National Oceanic and Atmospheric Administration (NOAA). (n.d.) National Weather Service: Radiosonde observations. Available: www.ua.nws.noaa.gov/factsheet.htm [accessed May 31, 2016].

O'Keefe, D. J. (2015). *Persuasion: Theory and research* (2nd ed.). Thousand Oaks, CA: SAGE.

Pedretti, E. G. (2004). *Perspectives on learning through research on critical issues-based science center exhibitions*. Hoboken, NJ: Wiley.

Petty, R. E., Wegener, D. T., & Fabrigar, L. R. (1997). Attitudes and attitude change. *Annual Review of Psychology, 48*(1), 609–647.

Placky, B., Maibach, E., Witte, J., Ward, B., Seitter, K. Gardiner, N., Herring, D., & Cullen, H. (2016). Climate matters: A comprehensive educational resource for broadcast meteorologists. *Bulletin of the American Meteorological Society*, doi: http://dx.doi.org/10.1175/BAMS-D-14-00235.1.

Randol, S. M. (2005). *The nature of inquiry in science centers: Describing and assessing inquiry at exhibits*. Unpublished doctoral dissertation, University of California, Berkeley.

Rowan, K. E. (1988). A contemporary theory of explanatory writing. *Written Communication, 5*(1), 23–56.

Rowan, K. E. (1990). Cognitive correlates of explanatory writing skill: An analysis of individual differences. *Written Communication, 7*(3), 316–341.

Rowan, K. E. (1999). Effective explanation of uncertain and complex science. In S. Friedman, S. Dunwoody, & C. L. Rogers (Eds.), *Communicating uncertainty: Media coverage of new and controversial science*, pp. 201–220. Mahwah, NJ: Erlbaum.

Rowan, K. E. (2003). Informing and explaining skills: Theory and research on informative communication. In J. O. Greene & B. R. Burleson (Eds.), *The handbook of communication and social interaction skills*, pp. 403–438. Mahwah, NJ: Erlbaum.

Sachatello-Sawyer, B., Fellenz, R. A., Burton, H., Gittings-Carlson, L., Lewis-Mahony, J., & Woolbaugh, W. (2002*). Adult museum programs: Designing meaningful experiences*. American Association for State and Local History Book series. Blue Ridge Summit, PA: AltaMira Press.

Samenow, J. (2012, June 12). Report: Climate warming has accelerated in U.S. since 1970, including Va., Md. *Washington Post*. Available: www.washington post.com/blogs/capital-weather-gang/post/report-climate-warming-has-accelerated-in-us-since-1970-including-in-va-md/2012/06/12/gJQAxr7bXV_blog.html?utm_term=.a2f4023fd8d9 [accessed March 10, 2017].

Sandman, P. M. (1993). *Responding to community outrage: Strategies for effective risk communication*. American Industrial Hygiene Association.

Slovic, P., & Peters, E. (2006). Risk perception and affect. *Current Directions in Psychological Science, 15*(6), 322–325.

154

Swain, K. A. (2007). Outrage factors and explanations in news coverage of the anthrax attacks. *Journalism and Mass Communication Quarterly*, *84*(2), 335–352.

Wilson, K. (2009). Opportunities and obstacles for television weathercasters to report on climate change. *Bulletin of the American Meteorological Society*, *90*(10), 1457–1465. doi: 10.1175/2009BAMS2947.1.

Witte, K. (1992). Putting the fear back into fear appeals: The extended parallel process model. *Communications Monographs*, *59*(4), 329–349.

Zhao, X. Z., Maibach, E. W., Gandy, J., Witte, H. J., Cullen, H., Klinger, B., Rowan, K., Witte, J., & Pyle, A. (2014). TV weathercasters as climate educators: Results of a field experiment. *Bulletin of the American Meteorological Society*. doi: http://dx.doi.org/10.1175/BAMS-D-12-00144.1.

8

NEWS COVERAGE OF CANCER RESEARCH

Does Disclosure of Scientific Uncertainty Enhance Credibility?

Chelsea L. Ratcliff, Jakob D. Jensen,
Katheryn Christy, Kaylee Crossley, and
Melinda Krakow

The news media are recognized as an essential channel for communicating health research and recommendations to the public (Atkin & Wallack, 1990; Jensen, Krakow, John, & Liu, 2013; Johnson, 1997). News stories can educate lay audiences about methods for preventing a myriad of health risks, including cancer, which is the second leading cause of death among Americans (Siegel, Miller, & Jemal, 2015; Stryker, Moriarty, & Jensen, 2008). However, whether or not the public trusts a source of risk information can influence how they interpret and respond to the risks (Malka, Krosnick, & Langer, 2009; Priest, Bonfadelli, & Rusanen, 2003; Siegrist, Connor, & Keller, 2012).

Prior research in the context of health journalism has identified a connection between perceived credibility and hedging (Jensen, 2008). In general, *hedged* language is language that employs modifying devices (hedges) to make tentative statements. In a scientific context, hedging is more aptly described as the disclosure of scientific uncertainty (Hyland, 1996). It is customary for scientific research published in peer-reviewed journals to include a discussion of study limitations and caveats, and for inferences to be made cautiously (i.e., with language of restrained possibility such as "could," "perhaps," and "might"; Reyna, 1981; Schwartz, Woloshin, & Welch, 1999).

When reporting scientific research to the public, a journalist can choose how much uncertainty to include. Sometimes the inclusion of hedging language is at direct odds with other news values. For example, although accuracy is a strong marker of quality in newswriting (Dudo, Dahlstrom, & Brossard, 2007; Kovach & Rosenstiel, 2007), journalists are expected to present information simply and clearly to make it easier for audiences to understand (see Bender, Drager, Davenport, & Fedler, 2009). Further, journalists are expected to appeal to audiences by presenting engaging material (Groot Kormelink & Costera Meijer, 2015). This tension can lead to the omission of uncertainty for the sake of clarity, novelty, or sensation value.

Journalists also choose whether to include disclosures of scientific uncertainty from the primary scientists responsible for a study, or alternately to invite unaffiliated scientists to comment. Casting a balanced view by interviewing multiple sources is a key tenet in journalism (Bender et al., 2009). Yet attempts to create balance in science coverage are frequently made by soliciting the point of view of an outside scientist *in place of* disclosure from the primary scientist. This may create the appearance that the primary scientist failed to acknowledge the uncertainty, or that scientists are dueling about the findings, either of which could inadvertently impact perceived credibility.

The current study examines whether certain practices in journalism could be systematically lowering public perceptions of credibility with regard to cancer research reports. Though likely unintentional, this could lead to biased processing and, potentially, dismissal of health information that is important in helping the public avoid health risks. We model this study on a prior experiment by Jensen (2008), which found a link between disclosure of scientific uncertainty attributed to the primary scientist and increased trustworthiness ratings for both the journalist and the primary scientist. We aim to see if Jensen's (2008) earlier findings hold (a) with updated news credibility measures (Yale, Jensen, Carcioppolo, Sun, & Liu, 2015), (b) in a sample that is more representative of the general public, and (c) in a more current media environment. Additionally, we explore whether source and amount of uncertainty influence public support for scientific research in general.

Capturing Perceptions of Credibility

In order to navigate the plethora of risks—including health risks—inherent in modern society, people often select other social actors in whom to trust (Kohring & Matthes, 2007). These are usually expert systems (such as news media, industry, scientists, and government) that individuals deem suitable to act on their behalf. Here, trust replaces knowledge, and individuals choose which information sources to trust based on certain criteria (Kohring & Matthes, 2007). *Credibility* is one such heuristic.

Operational definitions of credibility are complex and vary widely in the literature. Early trust and credibility research, which focused on communicators in general, identified two major subdimensions of credibility: *expertise* and *trustworthiness* (Hovland, Janis, & Kelley, 1959). Expertise was operationalized as believing an actor to be informed and intelligent, while trustworthiness reflected a belief that the actor was impartial and not intending to persuade (Hovland, Janis, & Kelley, 1959). McCroskey and Young (1981) proposed a refinement to these widely used measures of credibility, identifying three distinct factors that comprised expertise: being intelligent, competent, and an expert; and three distinct factors that comprised trustworthiness: being trustworthy, honest, and ethical.

News Credibility

In measuring perceived credibility of newspapers and TV news, Gaziano and McGrath (1986) grouped the following 12 items together as a single factor: fair, unbiased, tells the whole story, accurate, respects the privacy of people, looks out for the interests of people, is concerned about the well-being of the community, separates fact from opinion, can be trusted, is concerned about the public interest, is factual, and has well-trained reporters. Their rationale was that these concepts have typically been treated as indicators of credibility in past research.

Meyer (1988) outlined a simpler measure of credibility comprised of five items: fairness, accuracy, unbiased, can be trusted, and tells the whole story. While each of these essentially describes *believability*, according to Meyer, he argued that "[t]his redundancy provides a far more accurate measurement than could be made by one of these items alone" (p. 574). Meyer also suggested that community affiliation (e.g., being concerned about the well-being of the community and the public interest) is distinct from credibility and should be measured with a separate scale, though West (1994) later found that addition to be unreliable. West also noted that the Gaziano-McGrath measure appeared to have multiple underlying factors.

Abdulla Garrison, Salwen, Driscoll, and Casey (2005) used a variation of the Gaziano and McGrath (1986) scale, grouping the following 11 items into three main factors: balanced, accurate, fair, objective, reports the whole story (under the primary dimension of *balance*), honest, believable, trustworthy (under the primary dimension of *honesty*), and current, up-to-date, timely (under the primary dimension of *currency*). One major difference in Abdulla et al.'s modified credibility scale is the replacement of concepts related to intent toward the receiver (e.g., community affiliation, goodwill) with concepts related to currency. A 12th item, bias, was not included in Abdulla et al.'s final scale for newspaper credibility.

Recently, Yale and colleagues (2015) tested Abdulla et al.'s (2005) scale as a single second-order factor (all nine items combined), as opposed to examining the honesty, balance, and currency separately as three first-order factors. The new factor structure mitigated discriminant validity issues observed in the original scale, suggesting that when testing all three factors—balance, honesty, or currency—they should be tested as a single scale to measure credibility.

Some scholars distinguish between *source* credibility and *message* credibility with regard to evaluations of news. Kiousis (2001) suggested that source credibility focuses on communicator variables (e.g., the individual journalist, the news outlet) while message credibility focuses on message variables (e.g., the content of news article). A third level of credibility judgment is also evident: perceived credibility of the platform. For instance, Kiousis (2001) found credibility ratings to be higher for print news than online or TV news. However, Kiousis noted that to some extent these layers are intertwined in audiences' minds.

The terms "journalists" and "news media" are sometimes used interchangeably in the literature (Kohring & Matthes, 2007). Frequently when communication scholars refer to trust in news media, they are actually speaking about trust in sources, such as journalists (Jensen, 2008). After all, it is journalists who select topics and facts to report, are responsible for reporting the information accurately, and offer their assessment of the issue—key dimensions of news trust, according to Kohring and Matthes (2007). Yet Kiousis (2001) made the case that perceptions of credibility—across layers, from journalist to outlet to media platform—are likely intertwined. In the current study, we asked participants to judge the news article instead of the journalist. Our aim was to keep the focus of their assessment on the content of the article, rather than shifting their thoughts toward a judgment of the person who said it, in order to examine the effects of our message characteristic variables. However, it is plausible that credibility evaluations of the article transfer to evaluations of the journalist (and vice versa).

Scientist Credibility

Few attempts have been made to specifically measure perceived credibility of scientists. Examinations of trust in scientists and scientific institutions have typically been embedded within larger studies about public trust in expert institutions (e.g., scientists, industry, government, and nonprofits; see Malka, Krosnick, & Langer, 2009; Priest, Bonfadelli, & Rusanen, 2003; Siegrist, Connor, & Keller, 2012).

Earle and Siegrist (2006) proposed a general trust model that divides trust into morality-based and performance-based assessment, with the former influencing *social trust* and the latter influencing *perceived competence*. Siegrist, Connor, and Keller (2012) applied this to public trust in scientists and industry, suggesting that public trust in these groups can be examined in terms of perceived shared values and perceived competence. They proposed a multidimensional scale with items to capture subdimensions of social trust (honesty, concern for public health and the environment) and subdimensions of confidence (related to competence). Given these measures, trust and confidence factors may be closely related to perceived credibility of scientists and industry; however, this was specific to an environmental risk context.

Priest, Bonfadelli, and Rusanen (2003) examined trust in scientists along with industry, government, and other social institutions. They operationalized trust as "doing a good job for society," arguing that the measure taps into a dimension of social trust (p. 754). Siegrist, Connor, and Keller (2012), on the other hand, reasoned that trust and confidence are related but distinct concepts; trust is based on value similarity (i.e., intentions toward society) while confidence (i.e., competence) is based on past performance. Both of these appear to mirror the traditional key subdimensions of credibility—trustworthiness and expertise—although intentions toward society may be more closely related to goodwill.

In a series of studies conducted during 1971–1975, McCroskey and colleagues identified several dimensions of source credibility, including competence, character, sociability, extroversion, and composure. McCroskey and Young (1981) evaluated multiple types of expert sources, including organizations, peers, public figures, the media, and instructors. Their dimensions pertained more to speech communication cases, where factors such as composure, sociability, and character could be evaluated. A later credibility scale developed by McCroskey examined credibility as it pertained to experts (McCroskey & Teven, 1999) and has been one of the most widely used scales to assess perceptions of credibility via the subdimensions of expertise and trustworthiness.

Sjöberg (2001, p. 189) argued that competence has two sides: "One is knowing, the other is knowing the limits of one's knowledge." He suggested the latter is a consideration when evaluating a source's trustworthiness. In a science context, this aspect of competence—knowing the limits of one's knowledge—could be measured by a scientist's willingness to disclose uncertainty about her research, and potentially is a measure that audiences use to gauge scientist credibility.

Uncertainty and Credibility

In scientific research, uncertainty describes how well something (for instance, a study finding or a conclusion) is known (Peters & Dunwoody, 2016). It is not fully understood how lay audiences process uncertainty, and a growing body of literature has sought to understand audience reactions (Binder, Hillback, & Brossard, 2016; Guenther, Froehlich, & Ruhrman, 2015; Guenther & Ruhrman, 2016; Jensen et al., 2017; Kimmerle, Flemming, Feinkohl, & Cress, 2015; Niederdeppe et al., 2014; Post & Maier, 2016; Winter, Kramer, Rosner, & Neubaum, 2015). However, the concepts of uncertainty and credibility have previously been explored together (Jensen, 2008; Priest, Bonfadelli, & Rusanen, 2003), and there is reason to believe message characteristics—such as whether, and to what extent, uncertainty is disclosed—can influence perceived credibility (Hendriks, Kienhues, & Bromme, 2016a; Hendriks, Kienhues, & Bromme, 2016b).

Amount of Uncertainty

The inclusion of uncertainty in health news can take the form of hedging language, or presentation of the limitations and caveats of research findings. A common newswriting principle is streamlining word choice, or "cutting out the fat" (Bender et al., 2009, p. 99). For example, journalists are often instilled with a belief that most adverbs and adjectives are unnecessary (see Bender et al., 2009). Aiming for strong and simple phrasing could lead to the removal of hedging language.

Yet research suggests that scientific uncertainty may be appreciated by lay audiences as well as the scientific community. For example, after reading hedged news reports of cancer research, participants in one study were less fatalistic about cancer than their peers who read non-hedged reports (Jensen et al., 2011a). Fuller expressions of uncertainty may even serve as a heuristic for news consumers with lower quantitative literacy and/or lower scientific knowledge. As Schwartz, Woloshin, and Welch (1999, p. 128) explain, sensing that an article has incomplete or undisclosed data can give the impression of "an underlying attempt to persuade rather than inform." Perceived intention to persuade in turn can lower trust and credibility ratings (Hovland, Janis, & Kelley, 1959; Kohring & Matthes, 2007).

People have heuristics for assessing the credibility of information even when it is not fully understood (Chaiken & Maheswaran, 1994). Potentially, lay audiences evaluate the quality of scientific research claims in news articles by recognizing the inclusion (or omission) of ambivalent language, caution surrounding claims, and specific data to support conclusions. Indeed, a study by Dahlstrom, Dudo, and Brossard (2012) found that audiences give more weight to scientific stories about health risks when precise information is included, defined as "specificity of information about a risk's pervasiveness, potency, or effects" (p. 156).

Elimination of uncertainty can happen at many stages of the research communication process. Journalists may assume audiences prefer streamlined health information (Allan, 2011). Potentially, the belief is that powerful (i.e., certain) language will enhance trust in the communicator or in health research in general, and thus promote positive health beliefs and behaviors. Yet, as Dorothy Nelkin (1996, p. 1601) wrote, "Scientists, eager to promote their latest breakthrough, contribute to hyperbole" as well. Scientists may speak in overly certain terms about their research out of a belief that it will enhance their credibility or increase support from the public and decision-makers for their work (Star, 1983). Public relations professionals may further remove uncertainty as the information goes from journal article to press release (Nelkin, 1996).

Attempts to present research in a saleable way may be misguided. Although powerful language appears to heighten credibility in other contexts, such as business (Ober, Zhao, Davis, & Alexander, 1999) and public speaking (see Hosman, 2002), the effect might not hold when presenting health and medical research (Jensen, 2008). In fact, scholars have argued that using powerless language in science communication is a demonstration of objectivity (Popper, 1934/2002), which could in turn reflect on scientists' credibility. Potentially, a similar pattern would hold for science journalists, as well.

In light of prior research, we predict the following about uncertainty in news coverage of scientific studies:

H1a: Cancer news reports that include a higher amount of scientific uncertainty will associate with greater perceived credibility of the *journalist*, compared with low-uncertainty coverage.

H1b: Cancer news reports that include a higher amount of uncertainty will associate with greater perceived credibility of the *scientist* leading the study, compared with low-uncertainty coverage.

Source of Uncertainty

When journalists do include uncertainty in reports of scientific research, it is often by way of a counter point of view from an expert or scientist unaffiliated with the study. Casting a "balanced" view is a basic principle of newswriting, and seeking outside commentary is a common and generally constructive practice in journalism (Bennett, 1996). However, whether news audiences associate this kind of balance with quality or credibility may be context dependent (Jensen, 2008). In science reporting, the balance frame may have unintended consequences, giving the impression that the original scientists behind the study are ignorant of—or even attempting to mask—limitations in their research (Jensen, 2008). Additionally, it may create the appearance that scientists in the scientific community are pitted against each other and lack accordance on health research, even when this is not the case (Allan, 2011).

Some have suggested that the news media incorporate fringe counter-perspectives for the sake of sensationalism or to force balance where none exists (Dixon & Clarke, 2013). Journalists have been accused of treating discussions of scientific breakthroughs like "football matches" and giving equal weight to opposing viewpoints without scrutinizing the evidence behind them (Allan, 2011, p. 773). Onora O'Neill (2004, p. 269) writes that news consumers hear about highly publicized cases of "scandals, dereliction, cover up and even corruption in medicine and biomedical research"—some of which is founded, she says, but most of it is not. This suggests an already existing, biased lens through which news audiences may be processing news reports about scientific discoveries (Chingching, 2015). The dueling frame—disclosures of scientific uncertainty from an outside source, instead of the primary scientist responsible for the study—could further impact perceptions of scientist credibility. Regardless of whether the aim is to create an appearance of conflict and heighten a story's sensation value or simply to employ a balanced frame, we predict that source attribution of uncertainty will impact credibility:

H2a: Limitations disclosed by the primary scientist, as opposed to an outside scientist, will lead to greater perceived credibility of the *journalist*.

H2b: Limitations disclosed by the primary scientist, as opposed to an outside scientist, will lead to greater perceived credibility of the primary *scientist*.

Potentially, amount of uncertainty and source attributions interact to influence credibility judgements. Jensen (2008) found a small but significant interaction between amount and source of uncertainty such that greater uncertainty, when attributed to the primary scientist, increased credibility ratings for the journalist and the scientist. In the current study, we test whether the same uncertainty amount source interaction emerges with updated credibility measures and a population more representative of the general public.

H3a: A high amount of uncertainty attributed to the primary scientist, as opposed to an outside scientist, will lead to greater perceived credibility of the *journalist*.

H3b: A high amount of uncertainty attributed to the primary scientist, as opposed to an outside scientist, will lead to greater perceived credibility of the *scientist*.

Support for Scientific Research

Both uncertainty and perceived credibility could be related to public support for science. First, past research has shown that the communication of scientific uncertainty is related to public engagement with science (Retzbach & Maier, 2015; Retzbach, Otto, & Maier, 2016). If uncertainty is related to engagement with science, then it stands to reason that it could also be connected to support for the scientific enterprise. Moreover, support for scientific research seems to be relatively high. As an illustration, the National Science Foundation administers a survey every two years to assess US public opinion about the federal funding of scientific research. The survey has found Americans to be generally supportive of scientific research; most recently, 83% of Americans agreed or strongly agreed that the federal government should support scientific research that advances the frontiers of knowledge, even if it does not bring immediate benefits (National Center for Science and Engineering Statistics, 2014). Given that the majority of the public likely hears about scientific research through the news, perceptions of credibility in news coverage of health research could influence public support for science. This has not previously been examined. Thus, we investigate the following:

RQ1: Is there a relationship among how scientific uncertainty is disclosed in the news, perceived credibility, and support for science?

Method

Design

Participants were randomly assigned to one of 16 conditions in a 2 (uncertainty amount) × 2 (uncertainty source) × 4 (cancer news article) between-subjects experiment. The amount of uncertainty was either high or low. The source of uncertainty was either the primary scientist (the scientist responsible for the study described in the article) or an outside scientist (a scientist unaffiliated with the study). Four different news articles were manipulated on these variables. Individuals completed a pretest, read a single news article, and then completed a posttest. Participants were paid $10 for participating in the study.

Sample. Participants (N = 880) were recruited in seven shopping malls in the Midwest and randomly assigned to one of the 16 news article conditions. Jensen's (2008) initial study surveyed a convenience sample of college students and was considered to be a starting point for further research. Participants in the present study represent a greater diversity of educational backgrounds and thus may be more representative of the US population. Participants provided demographic information, including

164

age ($M = 35.92$, $SD = .16$; range: 18–84), sex (female: 66.10%), education (more than 12th grade: 53.30%), and race (83.2% Caucasian, 11.7% African American, 3.1% Hispanic, Latino, or Spanish Origin, 1.0% Asian or Pacific Islander, 1.8% American Indian or Native American, and 2.3% self-described as "other"; participants could check more than one category). The mean household income was $51,769 ($SD = $42,954).

Stimulus materials. All participants randomly received a news article on one of four cancer research topics embedded within a survey. Survey questions were the same for all participants. The article was manipulated to represent one of four possible uncertainty conditions: low-uncertainty/ primary scientist disclosure, high-uncertainty/primary scientist disclosure, low-uncertainty/dueling disclosure, high-uncertainty/dueling disclosure. Disclosure refers to uncertainty addressed by the scientist affiliated with the study (the primary scientist), while dueling refers to uncertainty addressed by an unaffiliated scientist.

Stimulus articles were developed by Jensen (2008) and involved the manipulation of real news articles gathered from the Lexis Nexis database. Search parameters included: US news articles from major papers or Midwest regional sources that contained "cancer research" or "cancer study" in the headline, lead paragraph(s), or key terms (Jensen, 2008). Using a random number generator, four articles were selected from these search results for inclusion in the study: two articles pertaining to research about cancer treatments (nanobombs, lung cancer treatment) and two pertaining to research in cancer prevention (Mediterranean diet, lycopene pills). See appendix for the full stimulus materials.

Survey Measures

Journalist credibility. After reading the article, participants were asked to evaluate the journalist's credibility. Journalist credibility was treated as a single second-order factor measured by nine items (accurate, honest, believable, balanced, report the whole story, objective, up-to-date, current, and timely; $M = 3.47$, $SD = .60$, $\alpha = .88$) using a five-point scale ranging from *strongly disagree* to *strongly agree* (Yale et al., 2015). These nine items were originally argued to represent the first-order factors of honesty, balance, and currency, but discriminant validity issues suggest that—when used together in the same analysis—they should be combined into a single scale (Yale et al., 2015). In other words, researchers have the option to use a single measure of credibility (all nine items combined) or to investigate hypotheses about a single first-order factor separately (e.g., an analysis that just includes the items representing the first-order factor of honesty). The current study utilizes the full scale, and also tests hypotheses related to the honesty factor ($M = 3.57$, $SD = .65$, $\alpha = .80$).

Scientist credibility. Participants were also asked to evaluate the primary scientist in the article. Expert source credibility has two underlying dimensions: expertise (intelligent, expert, competent; $M = 3.65$, $SD = .68$, $\alpha = .83$) and trustworthiness (trustworthy, honest, ethical; $M = 3.48$, $SD = .68$, $\alpha = .83$). These six items were assessed on five-point scales ranging from *strongly disagree* to *strongly agree* (McCroskey & Teven, 1999). Although McCroskey and Teven (1999) proposed "goodwill" as a third dimension of credibility, Jensen (2008) argued that goodwill is a separate construct and did not include it in the credibility scale used in his 2008 study. It was not included in the present study.

Support for scientific research. Participants were also asked about level of support for scientific research in general. Specifically, they reported how much they agree with the following statement: "Even if it brings no immediate benefits, scientific research that advances the frontiers of knowledge is necessary and should be supported by the Federal Government." Answers were given on a four-point scale ranging from *strongly disagree* to *strongly agree* ($M = 3.09$, $SD = .87$). This single-item measure comes from the Science and Engineering Indicators of the National Science Foundation, published by the National Center for Science and Engineering Statistics (NCSES, 2014).

Power analysis. G*Power was used to calculate power for the design (Faul, Erdfelder, Buchner, & Lang, 2009). Past studies have found small effects (Jensen, 2008; Jensen et al., 2011a). For a three-way ANOVA with 16 cells, the design was adequately powered (.84) to detect a small effect ($f = .10$). That said, researchers should be mindful of both Type I and Type II error when searching for small effects. Type I error is guarded against via replication. Type II error is countered by focusing on effect size rather than relying heavily on the p-value logic of null hypothesis testing.

Results

Five three-way ANOVAs were conducted to test hypotheses H1a–H3b and RQ1. Uncertainty and source were fixed factors and news article was treated as a random factor (per Jackson & Brashers, 1994). News article was treated as random as the variation on that factor (i.e., 4 random news articles) represents natural variability rather than specific levels of interest (Jackson & Brashers, 1994).

The first ANOVA included the single dimension journalist credibility measure from Yale and colleagues (2015) as the outcome variable to test H1a, H2a, and H3a. The small uncertainty × source interaction found in previous research manifested once again, $F(1, 3.15) = 6.44$, $p = .081$. No other factors or interactions were significant (see Table 8.1). Consistent with Jensen (2008), participants in the high uncertainty/primary scientist disclosure condition perceived journalists as more credible than did their peers

166

in the low uncertainty/primary scientist condition (size of the effect between conditions: $r = .10$; for means and standard deviations, see Table 8.2).

As a follow-up analysis, a second ANOVA was carried out using only the credibility items representing the subdimension of honesty. Using an older measure, Jensen (2008) found a significant uncertainty × source interaction for trustworthiness. Consistent with the first ANOVA and with Jensen (2008), the follow-up ANOVA revealed a small uncertainty × source interaction, $F(1, 3.18) = 7.58$, $p = .066$. Once again, the high uncertainty/primary scientist condition correlated with higher journalist honesty ratings compared to the low uncertainty/primary scientist condition (size of the effect between conditions: $r = .10$; for means and standard deviations, see Table 8.3).

H1b, H2b, and H3b postulated that high uncertainty disclosed by the primary scientist would also link with higher trustworthiness ratings for the primary scientist. The credibility of experts is thought to have two underlying dimensions: trustworthiness and expertise. Two ANOVAs were conducted, one with trustworthiness as an outcome and the other with expertise as an outcome. No significant main effects or interactions were observed (see Table 8.1).

Table 8.1 ANOVA Results by Outcome Variable

	Journalist's Credibility	Journalist's Trustworthiness	Scientist's Trustworthiness	Scientist's Expertise	Support for Research
Uncertainty	1.15	3.28	.00	1.25	.01
Source	.06	.02	.10	1.53	.69
Article	5.69†	4.35	.81	5.66**	4.06
Uncertainty × Source	6.44†	7.58†	.04	.15	.16

Note: F-ratios for all main effects and the uncertainty × source interaction.

†$p < .10$ **$p < .01$

Table 8.2 Uncertainty × Source Attribution Interaction on Journalist's Credibility

	Disclosure	Dueling
High Uncertainty	3.52 (.56)	3.47 (.52)
Low Uncertainty	3.41 (.62)	3.48 (.68)

Note: Means and standard deviations (in parentheses). Post-hoc tests reveal that high uncertainty disclosure is significantly different than low uncertainty disclosure ($p < .05$). No other means are significantly different.

Table 8.3 Uncertainty × Source Attribution Interaction on Journalist's Trustworthiness

	Disclosure	Dueling
High Uncertainty	3.63 (.62)	3.52 (.58)
Low Uncertainty	3.50 (.68)	3.56 (.72)

Note: Means and standard deviations (in parentheses). Post-hoc tests reveal that high uncertainty disclosure is significantly different than low uncertainty disclosure ($p < .05$). No other means are significantly different.

Using four different cancer news articles in the present experiment allowed us to generalize across articles. We were not interested in whether one topic generated more perceived credibility than another, but whether our factors would generalize above and beyond the variance that could be attributed to a particular article. The observed interaction in the high uncertainty by primary scientist condition occurred across all four articles.

RQ1 asked if uncertainty and source attribution were related to support for scientific research. No significant main effects or interactions were observed (see Table 8.1).

Discussion

Journalists are trusted as key translators of scientific research for the public. The news is an especially important avenue for educating people about cancer and other major health risks (Dudo, Dahlstrom, & Brossard, 2007; Jensen et al., 2013; Stryker et al., 2008). Yet current norms in news coverage of health research could systematically lower public trust in these reports. For example, journalists frequently minimize uncertainty when reporting scientific findings. They may alternatively disclose it in a dueling frame by soliciting comments from an outside source instead of the scientists responsible for the study (Jensen, 2008).

Using updated news credibility measures (Yale et al., 2015), the present experiment found that amount and source of uncertainty in cancer news articles significantly impacted audience perceptions of journalist credibility. Specifically, participants found the journalist more credible and trustworthy when the story contained a *higher* amount of uncertainty attributed to the *primary* scientist. The observed effect was small but significant and held across all four different cancer news articles. This suggests that the effect occurs systematically and was not due to features of a particular article or cancer topic.

The same conditions may affect credibility judgments for scientists, though it was not apparent in the current study. Jensen (2008) did find that high uncertainty disclosed by the primary scientist led to higher credibility ratings of both the journalist and the scientist. Thus, our study only partially replicates Jensen's earlier findings. Potentially, source and amount of uncertainty did not impact scientist credibility in our study because there are better measures that should be used to assess lay perceptions of scientist credibility (e.g., a scale specific to scientists). There is also the possibility of a small drip effect. Media effects are typically modest and often conceptualized as cumulative (Jensen, Bernat, Wilson, & Goonwardene, 2011b). Thus, subtle effects that are imperceptible during a single exposure can produce larger effects over time. It could be that omitting uncertainty in scientific news coverage, or disclosing it by way of a dueling frame, steadily undercuts journalists' credibility.

Public Health Implications

Public understanding of health is in jeopardy when journalists present medical discoveries as being more definite than they actually are (Allan, 2011; Schwartz, Woloshin, & Welch, 1999; Thiebach, Mayweg-Paus, & Jucks, 2015). To do so can "convey a false sense of the magnitude and certainty of the benefits of interventions, engendering unrealistic expectations" (Schwartz, Woloshin, & Welch, 1999, p. 131). Unhedged depictions of health risks, meanwhile, can cause undue fear (Schwartz, Woloshin, & Welch, 1999) and lead to fatalistic beliefs (Jensen et al., 2011a).

Minimizing scientific uncertainty could also increase skepticism in science and medicine. Past research has suggested that streamlining (e.g., reducing the amount of uncertainty) may set up research-based recommendations for backlash or rejection (Jensen et al., 2013). Communicating in certain terms about health and medical discoveries may create public confusion and even controversy by making the findings from multiple studies appear contradictory. A survey for the World Cancer Research Fund (WCRF) found that more than half of respondents believed "scientists were always changing their minds" about cancer causes and preventive measures (BBC, 2009). Indeed, sometimes news outlets report, seemingly back to back, that the very same things can cause cancer and cure it (Anderson, Brossard, & Scheufele, 2010). These apparent extremes are likely, at times, to be the result of streamlined study conclusions and omitted caveats. Disclosure of uncertainty in a dueling frame could also be a cause.

In view of the results of this and prior studies, it seems that lay audiences have come to interpret unhedged research claims as an indicator that the journalist or the scientist is overstating study findings. This, in turn, could harm trust in these important sources of health information. Several scholars have noted that trust in sources of risk information influences how people respond to reported risks (Malka, Krosnick, & Langer, 2009; Priest, Bonfadelli, & Rusanen, 2003; Siegrist, Connor, & Keller, 2012).

In the Context of an Evolving Media Environment

Because the news media have a latent influence on audience perceptions (Arendt, 2010), it is vital to examine connections among health risk perceptions, trust in information sources (e.g., scientists and journalists), and norms in science reporting (Jensen, 2008; Dahlstrom, Dudo, & Brossard, 2012). The current study examined print news articles. Although newspapers have garnered higher trust ratings than other news platforms in past research (Kiousis, 2001), the majority of Americans (57%) prefer to get their news from TV, followed by 38% who prefer online; only 20% get most of their news in print, according to a Pew Research Survey (Mitchell, Gottfried, Barthel, & Shearer, 2016). Nonetheless, examining trust in print news remains important, and findings from our study likely pertain to audience trust in TV, radio, and online news domains. Kiousis (2001) suggested that layers of news credibility—the news content, the journalist, the outlet, and the media platform—are intertwined. News consumers' criteria for assessing credibility may be constant across platforms and judgements of credibility may permeate across news media layers.

Growing concerns about fake news—fictional news stories circulated online (Barthel, Mitchel, & Holcomb, 2016)—could heighten audience skepticism toward news media. Roughly two-thirds of US adults who responded to a Pew Research Center survey claimed that fake news has caused a great deal of confusion about current events (Barthel, Mitchel, & Holcomb, 2016). This could signal an era in which journalists must strive harder to win audience trust. Careful reporting of cancer and other health risk research is an important area for consideration.

Limitations and Future Directions

The current study had a number of limitations. First, the length of the articles could have influenced perceptions of credibility. Articles in the high uncertainty conditions were one or two paragraphs longer. Potentially, some readers make heuristic judgments that more information is more trustworthy (although, longer articles in the high uncertainty/dueling conditions did not increase journalist credibility ratings). Second, the study only examined the impact of exposure to a single news article. Given the small but consistent significant effect, and the possibility that true impacts of exposure manifest cumulatively, it may be worthwhile for media effects scholars to study the effects of uncertainty disclosure with longitudinal study designs. Research should also continue to investigate how norms in news coverage impact scientist credibility, especially given the observed effect on journalist credibility.

Conclusion

Despite its limitations, this study makes an important contribution to credibility measurements. It replicated one major finding from Jensen (2008) with a diverse US sample that may be more representative of the population. Our results add to those of Jensen (2008) to indicate that amount of scientific uncertainty and source attributions can influence public trust in journalists. The results of our study indicate that lay audiences recognize a certain degree of uncertainty is inherent in the scientific process and in turn place greater trust in hedged research reports (or the journalists who write them).

While media are not always "exaggerating risk, whipping up hysteria and distorting reality" (Kitzinger, 1999, p. 55), this may be the perception among audiences. To counter skepticism and unintentional biases, journalists may consider which reporting practices, such as including scientific uncertainty in research reports, will foster favorable credibility judgements for both journalists and potentially also scientists.

References

Abdulla, R., Garrison, B., Salwen, M., Driscoll, P., & Casey, D. (2005). Online news credibility. In M. Salwen, B. Garrison, & P. Driscoll (Eds.), *Online news and the public*. Mahwah, NJ: Lawrence Erlbaum Associates.

Allan, S. (2011). Introduction: Science journalism in a digital age. *Journalism: Theory, Practice and Criticism, 12*(7), 771–777.

Anderson, A. A., Brossard, D., & Scheufele, D. A. (2010). The changing information environment for nanotechnology: Online audiences and content. *Journal of Nanoparticle Research, 12*(4), 1083–1094.

Arendt, F. (2010). Cultivation effects of a newspaper on reality estimates and explicit and implicit attitudes. *Journal of Media Psychology, 22*(4), 147–159.

Atkin, C. K., & Wallack, L. (1990). *Mass communication and public health: Complexities and conflicts* (Vol. 121). Newbury Park, CA: SAGE Publications.

Barthel M., Mitchel, A., & Holcomb, J. (2016). Many Americans believe fake news is sowing confusion. Pew Research Center. Available from www.journal ism.org/2016/12/15/many-americans-believe-fake-news-is-sowing-confusion (accessed on March 23, 2017).

BBC (2009, May 24). Britons "wary over cancer advice." Available from http://news.bbc.co.uk/2/hi/health/8059223.stm (accessed on December 15, 2015).

Bender, J. R., Drager, M. W., Davenport, L., & Fedler, F. (2009). *Reporting for the media* (9th ed.). New York: Oxford University Press.

Bennett, W. L. (1996). An introduction to journalism norms and representations of politics. *Political Communication, 13*, 373–384.

Binder, A. R., Hillback, E. D., & Brossard, D. (2016). Conflict or caveats? Effects of media portrayals of scientific uncertainty on audience perceptions of new technologies. *Risk Analysis, 36*(4), 831–846.

Chaiken, S., & Maheswaran, D. (1994). Heuristic processing can bias systematic processing: Effects of source credibility, argument ambiguity, and task importance on attitude judgment. *Journal of Personality and Social Psychology*, 66(3), 460–460.

Chingching, C. (2015). Motivated processing: How people perceive news covering novel or contradictory health research findings. *Science Communication*, 37(5), 602–634.

Dahlstrom, M. F., Dudo, A., & Brossard, D. (2012). Precision of information, sensational information, and self-efficacy information as message-level variables affecting risk perceptions. *Risk Analysis*, 32(1), 155–166.

Dixon, G. N., & Clarke, C. E. (2013). Heightening uncertainty around certain science: Media coverage, false balance, and the autism-vaccine controversy. *Science Communication*, 35(3), 358–382.

Dudo, A. D., Dahlstrom, M. F., & Brossard, D. (2007). Reporting a potential pandemic: A risk-related assessment of avian influenza coverage in U.S. newspapers. *Science Communication*, 28(4), 429–454.

Earle, T. C., & Siegrist, M. (2006). Morality information, performance information, and the distinction between trust and confidence. *Journal of Applied Social Psychology*, 36(2), 383–416.

Faul, F., Erdfelder, E., Buchner, A., & Lang, A.-G. (2009). Statistical power analyses using G*Power 3.1: Tests for correlation and regression analyses. *Behavior Research Methods*, 41(4), 1149–1160.

Gaziano, C., & McGrath, K. (1986). Measuring the concept of credibility. *Journalism Quarterly*, 63(3), 451–462.

Groot Kormelink, T., & Costera Meijer, I. (2015). Truthful or engaging? Surpassing the dilemma of reality versus storytelling in journalism. *Digital Journalism*, 3(2), 158–174.

Guenther, L., Froehlich, K., & Ruhrman, G. (2015). (Un)Certainty in the news: Journalists' decisions on communicating the scientific evidence of nanotechnology. *Journalism & Mass Communication Quarterly*, 92(1), 199–220.

Guenther, L., & Ruhrman, G. (2016). Scientific evidence and mass media: Investigating the journalistic intention to represent scientific uncertainty. *Public Understanding of Science*, 25(8), 927–943.

Hendriks, F., Kienhues, D., & Bromme, R. (2016a). Disclose your flaws! Admission positively affects the perceived trustworthiness of an expert blogger. *Studies in Communication Science*, 16(2), 124–131.

Hendriks, F., Kienhues, D., & Bromme, R. (2016b). Evoking vigilance: Would you (dis)trust a scientist who discusses ethical implications of research in a science blog? *Public Understanding of Science*, 25(8), 992–1008.

Hosman, L. A. (2002). Language and persuasion. In J. P. Dillard & M. Pfau (Eds.), *The persuasion handbook: Developments in theory and practice*. Thousand Oaks, CA: SAGE Publications.

Hovland, C. I., Janis, I. L., & Kelley, H. (1959). *Communication and persuasion: Psychological studies of opinion change* (3rd ed.). New Haven, CT: Yale University Press.

Hyland, K. (1996). Writing without conviction? Hedging in science research articles. *Applied Linguistics*, 17(4), 433–454.

Jackson, S., & Brashers, D. E. (1994). *Random factors in ANOVA*. Thousand Oaks, CA: SAGE Publications.

Jensen, J. D. (2008). Scientific uncertainty in news coverage of cancer research: Effects of hedging on scientists' and journalists' credibility. *Human Communication Research, 34*(3), 347–369.

Jensen, J. D., Carcioppolo, N., King, A. J., Bernat, J. K., Davis, L., Yale, R., & Smith, J. (2011a). Including limitations in news coverage of cancer research: Effects of news hedging on fatalism, medical skepticism, patient trust, and backlash. *Journal of Health Communication, 16*(5), 486–503.

Jensen, J. D., Bernat, J. K., Wilson, K., & Goonwardene, J. (2011b). The delay hypothesis: The manifestation of media effects over time. *Human Communication Research, 37*, 509–528.

Jensen, J. D., Krakow, M., John, K. K., & Liu, M. (2013). Against conventional wisdom: When the public, the media, and medical practice collide. *BMC Medical Informatics and Decision Making, 13* (Suppl 3), S4.

Jensen, J. D., Scherr, C. L., Brown, N., Jones, C., Christy, K., & Hurley, R. J. (2014). Public estimates of cancer frequency: Cancer incidence perceptions mirror distorted media depictions. *Journal of Health Communication, 19*, 609–624.

Jensen, J. D., Pokharel, M., Scherr, C. L., King, A. J., Brown, N., & Jones, C. (2017). Communicating uncertain science to the public: How amount and source of uncertainty impact fatalism, backlash, and overload. *Risk Analysis, 37*(1), 40–51.

Johnson, J. D. (1997). *Cancer-related information seeking*. Cresskill, NJ: Hampton Press.

Kimmerle, J., Flemming, D., Feinkohl, I., & Cress, U. (2015). How laypeople understand the tentativeness of medical research news in the media: An experimental study on the perception of information about deep brain stimulation. *Science Communication, 37*(2), 173–189.

Kiousis, S. (2001). Public trust or mistrust? Perceptions of media credibility in the information age. *Mass Communication & Society, 4*(4), 381–403.

Kitzinger, J. (1999). Researching risk and the media. *Health, Risk & Society, 1*(1), 55–69.

Kohring, M., & Matthes, J. (2007). Trust in news media development and validation of a multidimensional scale. *Communication Research, 34*(2), 231–252.

Kovach, B., & Rosenstiel, T. (2007). *The elements of journalism: What newspeople should know and the public should expect*. New York: Three Rivers Press.

Malka, A., Krosnick, J. A., & Langer, G. (2009). The association of knowledge with concern about global warming: Trusted information sources shape public thinking. *Risk Analysis, 29*(5), 633–647.

McCroskey, J. C., & Teven, J. J. (1999). Goodwill: A reexamination of the construct and its measurement. *Communications Monographs, 66*(1), 90–103.

McCroskey, J. C., & Young, T. J. (1981). Ethos and credibility: The construct and its measurement after three decades. *Communication Studies, 32*(1), 24–34.

Meyer, P. (1988). Defining and measuring credibility of newspapers: Developing an index. *Journalism & Mass Communication Quarterly, 65*(3), 567–574.

173

Mitchell, A., Gottfried, J., Barthel, M., & Shearer, E. (2016). The modern news consumer: News attitudes and practices in the digital era. Pew Research Center. Available from www.journalism.org/2016/07/07/the-modern-news-consumer (accessed on March 23, 2017).

National Center for Science and Engineering Statistics (NCSES). (2014). *Science and Engineering Indicators*. Available from www.nsf.gov/statistics/seind14/index.cfm/chapter-7/c7s3.htm (accessed on December 14, 2015).

Nelkin, D. (1996). An uneasy relationship: The tensions between medicine and the media. *The Lancet, 347*(9015), 1600–1603.

Niederdeppe, J., Lee, T., Robbins, R., Kim, H. K., Kresovich, A., Kirshenblat, D., Standridge, K., Clarke, C. E., Jensen, J. D., & Fowler, E. F. (2014). Content and effects of news stories about uncertain cancer causes and preventive behaviors. *Health Communication, 29*, 332–346.

Ober, S., Zhao, J. J., Davis, R., & Alexander, M. W. (1999). Telling it like it is: The use of certainty in public business discourse. *Journal of Business Communication, 36*(3), 280–296.

O'Neill, O. (2004). Accountability, trust and informed consent in medical practice and research. *Clinical Medicine, 4*(3), 269–276.

Peters, H. P., & Dunwoody, S. (2016). Scientific uncertainty in media content: Introduction to this special issue. *Public Understanding of Science, 25*(8), 893–908.

Popper, K. (2002). *The logic of scientific discovery*. New York: Routledge. (Originally published in 1934)

Post, S., & Maier, M. (2016). Stakeholders' rationales for representing uncertainties of biotechnological research. *Public Understanding of Science, 25*(8), 944–960.

Priest, S. H., Bonfadelli, H., & Rusanen, M. (2003). The "trust gap" hypothesis: Predicting support for biotechnology across national cultures as a function of trust in actors. *Risk Analysis, 23*(4), 751–766.

Retzbach, A., & Maier, M. (2015). Communicating scientific uncertainty: Media effects on public engagement with science. *Communication Research, 42*(3), 429–456.

Retzbach, J., Otto, L., & Maier, M. (2016). Measuring the perceived uncertainty of scientific evidence and its relationship to engagement of science. *Public Understanding of Science, 25*(6), 638–655.

Reyna, V. F. (1981). The language of possibility and probability: Effects of negation on meaning. *Memory & Cognition, 9*(6), 642–650.

Schwartz, L. M., Woloshin, S., & Welch, H. G. (1999). Risk communication in clinical practice: Putting cancer in context. *Journal of the National Cancer Institute Monographs, 25*(1), 124–133.

Siegel, R. L., Miller, K. D., & Jemal, A. (2015). Cancer statistics, 2015. *CA: A Cancer Journal for Clinicians, 65*(1), 5–29.

Siegrist, M., Connor, M., & Keller, C. (2012). Trust, confidence, procedural fairness, outcome fairness, moral conviction, and the acceptance of GM field experiments. *Risk Analysis, 32*(8), 1394–1403.

Sjöberg, L. (2001). Limits of knowledge and the limited importance of trust. *Risk Analysis, 21*(1), 189–198.

Star, S. L. (1983). Simplification in scientific work: An example from neuroscience research. *Social Studies of Science, 13*, 205–228.

Stryker, J. E., Moriarty, C. M., & Jensen, J. D. (2008). Effects of newspaper coverage on public knowledge about modifiable cancer risks. *Health Communication, 23*(4), 380–390.

Thiebach, M., Mayweg-Paus, E., & Jucks, R. (2015). "Probably true" says the expert: How two types of lexical hedges influence students' evaluation of scientificness. *European Journal of Psychology of Education, 30*(3), 369–384.

Yale, R. N., Jensen, J. D., Carcioppolo, N., Sun, Y., & Liu, M. (2015). Examining first- and second-order factor structures for news credibility. *Communication Methods and Measures, 9*(3), 152–169.

West, M. D. (1994). Validating a scale for the measurement of credibility: A covariance structure modeling approach. *Journalism Quarterly, 71*(1), 159–168.

Winter, S., Kramer, N. C., Rosner, L. & Neubaum, G. (2015). Don't keep it (too) simple: How textual representations of scientific uncertainty affect laypersons' attitudes. *Journal of Language and Social Psychology, 34*(3), 251–272.

9

EVALUATING ONLINE HEALTH INFORMATION SYSTEMS

Gary L. Kreps and Jordan Alpert

Introduction

Powerful new online health information systems have been shown to hold tremendous promise for enhancing the delivery and use of risk and health communication programs (Kreps, 2015; 2011b). Tremendous growth and widespread adoption of online health information systems, such as health information websites, interactive health decision support systems, and mobile health devices, have demonstrated great potential to enhance response to health and risk issues by supplementing and extending traditional channels for communication (Kreps, 2015). The use of new health information technologies can enable broad dissemination of relevant health information that can be personalized to the unique information needs of individuals facing health risks (Kreps, in press; Neuhauser & Kreps, 2008). These e-health communication channels can provide health care consumers and providers with the relevant health information they need to respond to serious health and risk issues exactly when and where they need the information (Krist, Nease, Kreps, Overholser, & McKenzie, 2016).

Unfortunately, many of the enthusiastic predictions about the amazing contributions of digital health programs for promoting response to risk and health issues have not reached fruition and the great potential of health information systems has resulted in limited returns (Kreps, 2014a; 2014b). Too often, health information technologies fail to communicate effectively with users due to problems with the ways the systems are designed and implemented with different audiences (Kreps, 2014b; Neuhauser & Kreps, 2010; 2008; 2003). To enhance the quality of online health and risk information systems, rigorous evaluation research needs to guide the design and refinement of these systems (Alpert, Krist, Aycock, & Kreps, 2016b; Kreps, 2002; 2014a; 2014c). It is necessary to conduct regular, rigorous, ongoing, and strategic evaluation of health and risk communication programs to guide development, refinement, and strategic planning (Green & Glasgow, 2006; Rootman et al., 2001).

Failure to engage in careful and concerted evaluation research is likely to doom the success of online health and risk communication systems (Kreps, 2002; 2014a). Evaluation research answers important questions about the specific influences online health communication programs have on different audiences, identifying which audiences are paying attention to the programs and what they are learning from the programs (Kreps, 2014a; Kreps & Neuhauser, 2013). Rigorously collected evaluation data can help identify when online health and risk communication programs are having any unintended influences, including boomerang and iatrogenic (negative) effects (Cho & Salmon, 2007; Rinegold, 2002). Poorly designed health and risk communication programs have had negative influences on key audiences, such as with the infamous National Youth Anti-Drug Media Campaign, which instead of combating the risk of widespread youth drug abuse, actually served to increase at-risk youths' interest in using illegal drugs (Hornik, Jacobsohn, Orwin, Piesse, & Kalton, 2008). Well-conducted evaluation research can help explain why health and risk communication programs work and don't work, as well as which parts of these programs work most effectively (Kreps, 2014a).

Formative Research

Formative evaluation research is conducted prior to the introduction of health and risk communication information systems to guide the design of these programs (Kreps, 2002; 2014a). Formative evaluation helps health information system designers answer key questions about the goals and purposes of the programs they are developing. The process of revealing formative evaluation data can clarify what system designers want to accomplish with specific health and risk communication programs, which audiences they want to reach and influence, and what they want audience members to do in response to these digital information system programs.

Formative data can provide essential information to system designers about the audiences they want to reach, such as what health and risk issues audience members are likely to be interested in, what audience members currently know about key health and risk issues, and which messages are likely to make sense to and resonate with different audiences. Formative evaluation data can be used to establish measurable goals and outcomes for online health and risk information programs. Formative data can be used to establish baselines for establishing current levels of knowledge about health and risk issues, as well as to identify key health and risk activities to track over time. Formative evaluation research can guide the adoption of relevant theories and intervention strategies to guide development and implementation of health and risk information systems. Furthermore, good formative evaluation research can also help ensure that health and risk communication programs are sensitive to unique audience needs, cultural orientations, literacy levels, and expectations (Kreps, 2014a; Neuhauser & Paul, 2011).

There are two primary and interrelated forms of formative evaluation research that are critically important to the design of health and risk information systems: needs analysis and audience analysis. *Needs analysis* is conducted to help systems designers develop a full understanding of the scope of health and risk issues, relevant behaviors, and current levels of knowledge about specific health and risk issues confronting different audiences. Needs analysis data helps system designers focus on the most relevant health and risk issues with their programs and provide audiences with the most useful and up-to-date health and risk information. It helps system designers determine the gaps between what is currently being done to respond to serious health and risk issues within different communities and what needs to happen to promote improved health and well-being.

Needs analysis data can often be most effectively collected through use of multiple research methods. Sometimes it is best to begin by observing existing data sets. For example, the use of archival analysis of existing data sets and materials, such as review of relevant epidemiological studies about disease incidence and outcomes, evaluation of previously conducted key audience surveys about knowledge and experiences concerning health and risk issues confronting different communities, and content analysis of public and private health utilization records and research reports concerning best practices for addressing specific health issues, can provide a wealth of relevant information for guiding the design and implementation of relevant digital health and risk communication programs (Alpert, Krist, Aycock, & Kreps, 2016c, Kreps, 2011a; 2014a). Sometimes, when there is insufficient data already collected about specific health and risk issues, new data needs to be collected to fully evaluate the health issues within specific communities. New needs analysis data can be collected using multiple methods, including use of self-report and observational measures, such as conducting surveys, interviews, and direct observations. Both quantitative and qualitative needs data can help health and risk information system designers develop a full understanding about relevant health issues.

Situation analysis is a form of needs analysis that examines the history and extent of specific health and risk issues within communities, focusing on how widespread the health and risk issues are, who the health issues affect, how the issues have been responded to in the past, and which recommendations have been made for ideal ways to address the health and risk issues. Channel analysis is a form of needs analysis that focuses on examining the current health and risk information systems being used within communities and how effective these channels have been in disseminating relevant health and risk information. SWOT analysis (strengths, weaknesses, opportunities, and threats) is a needs analysis framework that focuses on identifying and analyzing the internal and external factors that can have an impact on addressing community health and risk issues (van Wijngaarden, Scholten, & van Wijk, 2010). Needs analysis is essential for helping systems developers understand the nature of the health and risk issues that information systems are designed to address. It also indicates the kinds of information needed to address key health and risk issues.

Audience analysis is another form of needs analysis that focuses on providing information about the different key populations that health and risk information systems designers want to reach and influence. Audience analysis should provide system designers with information about which groups of people are at greatest risk for different health threats, what they currently know about key health threats, and what these audiences still need to know. It tells system designers what beliefs, attitudes, and values key audiences hold relevant to the health and risk issues that need to be addressed, how the audiences have responded to similar health and risk issues in the past, which different channels of communication they use for accessing health and risk information, and how effective these channels have been at providing them with accurate, relevant, and up-to-date health and risk information. Audience analysis also provides data about the most relevant communication characteristics of different key audiences, such as the primary languages they speak, their health literacy levels, their levels of trust in different information sources, and their receptivity to information about different health and risk issues. Audience analysis data are essential for guiding the design of responsive health and risk information systems.

Audience analysis data help system designers segment the most relevant and homogenous audiences for different health and risk information systems, so the information systems can be designed to be meaningful and influential for these key populations. This means that health information systems are typically best designed for specific audiences, illustrating the popular maxim that "one size does not necessarily fit every audience" (Kreps, 2012). Audience analysis data are generally collected by conducting interviews, focus groups, and surveys to gather self-report information from different populations. Sometimes key documents are analyzed, such as websites, online posts, letters, and newspapers through content analysis to examine key audience beliefs and attitudes about salient health and risk issues. Secondary analysis of relevant surveys, such as examination of data from the Health Information National Trends Survey (HINTS), can also provide relevant audience analysis data (Finney Rutten, Hesse, Moser, & Kreps, 2011; Hesse et al., 2005). In addition, observational data can provide insightful audience analysis data for guiding design of health and risk information systems. Formative evaluation research provides rationale and direction for the design of health and risk information systems that address important issues, provides relevant and up-to-date health and risk information, and reflects the unique cultures, communication orientations, and health information needs of intended audiences (Kreps, 2014a).

As the use of social media has become a vital channel for conducting online health communication campaigns, these media can also be leveraged as a powerful tool during formative evaluation research. In general, web-based tools and channels, including the use of popular social media systems like Facebook and Twitter, have advantages over in-person methods because these digital channels can transcend normal physical barriers (geographical distance and time constraints), making searchable content convenient to access and encouraging interactivity (Chu & Chan, 1998; Kreps, in-press). Social media reaches large and specific audiences that share common interests. Evidence suggests that up to 60% of public health departments employ at least one social media application, with nearly 90% using Twitter and 56% using Facebook (Thackeray, Neiger, Smith, & Van Wagenen, 2012). Facebook is the most popular social network for individual use, including use by 62% of adults 65 and older (Greenwood, Perrin, & Duggan, 2016). Other applications like Twitter, Pinterest, and Instagram are gaining popularity and tend to be used more by online adults ages 18–29, showing increasing potential for use to communicate health and risk information (Greenwood et al., 2016).

Eliciting feedback or input from social media users can be collected by reviewing websites, blogs, or social networking groups (Burke-Garcia, Berry, Kreps, & Wright, 2017). For instance, collecting needs or audience analysis from a key population segment that possesses relevant experience with a particular health and risk topic can be accomplished by posting a question on a Facebook wall to trigger a discussion (Neiger et al., 2012). This method is particularly effective to gather insights from hard-to-reach populations or when stigmatized issues are concerned. For instance, a discussion was created on a popular social networking website to understand teenagers' HIV risk prevention strategies (Levine et al., 2011). This technique enabled the researchers to capture the exact language used by teenagers to use in creating appropriate risk prevention messages, and was a convenient and low cost means for collecting valuable health communication insights.

Process Evaluation Research

To ensure that online health information systems achieve their health communication goals, it is important to test key program components during the roll-out and use of digital health and risk communication interventions process evaluation research (Moore et al., 2014). Health and risk information programs need to be carefully assessed to determine their suitability and effectiveness with different audiences for addressing specific health and risk issues. User responses can be tracked to determine whether health and risk information programs are working well with different audiences. Tests are often conducted to determine how effective the message strategies and the communication channels used are for disseminating health and risk messages. Field tests are often conducted to determine how well the digital health and risk intervention programs have been implemented in key settings. User responses to programs can be tracked over time, especially after refinements are made to the programs to illustrate program usage trends. Digital health and risk information programs can also be tested experimentally to determine how acceptable and usable they are for key audience representatives. These tests often generate user recommendations for refining health and risk communication program features that can be implemented to improve intervention programs. Process evaluation is essential for identifying strategies to improve the quality and delivery of online health and risk communication systems.

Process evaluation data can be collected with user-response systems, such as questionnaires, interviews, or focus groups, that ask representative program participants about their experiences using the health information system, as well as elicit their evaluations of the strengths and weaknesses of program components. These tools are sometimes referred to as user satisfaction surveys. The Critical Incident Method is an especially useful and sophisticated qualitative user-response system for process evaluation that asks representative users about the best and worst elements in health and risk information systems, providing insightful data leading to in-depth recommendations for emphasizing the strongest parts and refining the weakest elements of health and risk information systems (Alpert, Kreps, Wright, & Desens, 2015).

Message testing experiments are also often used to assess user responses to health and risk messages, examining how much users liked the messages, as well as how informative, how believable, and how influential the messages were. System users are typically asked to provide suggestions for revising the health and risk messages to make them clearer, more interesting, and more influential. A/B testing is a message testing strategy that compares two versions of a webpage or digital health and risk communication application against each other to determine which one performs better. Sometimes eye-tracking tests are conducted to determine which messages respondents focus on and which messages they find most arousing. There are also standardized text analysis programs that are used to assess readability levels of health and risk communication system content, such as use of the CDC's Clear Communication Index (Alpert, Desens, Krist, & Kreps, 2016a).

Usability tests are often conducted to determine how well different representative users can navigate online health and risk information systems (Kreps, 2014a; Nielsen, 1994; 1999). Representative system users are asked during usability tests to demonstrate how they use the system, showing how they can navigate health and risk communication systems to find specific information on the systems. Researchers often will ask system users to comment on how easy or difficult it is for them to find information and navigate the health and risk communication systems during the usability tests, inviting respondents to suggest better ways to design the information systems to make them easier and more effective to use. The data provided from the usability tests can reveal hidden system flaws and suggest strategies for refining health and risk communication system design. For instance, a digital exercise simulation called BringItOn, which was designed by Albu, Atack, and Srivastava (2015) to increase users' physical activity levels to promote health, recovery, or rehabilitation, was subjected to usability testing that included heuristic expert analysis and think-aloud verbal protocol. Heuristic analysis involves having an expert, in this case a software engineer, evaluate an application and compare it to industry best practices (Nielsen, 1994). The think-aloud verbal protocol involves asking a user to describe decision-making criteria used during a problem-solving task (Fonteyn, Kuipers, & Grobe, 1993). Based on these data gathered through these methods, BringItOn revised the software to better fit the needs and wants of participants.

In addition to usability tests, system usage data are tracked to identify who uses the health and risk information system, how often they use the system, and how much time they spend interacting with the system (Kreps, 2002). Tracking data can often be collected unobtrusively through analysis of system use and billing records. Also, website usage metrics and surveys can be tracked to measure levels of reach and engagement. This type of process evaluation tracking was utilized in the FaceSpace Sexual Health Promotion Project, with the metrics providing objective data about audience usage of the system and the timing of their engagement with the system (Nguyen et al., 2013). Survey data were gathered to explain users' online and sexual behaviors, while team meeting notes kept records of the challenges associated with conducting a sexual health promotion program using social media (Nguyen et al., 2013). While usage data are interesting, it is often necessary to question users directly to find out why they use the system, how well the system works for them, and whether the information they accessed from the system influenced their health decisions, behaviors, and outcomes (Kreps, 2014a; Webb, Campbell, Schwartz, & Sechrist, 1972). Process evaluation research is critically important for tracking user responses to health and risk information systems over time and for providing evidence for refining system components to effectively meet the needs of system users (Kreps, 2002).

Summative Evaluation Research

Summative evaluation research is used to measure overall influences and outcomes from online health and risk information systems. Summative research is conducted after the health and risk information system has been in use for a substantial period of time to document the positive and negative influences the information system has had on addressing key health issues. Many of the evaluation research methods that were used in conducting both formative and process evaluation research on health and risk information systems are conducted again to compare system performance over time. By comparing baseline (pre-test) data on audience member's beliefs, attitudes, knowledge, behaviors, and health status with outcomes (post-test) data on these same factors, a quasi-experimental, pre-post field test can be conducted to assess changes that have occurred during use of the health and risk information system. These changes can be compared to measures of comparison groups that did not have access to the health and risk information system to illustrate whether changes that occurred with the test group were related to system use. The summative evaluation data that are collected can provide important measures about the overall usefulness of online health and risk communication programs for addressing important issues and promoting public health (Kreps, 2002; 2014a; Nutbeam, 1998).

Summative data are collected to examine overall patterns of health and risk information program use, user satisfaction with programs, message exposure and retention from the programs, changes in key outcome variables (such as learning, relevant health behaviors, health services utilization, and health status) related to the intervention, as well as to provide economic analyses of program costs and benefits (cost-benefit analysis). Summative research also identifies strategies for sustaining the best health and risk communication intervention programs over time. Strong summative evaluation data can be very influential in determining the overall value of the health and risk information systems, identifying specific directions for improving these digital systems, and securing support for establishing program sustainability and institutionalization (Kreps, 2014a).

A good way to bolster summative evaluation of online social media–based health communication programs is to utilize social media tracking web analytics to identify key program performance indicators (KPIs). KPIs are metrics that assess pre-established goals of a social media program (Sterne, 2010). Metrics such as the number of clicks, shares, mentions, and followers can be used to gauge a variety of KPIs, like improved levels of interaction and awareness. Other KPIs include exposure (the number of times content on social media is viewed), reach (the number of people who have contact with the social media application), and engagement (participation in creating, sharing, and using content) (Neiger et al., 2012).

183

Based on a campaign's goals, KPIs should be identified and defined during the formative and process evaluation research stages. To monitor KPIs, typically a social media performance dashboard is used, which is an insight tool that monitors media performance and provides guidance for digital health and risk communication program enhancement and optimization (Murdough, 2009).

Social media provides a wealth of information that could be evaluated both quantitatively and qualitatively. Summative evaluation dashboards can be used to evaluate reach, discussions, and general outcomes. Reach focuses on several factors, including: the volume of mentions, where mentions are occurring (e.g., Twitter, social networks, blogs, discussion forums) and the social influence of individuals discussing the issue (Murdough, 2009). Discussions identify the main topics or themes, the tone of discussions (e.g., positive or negative), and whether sentiment concerning the health and risk issues has changed (Murdough, 2009).

Conclusion and Future Directions

Evaluation research should be an indispensable part of the development and refinement of every online health and risk communication information system (Kreps, 2014a; Rootman et al., 2001). Such research enables system developers to utilize user experience in designing and refining health information systems. This process is known as participatory or user-centered design (Nuehauser, 2001; Neuhauser et al., 2007; Neuhaser & Kreps, 2011; 2014). User-centered design not only helps direct the development of sophisticated, user-friendly digital health and risk communication systems, but it also encourages overall user involvement with the information systems (Neuhauser, 2001). The best health and risk communication information systems are designed to involve intended system users, reflecting the experiences and insights of these system users (Neuhauser et al., 2007).

Evaluation researchers should carefully identify available sources of audience analysis data when assessing health and risk communication systems. What do we already know about key audiences for these health and risk programs? Are there natural sources of information about key events that can be used to inform health and risk system evaluation efforts, such as the use of medical billing records, public records, or message transcripts? Health and risk information system designers can often fruitfully design and build-in user-response mechanisms for online programs to provide regular user feedback about program use. Researchers should carefully identify relevant data about key audience attributes and behaviors to use as benchmarks for later comparisons after the use of health and risk communication programs, both from established data sources or from newly collected data, to establish key baselines and track changes (hopefully improvements in these key indicators) over time. Usability tests should be conducted regularly to determine the suitability of digital health and risk communication programs for different groups of users. Researchers should also work closely with key representatives from targeted audiences to conduct user-centered design and community participative evaluation research to examine audience responses to digital health and risk communication programs (Neuhauser et al., 2007). Data from evaluation research should be applied to refining and improving all digital health and risk communication programs.

References

Albu, M., Atack, L., & Srivastava, I. (2015). Simulation and gaming to promote health education: Results of a usability test. *Health Education Journal*, 74(2), 244–254.

Alpert, J. M., Kreps, G. L., Wright, K. B., & Desens, L. C. (2015, May). *Humanizing patient-centered health information systems: Critical incidents data to increase engagement and promote healthy behaviors.* Presented to the International Communication Association conference, San Juan, Puerto Rico.

Alpert, J., Desens, L., Krist, A., & Kreps, G. L. (2016a). Measuring health literacy levels of a patient portal using the CDC's Clear Communication Index. *Health Promotion Practice*, 18(1), 140–149. doi: 10.1177/1524839916643703.

Alpert, J. M., Krist, A. H., Aycock, B. A., & Kreps, G. L. (2016b). Designing user-centric patient portals: Clinician and patients' uses and gratifications. *Telemedicine and e-Health*, advance online publication. doi:10.1089/tmj.2016.0096.

Alpert, J. M., Krist, A. H., Aycock, B. A., & Kreps, G. L. (2016c). Applying multiple methods to comprehensively evaluate a patient portal's effectiveness to convey information to patients. *Journal of Medical Internet Research*, 18(5), e112. doi: 10.2196/jmir.5451.

Burke-Garcia, A., Berry, C., Kreps, G. L., & Wright, K. (2017). The power and perspective of mommy-bloggers: Formative research with social media opinion leaders about HPV vaccination. *Proceedings of the Hawaii International Conference on System Sciences*, HICSS-50, pp. 1932–1941. IEEE Computer Society Digital Library. URI: http://hdl.handle.net/10125/41388.

Cho, H., & Salmon, C. T. (2007). Unintended effects of health communication campaigns. *Journal of Communication*, 57(2), 293–317.

Chu, L. F., & Chan, B. K. (1998). Evolution of web site design: implications for medical education on the Internet. *Computers in Biology and Medicine*, 28(5), 459–472.

Finney Rutten, L., Hesse, B., Moser, R., & Kreps, G. L. (Eds.) (2011). *Building the evidence base in cancer communication.* Cresskill, NJ: Hampton Press.

Fonteyn, M. E., Kuipers, B., & Grobe, S. J. (1993). A description of think aloud method and protocol analysis. *Qualitative Health Research*, 3(4), 430–441.

Green, L. W., & Glasgow, R. E. (2006). Evaluating the relevance, generalization, and applicability of research: Issues in external validation and translation methodology. *Evaluation and the Health Professions*, 29(1), 126–153.

Greenwood, S., Perrin, A., & Duggan, M. (2016, November 11). Social media update 2016. Retrieved March 16, 2017, from www.pewinternet. org/2016/11/11/social-media-update-2016/.

Hesse, B. W., Nelson, D. E., Kreps, G. L., Croyle, R. T., Arora, N. K., Rimer, B. K., & Viswanath, K. (2005). Trust and sources of health information. The impact of the Internet and its implications for health care providers: Findings from the first Health Information National Trends Survey. *Journal of the American Medical Association (JAMA) Internal Medicine* (formerly *Archives of Internal Medicine*), 165(22), 2618–2624.

Hornik, R., Jacobsohn, L., Orwin, R., Piesse, A., & Kalton, G. (2008). Effects of the National Youth Anti-Drug Media Campaign on youths. *American Journal of Public Health*, 98(12), 2229–2236.

Kreps, G. L. (in press). Strategic design of online information systems to enhance health outcomes through communication convergence. *Human Communication Research*.

Kreps, G. L. (2002). Evaluating new health information technologies: Expanding the frontiers of health care delivery and health promotion. *Studies in Health Technology and Informatics*, 80, 205–212.

Kreps, G. L. (2011a). Methodological diversity and integration in health communication inquiry. *Patient Education and Counseling*, 82, 285–291.

Kreps, G. L. (2011b). The information revolution and the changing face of health communication in modern society. *Journal of Health Psychology*, 16, 192–193.

Kreps, G. L. (2012). Consumer control over and access to health information. *Annals of Family Medicine*, 10(5). Retrieved from www.annfammed.org/con tent/10/5/428.full/reply#annalsfm_el_25148.

Kreps, G. L. (2014a). Evaluating health communication programs to enhance health care and health promotion. *Journal of Health Communication*, 19(12), 1449–1459. doi: 10.1080/10810730.2014.954080.

Kreps, G. L. (2014b). Achieving the promise of digital health information systems. *Journal of Public Health Research*, 3(3), 421, 128–129. doi: 10.4081/ jphr.2014.471.

Kreps, G. L. (2014c). Epilogue: Lessons learned about evaluating health communication programs. *Journal of Health Communication*, 19(12), 1510–1514.

Kreps, G. L. (2015). Communication technology and health: The advent of ehealth applications. In L. Cantoni & J. A. Danowski (Eds.). *Communication and Technology*, Vol. 5 of *Handbooks of Communication Science*, pp. 483–493, (P. J. Schulz & P. Cobley, General Editors). Berlin, Germany: De Gruyter Mouton Publications.

Kreps, G. L., & Neuhauser, L. (2010). New directions in ehealth communication: Opportunities and challenges. *Patient Education and Counseling*, 78, 329–336.

Kreps, G. L., & Neuhauser, L. (2013). Artificial intelligence and immediacy: Designing health communication to personally engage consumers and providers. *Patient Education and Counseling*, 92, 205–210.

Krist, A. H., Nease, D. E., Kreps, G. L., Overholser, L., & McKenzie, M. (2016). Engaging patients in primary and specialty care. In Hesse, B. W., Ahern, D. K., & Beckjord, E. (Eds.), *Oncology informatics: Using health information technology to improve processes and outcomes in cancer care* (pp. 55–79). Amsterdam, The Netherlands: Elsevier.

Levine, D., Madsen, A., Wright, E., Barar, R. E., Santelli, J., & Bull, S. (2011). Formative research on MySpace: Online methods to engage hard-to-reach populations. *Journal of Health Communication*, 16(4), 448–454.

Moore, G., Audrey, S., Barker, M., Bond, L., Bonell, C., Cooper, C., Hardeman, W., Moore, L., O'Cathain, A., Tinati, T., Wight, D., & Baird, J. (2014). Process evaluation in complex public health intervention studies: The need for guidance. *Journal of Epidemiological Community Health*, 68, 101–102.

Murdough, C. (2009). Social media measurement: It's not impossible. *Journal of Interactive Advertising*, 10(1), 94–99.

Neiger, B. L., Thackeray, R., Van Wagenen, S. A., Hanson, C. L., West, J. H., Barnes, M. D., & Fagen, M. C. (2012). Use of social media in health promotion purposes, key performance indicators, and evaluation metrics. *Health Promotion Practice*, 13(2), 159–164.

Neuhauser, L. (2001). Participatory design for better interactive health communication: A statewide model in the USA. *Electronic Journal of Communication*, 11(3).

Neuhauser, L., Constantine, W. L., Constantine, N. A., Sokal-Gutierrez, K., Obarski, S. K., Clayton, L., Desai, M., Sumner, G., & Syme, S. L. (2007). Promoting prenatal and early childhood health: Evaluation of a statewide materials-based intervention for parents. *American Journal of Public Health*, 97(10), 813–819.

Neuhauser, L., and Kreps, G. L. (2003). Rethinking communication in the e-health era. *Journal of Health Psychology*, 8, 7–22.

Neuhauser, L., & Kreps, G. L. (2008). Online cancer communication interventions: Meeting the literacy, linguistic, and cultural needs of diverse audiences. *Patient Education and Counseling*, 71(3). 365–377.

Neuhauser, L., & Kreps, G. L. (2010). Ehealth communication and behavior change: Promise and performance. *Journal of Social Semiotics*, 20(1), 9–27.

Neuhauser, L., & Kreps, G. L. (2011). Participatory design and artificial intelligence: Strategies to improve health communication for diverse audiences. In N. Green, S. Rubinelli, & D. Scott. (Eds.), *Artificial intelligence and health communication* (pp 49–52). Cambridge, MA: AAAI Press.

Neuhauser, L., & Kreps, G. L. (2014). Integrating design science theory and methods to improve the development and evaluation of health communication programs. *Journal of Health Communication*, 19(12), 1460–1471.

Neuhauser, L., & Paul, K. (2011). Readability, comprehension and usability. In *Communicating risks and benefits: An evidence-based user's guide*. Silver Spring, MD: U.S. Department of Health and Human Services. Bethesda, MD: Food and Drug Administration.

Neuhauser, L., Schwab, M., Obarski, S. K., Syme, S. L., & Bieber, M. (1998). Community participation in health promotion: Evaluation of the California Wellness Guide. *Health Promotion International*, 13(3).

Nguyen, P., Gold, J., Pedrana, A., Chang, S., Howard, S., Ilic, O., Hellard, M., & Stoove, M. (2013). Sexual health promotion on social networking sites: A process evaluation of the FaceSpace project. *Journal of Adolescent Health*, 53(1), 98–104.

Nielsen, J. (1994). *Usability engineering*. Amsterdam, The Netherlands: Elsevier.

Nielsen, J. (1999). *Designing Web usability: The practice of simplicity*. Indianapolis, IN: New Riders Publishing.

Nutbeam, D. (1998). Evaluating health promotion—progress, problems, and solutions. *Health Promotion International, 13*, 27–44.

Rinegold, D. J. (2002). Boomerang effects in response to public health interventions: Some unintended consequences in the alcoholic beverage market. *Journal of Consumer Policy, 25*, 27–63.

Rootman, I., Goodstadt, M., McQueen, D., Potvin, L., Springett, J., & Ziglio, E. (Eds.). (2001). *Evaluation in health promotion: Principles and perspectives.* Copenhagen, Denmark: WHO.

Sterne, J. (2010). *Social media metrics: How to measure and optimize your marketing investment.* Hoboken, NJ: John Wiley & Sons.

Thackeray, R., Neiger, B. L., Smith, A. K., & Van Wagenen, S. B. (2012). Adoption and use of social media among public health departments. *BMC Public Health, 12*(1), 242.

van Wijngaarden, J. D. H., Scholten, G. R. M., & van Wijk, K. P. (2010). Strategic analysis for health care organizations: The suitability of the SWOT-analysis. *International Journal of Health Planning and Management.* Retrieved from www.researchgate.net/profile/Jeroen_Wijngaarden/publication/45094861_Strategic_analysis_for_health_care_organizations_the_suitability_of_the_SWOT-analysis/links/541fc9860cf203f155c25f28.pdf.

Webb, E. J., Campbell, D. T., Schwartz, R. D., & Sechrist, L. (1972). *Unobtrusive measures: Nonreactive research in the social sciences.* New York: Rand McNally & Company.

Part III

SITUATING THEORY IN RISK AND HEALTH COMMUNICATION CONTEXTS

10

EXAMINING PRINT COVERAGE OF THE KEYSTONE XL PIPELINE

Using the Social Amplification of Risk Framework

Michel M. Haigh

Using the Social Amplification of Risk Framework

On November 6, 2015, President Barack Obama announced the administration had rejected TransCanada's bid to build the northern section of the Keystone XL pipeline (KXL) (Carpenter, 2015). This was the end to a seven-year battle between politicians, environmentalists, and the energy industry.[1]

The debate started in September 2008 when TransCanada filed an application with the US Department of State to build the KXL pipeline. The pipeline would cross an international border, which is why the US Department of State had to approve it. In January 2012, President Obama rejected the initial 1,700-mile version of the pipeline that would travel from Alberta, Canada, to Port Arthur, Texas. In response, TransCanada split the project in two. The *northern section* would travel 875 miles from Alberta, Canada, to Steele City, Nebraska (Koch, 2014). The *southern section* of the pipeline would run from Cushing, Oklahoma, to the Gulf Coast. The proposed KXL was going to carry 830,000 barrels of oil per day and create 42,000 jobs. TransCanada said the pipeline would also transport oil production from the Bakken formation in North Dakota and Montana (Keystone XL opposition turns to beetle . . . , 2013).

The southern section known as the Gulf Coast pipeline began supplying oil in January 2014. Because the southern section did not cross a national border, it did not require State Department approval (Mufson, 2014). Obama rejected the building of the northern section in November 2015.

Public support for the KXL varied. In a 2013 poll conducted by the Pew Research Center, more than 65% of adults supported the KXL. By 2014, a poll conducted by *USA Today*, Stanford University, and the nonpartisan group Resources for the Future, found only 56% of adults supported the KXL project (Koch, 2014). The Energy Collective (Droitsch, 2014) wrote a piece and attributed the shift in public opinion to people learning more about the KXL. "There is growing awareness by Americans about the risks tar sands poses to climate, health and water . . . the more they ask for clean energy alternatives. Once people learn Keystone XL is not a generic pipeline carrying conventional oil but instead that it will carry tar sands, a uniquely corrosive and acidic mixture that will ruin water supplies when spilled," public support wanes (paragraph 4).

When rejecting the pipeline, President Obama said, "This pipeline would neither be a silver bullet for the economy as promised by some, nor the express lane to climate disaster proclaimed by others" (as cited in Carpenter, 2015, paragraph 8). The current study examines seven years of newspaper coverage at both the national and state (local) level to understand the story of the KXL. There are a number of different ways to frame the story about the KXL. This study examined if stories reflected more on the risks or benefits of the KXL, what frames were employed, and if the story varied at the national and local level of coverage. A longitudinal study was conducted to determine how the coverage changed over time.

Literature Review

Two frameworks guided this study, because they address the link between the media and policy—the social amplification of risk framework (SARF) and agenda setting.

Social Amplification of Risk Framework (SARF)

Kasperson et al. (1988) developed SARF to provide an integrative theoretical framework that would connect studies on risk from a number of theoretical perspectives including media research, psychometric and cultural schools, and organizational responses. "The social amplification of risk denotes the phenomenon by which information processes, institutional structures, social-group behavior, and individual responses shape the social experience of risk" (Kasperson et al., 1988, p. 181). They argue there is no "absolute" or "socially determined" risk. Risk depends on the public response influenced by information made available to them.

The SARF model starts with *risk events*—actual or hypothesized. The next part of the model is *amplification and attenuation*. Many variables amplify the risk. The variables include *sources of information* (e.g., personal experience, direct or indirect communication), *information channels* (e.g., individual senses, information social networks, and professional information brokers), *social stations* (e.g., opinion leaders, government agencies, news media), *individual stations* (e.g., decode message, rely on heuristics, evaluate and interpret), and *institutional and social behavior* (e.g., attitude change and social action). The amplification increases/decreases the amount of information society has available and the salience of the issue. This social amplification creates *ripple effects* (Kasperson et al., 1988).

These ripple effects may include the impact of risk on markets, community opposition, and loss of trust. Ripple effects also indicate stakeholder groups and the local community (those who can be impacted by the risk) may start to take action.

The current study is interested in the social amplification of risk. Specifically, it examines the social station of the news media. Singer and Endreny (1993) state the media report on risk events and not necessarily on risk issues. Whereas, Wilkins (1987) and Wilkins and Patterson (1987) state the media frame the risk discourse. "There can be no doubt that the mass media are an important element in communication systems, the processing of risk in amplification stations . . . [and] how risk problems are framed" (Kasperson, Kasperson, Pidgeon, & Slovic, 2003, p. 22).

Agenda Setting and Framing

In the original agenda setting study, McCombs and Shaw (1972) assume issues emphasized in news coverage influence the issues discussed in society. There are three research traditions for studying agenda setting, including the policy, media, and public agendas. Policy agenda setting examines how an issue arrives on the policy agenda. The media agenda is investigated to determine what makes the news. The final research tradition is the public agenda setting process (Dearing & Rogers, 1996). After more than 40 years of research, agenda setting has evolved to include multiple levels. The first level of agenda setting explains the transfer of object salience from the media to the public agenda (Ghanem, 1997). The second level of agenda setting examines the "way an issue or other object is covered in the media" (Ghanem, 1997, p. 4). It is important to understand how an issue is covered because this impacts the importance of the issue on the public agenda. This second level of agenda setting is often called framing.

Framing. Entman (1993) states, "Frames select and call attention to particular aspects of the reality described, which logically means that frames simultaneously direct attention away from other aspects" (p. 54). Media frames can be broken into four major dimensions: the topic of a news item (what is presented in the frame), presentation (size and placement), cognitive attributes (details of what is included), and affective attributes (tone or picture) (Willnat, 1997).

The cognitive and affective attributes of frames will influence how the public perceives an issue and its consequences. Individuals make their decisions about an issue by what is discussed in the media even though they lack all of the details (Jasperson, Shah, Watts, Faber, & Fan, 1998). Omitting definitions, problems, evaluations, and recommendations changes the information the public has available (Entman, 1993).

Each news story is unique because of the frame and the details omitted. The words and images used in news stories activate thoughts in readers (Taber, Lodge, & Glather, 2001). Readers use this information to build a knowledge network to employ when they want to discuss the topic (Entman, 2004).

There are many different types of frames. For example, *episodic frames* approach stories as a case study, event-oriented, and concrete instances; whereas, *thematic frames* place the issue in a larger more general context and provide background information. The use of an episodic or thematic frame impacts the attribution of responsibility. Episodic stories lead to individuals attributing responsibility to other individuals, and thematic frames lead to societal responsibility (Iyengar, 1991). When applying the SARF model, framing is the amplification and attenuation process carried out through the social station of the media system (Kasperson et al., 2003).

Nisbet and Huge (2007) examined frames used to discuss plant biotechnology. They developed several types of frames applicable in science communication research. The political strategy frame discusses the political debate about science issues. Most of the stories will discuss the actions of presidents, members of congress, or other political agencies. The public engagement/education frame is employed in stories discussing poll results, public opinion, awareness, or education of individuals about the issue (Nisbet & Huge, 2007).

Haigh (2010) found the US economy and political strategy frames were the most common frames employed to discuss alternative energy. Stories about alternative energy were very thematic. She concluded the information individuals had available to make decisions was policy-based since that was the dominant type of story frame.

Kasperson et al. (1988) said social amplification creates ripple effects. In other words, the social station of the media produces ripple effects by the way it frames the story. In the current study, the media create ripple effects by the frames it employs when discussing the KXL. The ripple effects may encourage stakeholder groups and the local community to get involved, which lead to regulatory changes. The original framework included four pathways to amplification. However, Kasperson et al. (2003) state there is now a fifth, defined as "high or growing social distrust of responsible institutions. Risk control efforts have frequently gone awry due to a lack of openness and "transparency" (p. 31). The current study examines how the US government and the energy industry were depicted in news coverage to determine what information the public had available to make decisions about the KXL. The study also examined if local and national media told the KXL pipeline story differently. States directly impacted by the KXL may focus on the direct impact of the pipeline and the risks associated with it being built; whereas the national media may discuss the impact of the KXL on the nation as a whole.

The current study examines how the media told the story of the KXL in order to determine if the media discussed the risk involved. It employs the frame categories developed by Nisbet and Huge (2007) and Haigh (2010) to see if the media focused on the economy, the public, the environment, or government policies when telling the KXL story.

Because the KXL is a national issue, thematic frames may be more common because they tend to place the issue in a larger context and provide background information. Haigh (2010) found thematic frames were the most common frames used when discussing alternative energy, so the same may be true here. She also found the frame used to discuss alternative energy varied from the national newspapers to the local newspaper coverage (e.g., differed in US economy frame and the type of alternative energy discussed). The tone of coverage and depiction of the energy industry also varied over time. Therefore, the following hypotheses and research questions are posited:

H1: Newspaper stories will use a dominant thematic frame to discuss the KXL, and nominal level frames will focus on: the US economy, the environment, political strategies, and public engagement.

RQ1: Which category of risk *and* benefit (human, environmental, or social/economical) will be discussed more frequently in the KXL stories?

RQ2: How will the media depict the: a) US energy industry, and b) US government in print stories discussing the KXL?

RQ3: What are the differences between the local and national coverage of the KXL?

RQ4: Did newspaper coverage of the KXL vary over time?

Method

Sampling Method and Unit of Analysis

The unit of analysis in this study was a newspaper article ($N = 629$). Newspaper articles from September 1, 2008 to February 1, 2015 were coded. September 1, 2008 was the start date because it was during the month of September that TransCanada first asked the State Department for a permit to build the KXL. The end date for the study was February 1, 2015 because it was roughly two weeks after the State of the Union address.

Stories were gathered from *The New York Times*, *The Wall Street Journal*, *The Washington Post*, *USA Today*, and the *Los Angeles Times*. *The New York Times*, *The Wall Street Journal*, *USA Today*, and *The Washington Post* were selected because of their national influence. As "newspapers of record," these publications shape the agendas of other media outlets. The *Los Angeles Times* was chosen because of its status as a leading West Coast paper. The specific papers selected have the largest circulation in those states. After the national newspaper coverage was collected, *two daily papers* from each of the states the KXL would travel through were also selected (Montana, North Dakota, South Dakota, Nebraska, Kansas, Oklahoma, and Texas).

Articles from September 1, 2008 to February 1, 2015 were collected from all papers. Access World News/Newsbank and LexisNexis Academic Universe provided the full text articles. "Keystone XL" or "Keystone pipeline" were used as the search terms in headlines and lead paragraphs. Only articles printed in the specified time frame with some combination of these words in the headline or lead paragraph were actually included in the sample. Editorials, letters, and op-eds were not included in the final data analysis.

Coder Training

A written coding instrument was developed to code the sample ($N = 629$). The coding instrument explained the procedures the independent coders should utilize. There were several nominal level frame categories, interval-level scales, and categories of demographic information (publication, date, and year) coded. Five undergraduate students were recruited to evaluate the content of the newspaper articles. Several one-hour training sessions were held. After practicing together, 10% ($n = 63$) of the sample was randomly selected and coded independently. Coders established a high degree of standardization during the training phase. Coders were not retrained and intercoder reliability was not examined after the initial 63 articles were coded because coders established a high degree of reliability.

Employing Rosenthal's (1984, 1987) formula for interval level data and multiple coders, intercoder reliabilities ranged from .86 to .99 for the interval level scales employed (tone, overall frame, depiction of the US government, and depiction of the energy industry). Next, the research assistants were trained to use the Nisbet and Huge (2007) and Haigh (2010) frame categories (see Variables Measured section for frame categories) coded for present or absent. For the nominal level frame categories Krippendorff's alpha ranged from .80 to .99.

Variables Measured

Independent Variable. The independent variable in this study was the year the article was published. The years examined included 2008 ($n = 8$), 2009 ($n = 31$), 2010 ($n = 38$), 2011 ($n = 138$), 2012 ($n = 139$), 2013 ($n = 110$), 2014 ($n = 125$), and 2015 ($n = 40$). *Location of the paper* (national $n = 223$; or state $n = 406$) was also coded.

Dependent Variables. Overall tone of article was assessed using a global attitude measure adapted from Burgoon, Miller, Cohen, and Montgomery (1978). Haigh (2010, 2014) used this measure in previous content analyses research to measure tone of newspaper articles. It consisted of six, 7-interval semantic differential scales: good/bad, positive/negative, wise/foolish, valuable/worthless, favorable/unfavorable, and acceptable/unacceptable ($\alpha = .98$; $M = 3.88$, $SD = .51$).

Story frame. A single item, 7-interval scale was used to measure the extent an article employed episodic or thematic framing, where 1 = thematic and 7 = episodic ($M = 2.65$, $SD = 1.44$) (Haigh, 2010, 2014).

Frames Employed. The frames developed by Nisbet and Huge (2007) and Haigh (2010) were employed. The nominal level frames coded included: political strategy, public engagement/education, the US economy, and environmental frame. The frames were coded as present or absent.

Risk/benefit. Coders also coded the stories for risks/benefits of the KXL. The types of risk coded included: human, environmental, and social/economic. Each type of risk was coded as present or not present in the story. The benefits of the KXL coded were: human, environmental, and social/economic; they were coded as present or absent.

Depiction of the US energy industry was assessed using the Individualized Trust Scale (ITS) initially developed by Wheeless and Grotz (1977). The scale consisted of four, 7-interval semantic differential scales. Specific scale items included: trusting/untrusting, candid/deceptive, sincere/insincere, and honest/dishonest ($\alpha = .99$; $M = 3.82$, $SD = .56$). Haigh (2010) previously employed this measure in a content analyses project examining alternative energy. This scale was also used to examine *depiction of the US government* ($\alpha = .98$; $M = 3.89$, $SD = .60$).

Results

Hypothesis 1 predicted that the dominant frames used to discuss the KXL would be thematic and feature the US economy frame, the environmental frame, the political strategy frame, and the public engagement frame. Descriptive statistics were used to examine the frame categories. Stories discussing the KXL were thematic in nature ($M = 2.65$, $SD = 1.44$). The environmental frame (59.6%) was the most common frame employed. Followed by: the US economy frame (45.9%), the political strategy frame

(45.9%), and public engagement/education frame (10%). Hypothesis 1 was supported.

Research Question 1 asked which category of risk and benefit (human, environmental, or social/economic) would be discussed more frequently in the KXL stories. Descriptive statistics indicated environmental risk was the most common risk discussed (11.8%). Human risk (5.9%) was discussed more often than the social/economic risk (4.5%) involved with the KXL. When discussing the benefits of the KXL, social/economic benefits were discussed most frequently (30.2%). The human benefits of building the KXL were also discussed (29.7%), but the environmental benefits of the pipeline were rarely discussed (2.4%).

Research Question 2 asked how the media depicted the US government and energy industry in print stories discussing the KXL. A one-sample t-test indicated the sample mean of $M = 3.82$, $SD = .56$, for the *depiction of the energy industry* was significantly different than neutral (test value of 4.0) $t (628) = -7.95$, $p < .001$. The *energy industry* was depicted negatively in newspaper stories. The analysis indicates the sample mean for the variable depiction of the *US government* $M = 3.89$, $SD = .56$ was significantly different from 4.0 $t (224) = -2.94$, $p < .001$. Therefore, newspaper coverage depicted the *US government* negatively when discussing the KXL.

Research Question 3 asked if there were differences between the local and national coverage of the KXL. Frequencies show there were more stories about the KXL in the state newspapers ($n = 406$) compared to the national newspapers ($n = 223$). An analysis of variance (ANOVA) was conducted on the independent variable of *location of paper* and the dependent variables: overall frame, tone, depiction of the US government, and depiction of the US energy industry. Statistically significant differences were found for the dependent variables: *overall tone* $F (1, 628) = 6.70$, $p =.01$, $\alpha = .01$; and *overall frame* $F (1, 628) = 32.80$, $p =.000$, $\alpha = .05$. There were no statistically significant differences found for depiction of the US government or US energy industry.

Table 10.1 Frames Employed to Discuss Keystone XL

Frame Type	Not Present	Present
Environmental	40.4%	59.6%
U.S. Economy	54.1%	45.9%
Public Engagement	90.0%	10.0%
Political Strategies	54.1%	45.9%

Notes: Coders coded if the frame was 0 = not present, 1 = present. Percents are shown for each category. The frame categories were originally developed by Nisbet and Huge (2007) and Haigh (2010).

State newspapers (local coverage) were slightly less negative in tone (M = 3.92, SD = .52) than national newspapers (M = 3.81, SD = .48) when discussing the KXL. State newspapers (local coverage) used a more thematic frame when discussing the KXL pipeline (M = 2.41, SD = 1.40) than national newspapers (M = 3.08, SD = 1.42) when discussing the KXL. The state newspapers portrayed the US government (M = 3.92, SD = .58) slightly less negatively than the national newspapers (M = 3.84, SD = .54) because 4.0 would be considered neutral on the 7-point scale. State newspapers (M = 3.83, SD = .57) and national newspapers (M = 3.82, SD = .55) did not vary significantly on the depiction of the US energy industry or US government.

When examining the differences between the two types of newspapers for nominal frames and the coverage of risk/benefits, chi-square analyses were conducted. Only the significant differences are reported. Local newspapers were more likely to employ the *political frame* χ^2 (1, N = 629) = 29.62, p = .00; and the *environmental frame* χ^2 (1, N = 629) = 3.46, p = .06 when discussing the KXL pipeline compared to national newspapers.

Local newspapers were more likely to discuss the *social benefits* χ^2 (1, N = 629) = 6.13, p = .01; and *human benefits* χ^2 (1, N = 629) = 5.37, p = .02 of the KXL compared to national newspapers. The papers did not vary in discussing the types of benefits of the KXL (environmental, human, social).

Research Question 4 asked if newspaper coverage of the KXL varied over time. An analysis of variance (ANOVA) was conducted on the independent variable of *year* and the dependent variables: overall frame, tone, depiction of the US government, and depiction of the US energy industry. Statistically significant differences were found for the dependent variables: *overall frame* $F(1, 628)$ = 4.08, p =.00, α = .04; and *depiction of the energy industry* $F(1, 628)$ = 3.00, p =.00, α = .03. There were no statistically significant differences found for depiction of the US government ($F(1, 628)$ = 1.05, p =.40, α = .03) or overall tone of coverage ($F(1, 628)$ = .22, p =.98, α = .00). Tukey HSD post hoc tests were conducted to find specific significant differences. When looking at the years of coverage, 2009 is the year where the overall frame was the most thematic (M = 1.48, SD = 1.09). There were statistically significant differences in the mean of overall frame when comparing the year 2009 to the later years (2010–2015). When looking at the depiction of the energy industry, the statistically significant differences were found for the year 2011. There were significant differences for the year 2011 (M = 3.70, SD = .62) compared to 2009 (M = 4.03, SD = .71) and 2014 (M = 3.93, SD = .53). The energy industry was depicted *most negatively* in 2013 (M = 3.74, SD = .55) and *more positively* in 2009 (M = 4.00, SD = .34).

Tone of coverage was most negative in 2010 (M = 3.80, SD = .92). It was most positive in 2011 (M = 4.01, SD = .35) when discussing the KXL.

Depiction of the US government was *most negative* in 2015 ($M = 3.76$, $SD = .55$) and *most positive* in 2010 ($M = 4.10$, $SD = .32$) with 4.0 representing neutral on the 7-point scale.

When examining the differences in nominal frames and the coverage of risk/benefits, chi-square analyses were conducted. Only the significant differences are reported. There were significant differences for the *political frame* $\chi2$ (7, $N = 629$) $= 80.24$, $p = .00$; and the *environmental frame* $\chi2$ (7, $N = 629$) $= 31.50$, $p = .00$. The use of the *political frame* was most common in 2014 (83 stories employed this frame) and it was not used at all in 2008. The *environmental frame* was employed most often in 2011 (93 stories employed this frame) and only two times in 2008. When looking

Table 10.2 Stories Employing Different Frames to Discuss Keystone XL Over Time

Frame Type	Environmental	U.S. Economy	Public Engagement	Political Strategies
Year				
2008	2	3	1	0
2009	12	12	1	5
2010	25	18	2	8
2011	93	55	19	47
2012	77	75	15	64
2013	82	47	15	49
2014	68	55	10	83
2015	16	24	0	33
Total	375	289	63	289

Note: The actual total number of stories employing the frame is reported.

Table 10.3 Differences in Dependent Variables from 2008–2015

	Tone	Depiction of Energy Industry	Depiction of U.S. Government	Frame
Years				
2008	3.88 (.35)	3.88 (.83)	4.00 (.20)	1.65 (1.06)
2009	3.93 (.57)	4.03 (.71)	4.00 (.20)	1.48 (1.09)
2010	3.84 (.55)	3.82 (.51)	4.10 (.31)	2.73 (1.40)
2011	3.86 (.49)	3.67 (.61)	4.00 (.46)	2.69 (1.39)
2012	3.87 (.46)	3.81 (.52)	3.91 (.60)	2.77 (1.56)
2013	3.87 (.56)	3.81 (.54)	3.97 (.59)	2.62 (1.22)
2014	3.91 (.51)	3.92 (.52)	3.79 (.61)	2.74 (1.48)
2015	3.92 (.53)	3.92 (.35)	3.76 (.55)	2.92 (1.48)
Totals	3.88 (.51)	3.82 (.56)	3.89 (.56)	2.65 (1.4)

at the pattern of risk/benefit coverage, the only significant difference was found for the *environmental risk* χ^2 (7, $N = 629$) = 14.50, $p = .04$. Environmental risk was discussed most often in 2013 (21 mentions) compared to not being present during the 2008 coverage. Tables 10.2–10.3 show the means and standard deviations and the number of mentions.

Discussion

The current study examined seven years of newspaper coverage at both the national and state levels discussing the KXL. This study looked at the risks media discussed in news stories, the frames employed, and if the story varied in different locations over time.

Hypothesis 1 found stories discussing the KXL were thematic. This finding mirrors Haigh's (2010) finding about newspaper stories discussing alternative energy. The types of frames employed when discussing the KXL were also similar to the frames used to discuss alternative energy (Haigh, 2010). Iyengar (1991) stated thematic frames tend to lead to societal responsibility. Reporters telling the story at the national or local level did not try to personalize the KXL story by employing episodic frames.

Newspapers used the environmental frame most often in stories about the KXL. The US economy frame, the political strategy frame, and public engagement/education frame were also employed. Kasperson, Jhaveri, and Kasperson (2001) discuss risk amplification and stigmatization. When the information flows from the media, and the media frames the information in such a way, it will impact the public perceptions of the nature of risk, which will eventually lead to the public looking at the impact of the risk on society (e.g., the local economy or other places). The frames used when discussing the KXL indicate the public will understand the environmental risk. The frames used support the idea of the amplification and attenuation component of the SARF. Most of the frames were concerned with one of the different variables in the framework including *social stations* (e.g., opinion leaders, government agencies) and *institutional and social behavior* (e.g., attitude change or political changes) (Kasperson et al., 2003).

Research Question 1 found environmental risk was the most common risk discussed in newspaper stories about the KXL. The media discussed the environmental impact the KXL might have more so than focusing on the human or economic risk involved with the KXL. Because the KXL was originally supposed to stretch from one US border to the other, it covered a lot of physical area. The focus on environmental risk supports the Energy Collective's (Droitsch, 2014) claim Americans were becoming more concerned with the impact the tar sands (what the KXL was carrying) would have on climate, health, and water. The "ripple effects"—getting people engaged in the risk discussion—eventually led to impacts. The media focus on the environment matches the impacts Kasperson et al.

(2003) identify. They identify "regulatory actions, organizational change, increase or decrease in physical risk, community concern, and loss of confidence in institutions" (p. 14) in the updated SARF.

TransCanada said the KXL would bring jobs and boost the economies in the states where it would pass (North Dakota, South Dakota, Nebraska, Kansas, Oklahoma, Texas). However, the media in those states did not cover the KXL as having the potential to boost the economy through the creation of new jobs (Keystone XL opposition turns to beetle . . . , 2013).

Research Question 2 asked how the media depicted the US government and energy industry in print stories discussing the KXL. The energy industry and the US government were depicted negatively in newspaper stories. These findings support Kasperson et al.'s (2003) conclusion that there is a "high or growing social distrust of responsible institutions" (p. 31). As Ruckelshaus (1996) states, "The more mistrust by the public, the less effective government becomes at delivering what people want and need. . . . The more ineffective government becomes, the more people mistrust it" (p. 2). Trust is an important part of the social amplification and attenuation part of the SARF. Kasperson et al. (2003) state understanding trust is a significant part of understanding how social (e.g., news media) and individual stations process risk. In the case of the KXL, the public would probably not have confidence in the US government or the energy industry because they were depicted negatively over the seven-year period. If the public lacks trust in the US government or the energy industry, they are probably more concerned with the risk the KXL introduces to the local community rather than the benefits. Public support for the KXL started to decline over time, and it took the US government seven years to decide about the KXL. The public may have grown weary waiting for a decision.

Research Question 3 asked about the differences between the local and national coverage of the KXL. State newspapers were slightly less negative than national newspapers. This could be due to the fact that state media could discuss the impact the KXL would have locally, and that would be hard for the national media to do. The national newspapers portrayed the US government slightly more negatively than the state newspapers. This finding could be explained by the fact state newspapers would want to keep the KXL coverage "local" and the national newspapers would frame the story from a national perspective.

Research Question 4 asked if newspaper coverage of the KXL varied over time. Tone of coverage was most negative in 2010. During 2010, the Department of State held 21 public comment meetings in communities along the KXL route. It is important to note the public engagement frame was not employed more often when these meetings were being held. This frame was only found in two of the stories from 2010. The public engagement frame was used most often in 2011 when news coverage was neutral.

The depiction of the US government was most negative in 2015 and most positive in 2010. The political frame was not used in 2010. When the depiction of the US government was most negative (2015), that's when the political strategy frame was used more often.

The energy industry was depicted most negatively in 2013 and more positively in 2009. The environmental frame was not employed as often in 2009. The environmental frame was used most often in 2011 and 2013. These findings indicate the frames employed may have impacted how the US energy industry and government were depicted. This confirms Kitzinger's (1999) statement that "comparisons between media coverage at different points in time, several years apart, also add important perspectives. Studies adopting this method demonstrate how coverage shifts under different historical conditions" (p. 59).

Limitations, Future Directions, and Practical Implications

The current study did not examine op-eds, letters to the editor, or editorials about the KXL. Additional research should examine those types of pieces to see if the policy agenda was influenced by the content presented there. Additional research could also examine public comments made on the online news articles to see what media consumers were commenting about.

The media environment is changing, but the current study looked at a traditional form of mass communication—the newspaper. However, there are a number of other media platforms that could also be examined. Local broadcast news transcripts as well as national news transcripts could be studied to understand the frames being employed and the tone of coverage used in broadcast stories. Social media platforms could also be examined to see what the public was saying about President Obama's decision to reject the KXL.

There is also the missing link of examining the public agenda and public opinion data to determine if media coverage made the KXL more salient, and what exactly was being discussed in the media when public support declined. Calsamiglia and Ferrero (2003) state that "scientific voices have a limited role in the press, much less weight than those of political actors." Scientists are qualified sources because of their job titles, but are often portrayed as lacking specific knowledge (p. 170). The sources cited in the newspaper stories about the KXL should be examined. The type of source quoted (e.g., a scientist, a politician, an economist), if the person was local or national, and the type of industry the source worked in could determine how credible the public found the source cited. Understanding how science issues are covered in broadcast, print, and social media is important to understand how public opinion about science issues changes over time.

Conclusion

This is one of the only studies examining longitudinal coverage of the KXL. The story of the KXL varied over time. The frames employed focused on the environmental aspect of the pipeline, the public engagement, and political strategies tied to the pipeline. By employing the SARF, the study was able to use one of the *social stations* (e.g., news media) to examine the information flow (e.g., framing), as well as the *institutional and social behavior* (e.g., politicians) and the impact of discussing risk (e.g., policy changes).

Note

1 In January of 2017, President Donald Trump signed an executive order supporting the KXL. TransCanada has to reapply for the permit, and the US State Department will have to study the application and approve it. This chapter was completed prior to the executive order being signed, but it is important to note the debate over the KXL is not over.

References

Burgoon, M., Miller, M. D., Cohen, M., & Montgomery, C. L. (1978). An empirical test of a model of resistance to persuasion. *Human Communication Research*, 5(1), 27–39. doi: 10.1111/j.1468-2958.1978.tb00620.

Calsamiglia, H., & Ferrero, C. L. (2003). Role and position of scientific voices: Reported speech in the media. *Discourse Studies*, 5(2), 147–173. doi: 10.1177/1461445603005002308.

Carpenter, Z. (2015, November 6). President Obama says no to Keystone XL. *The Nation*. Available at: www.thenation.com/article/breaking-president-obama-says-no-to-keystone-xl/. Last accessed on January 31, 2017.

Dearing, J. W., & Rogers, E. (1996). *Agenda-setting* (Communication Concepts, Vol. 6). Thousand Oaks, CA: SAGE Publications.

Droitsch, D. (2014, January 30). New poll on Keystone XL tar sands pipeline indicating growing opposition, waning support. The Energy Collective. Available at: www.theenergycollective.com/danielle-droitsch/334201/new-poll-keystone-xl-tar-sands-pipeline-indicating-growing-opposition-pipel. Last accessed on January 31, 2017.

Entman, R. (1991). Framing U.S. coverage of international news: Contrasts in narratives of the KAL and Iran air incidents. *Journal of Communication*, 41(4), 6–27. doi: 10.1111/j.1460-2466.1991.tb02328.x.

Entman, R. (1993). Framing: Toward clarification of a fractured paradigm. *Journal of Communication*, 43(4), 51–58. doi: 10.1111/j.1460-2466.1993.tb01304.x.

Entman, R. (2004). *Projections of power: Framing news, public opinion, and U.S. foreign policy*. Chicago, IL: University of Chicago Press.

Ghanem, S. (1997). Filling in the tapestry: The second level of agenda setting. In M. McCombs, D. Shaw, & D. Weaver (Eds.), *Communication and democracy: Exploring the intellectual frontiers in agenda-setting theory* (pp. 3–14). Mahwah, NJ: Lawrence Erlbaum.

Haigh, M. M. (2010). Newspapers use three frames to cover alternative energy. *Newspaper Research Journal, 31*(2), 47–63.

Haigh, M. M. (2014). Afghanistan war coverage more negative over time. *Newspaper Research Journal, 35*(3), 38–51.

Iyengar, S. (1991). *Is anyone responsible? How television frames political issues.* Chicago, IL: The University of Chicago Press.

Jasperson, A. E., Shah, E. V., Watts, M., Faber, R. J., & Fan, D. P. (1998). Framing and the public agenda: Media effects on the importance of the federal budget deficit. *Political Communication, 15*(2), 205–224. doi: 10.1080/10584609809342366.

Kasperson, R. E., Renn, O., Slovic, P., Brown, H. S., Emel, J., Goble, R., Kasperson, J. X., & Ratick, S. (1988). The social amplification of risk: A conceptual framework. *Risk Analysis, 8*(2), 177–187. doi: 10.1111/j.1539-6924.1988.tb01168.x.

Kasperson, R. E., Jhaveri, N., & Kasperson, J. X. (2001). Stigma, places, and the social amplification of risk: Toward a framework of analysis. In J. Flynn, P. Slovic, & J. Kunreuther (Eds.), *Risk, media and stigma: Understanding public challenges to modern science and technology* (pp. 9–28). London: Earthscan.

Kasperson, J. X., Kasperson, R. E., Pidgeon, N., & Slovic, P. (2003). The social amplification of risk: Assessing fifteen years of research and theory. In N. Pidgeon, R. E. Kasperson, & P. Slovic (Eds.), *The social amplification of risk* (pp. 13–46). Cambridge, UK: Cambridge University Press.

Keystone XL opposition turns to beetle in the effort to block the $7 billion project, its thousands of jobs, and energy security. (2013, March 6). United Sates House Committee on Energy and Commerce. Available at: http://energycommerce.house.gov/content/keystone-xl.

Kitzinger, J. (1999). Researching risk and the media. *Health, Risk & Society, 1*(1), 55–69. doi: 10.1080/13698579908407007.

Koch, W. (2014, January 28). *USA Today* poll: Slight majority backs Keystone pipeline. *USA Today.* Available at: www.usatoday.com/story/news/nation/2014/01/28/keystone-pipeline-poll/4935083/. Last accessed on January 31, 2017.

McCombs, M. E., & Shaw, D. L. (1972). The agenda-setting function of mass media. *Public Opinion Quarterly, 36*(2), 176–187. Available at: www.jstor.org/stable/2747787.

Mufson, S. (2014, January 21). Keystone pipeline's southern leg to begin transporting oil to U.S. Gulf Coast. *The Washington Post.* Available at: www.washingtonpost.com/business/economy/oil-to-begin-flowing-in-southern-leg-of-keystone-pipeline/2014/01/21/ffe35abc-82bb-11e3-bbe5- 6a2a3141e3a9_story.html. Last accessed on January 31, 2017.

Nisbet, M. C., & Huge, M. (2007). Where do science debates come from? Understanding attention cycles and framing. In D. Brossard, J. Shanahan, & T. C. Nesbitt (Eds.), *The public, the media, & agricultural biotechnology* (pp. 193–230). Cambridge, MA: CABI.

Rosenthal, R. (1984). *Meta-analytic procedures for social research.* Beverly Hills, CA: SAGE.

Rosenthal, R. (1987). *Judgment studies: Design, analysis, and meta-analysis.* Cambridge, UK: Cambridge University Press.

Ruckelshaus, W. (1996, November 15). *Trust in government: A prescription for restoration.* The Webb Lecture to the National Academy of Public Administration. Washington, DC.

Singer, E., & Endreny, P. (2003). *Reporting on risk: How the mass media portray accidents, diseases, other hazards.* New York: Russell Sage Foundation.

Taber, C. S., Lodge, M., & Glathar, J. (2001). The motivated construction of political judgments. In J. H. Kuklinski (Ed.), *Citizens and politics: Perspectives from political psychology* (pp. 198–226). New York: Cambridge University Press.

Wheeless, L. R., & Grotz, J. (1977). The measurement of trust and its relationship to self-disclosure. *Human Communication Research, 3*(3), 250–257. doi: 10.1111/j.1468-2958.1977.tb00523.x.

Wilkins, L. (1987). Shared vulnerability: The mass media and American perception of the Bhopal disaster. Westport, CT: Greenwood Press.

Wilkins, L., & Patterson, P. (1987). Risk analysis and the construction of news. *Journal of Communication, 37*(3), 80–92. doi: 10.1111/j.1460-2466.1987.tb 00996.x.

Willnat, L. (1997). Agenda setting and priming: Conceptual links and differences. In M. McCombs, D. L. Shaw, & D. Weaver (Eds.), *Communication and democracy: Exploring the intellectual frontiers in agenda-setting theory* (pp. 51–66). Mahwah, NJ: Erlbaum.

11

TERRORISM, RISK COMMUNICATION, AND PLURALISTIC INQUIRY

Kevin J. Macy-Ayotte

> Risk communication can be defined as the exchange of information among interested parties about the nature, magnitude, significance, or control of a risk.
>
> (Covello, 1992, p. 359)

Communication about the causes, consequences, and control of danger has long been part of human society. Although the stakeholders Covello (1992) enumerated, i.e. "government agencies, corporations or industry groups, unions, the communications media, scientists, professional organizations, public interest groups, communities, and individual citizens" (p. 359), have a decidedly modern character, Palenchar (2009) noted that speculation about the probability of dangerous events can be traced back to the time of the Babylonians. The more formal emergence of risk communication as a distinct, if not fully coherent, area of scientific and academic inquiry can be traced to the mid-20th century concern with industrial hazards and the then-novel dangers of nuclear technology. To some extent, from that early interest through today, the analysis of risk has always been multidisciplinary in the sense that different fields (chemistry, engineering, meteorology, medicine, etc.) each dealt with potentially hazardous phenomena, and various academic disciplines (psychology, public health, communication, and more) have contributed research offering insights on ways to disseminate information about risks to various stakeholders. There is ample evidence of the opportunity for such disciplinary pluralism—scholars from psychology, public health, communication studies, international relations, and many other disciplines all publish research relevant to the study of risk communication, but the potential contributions of all are rarely considered in any particular article.

Communicating the Risk of Terrorism

Although of some limited interest during the final two decades of the Cold War between the United States and the Soviet Union, communication about terrorism threats did not receive much focused attention from risk communication scholars until the September 11, 2001 terrorist attacks. Following shortly after, the dissemination of anthrax spores in US mail in October and November 2001 further demonstrated the importance of communicating effectively with the public about the risks associated with bioterrorism. In particular, the difficulties—and in some cases failures—of communication by the Centers for Disease Control and other government agencies about risk to the public and appropriate protective measures have been well documented (Becker, 2005; Vanderford, 2003). Recognizing the potential benefit of applying expertise in communication processes to the increasing range of terrorist threats, Sparks, Kreps, Botan, and Rowan (2005) argued that "communication scholars need to become involved in providing research-based expertise both theoretically and methodologically for constructing, tailoring, and evaluating messages in terrorism contexts" (p. 1). Nearly a decade later, however, Ruggiero and Vos (2013) observed that "relatively little attention has been paid to the topic [of terrorism risk communication] in communication journals" (p. 163).

Ruggiero and Vos' (2013) worry about the dearth of communication research on terrorism risks serves as a useful starting point for reflection upon both the continuing need for such research and the danger of theoretical and methodological narrowness, sometimes outright parochialism, in existing research on terrorism risk communication. To begin with, Ruggiero and Vos note that the majority of articles in their survey relied upon empirical methodologies, itself documentation of the preference for, or at least primary visibility of, quantitative research over humanistic (e.g., rhetorical and critical) methods of inquiry.

However, Ruggiero and Vos' own methodology is illustrative of potentially problematic assumptions about what counts as legitimate terrorism risk communication research. Their review of scholarship on terrorism and communication found 435 articles altogether that the literature review authors then culled to 193 by sorting for "scientific articles" as well as other criteria (p. 154). Although the authors specify their exclusion of opinion pieces and commentary, the criteria for an article to qualify as "scientific" were not explicitly articulated. European scholars sometimes label research as "scientific" in fields such as philosophy that would likely be described as "humanistic" in the United States. While the European descriptor of "scientific" connotes systematic analysis, in the US it is generally reserved for quantitative (and less commonly, qualitative) empirical research. But a careful examination of the exemplars mentioned by Ruggiero and Vos suggests they employed criteria that filtered out certain theoretical and methodological approaches as unscientific. The categories identified by the authors for their summary literature review include the role of cultural knowledge and popular culture in influencing perceptions of terrorism risk (p. 158), as well as a category for "leadership communication and rhetoric" (p. 159) containing research on President George W. Bush's "public communication and crisis rhetoric" regarding the September 11, 2001, terrorist attacks. However, the examples cited do not include any of the widely recognized scholars (e.g., Dana Cloud, Jeremy Engels, Stephen Hartnett, Robert Ivie, Roger Stahl, and Carol Winkler) who regularly publish in communication journals on the topic of terrorism. It is possible that critical and rhetorical scholarship on communication about terrorism was not actively excluded but simply missed in the initial survey, but this too would demonstrate a methodological assumption substantially limiting what counts as risk communication research.

The absence of rhetorical approaches to the study of risk communication in general is not new, whether because few scholars employed rhetorical methods or because editors and reviewers have found such work less worthy of publication (Grabill & Simmons, 1998). In the case of terrorism preparedness exercises, federal government planning similarly tends to presume the empirical quantifiability of risk. For example, Danisch (2011) described the Department of Homeland Security's "primary method of risk management" where "event trees and decision analysis are added to 'multi-attribute analysis'" (p. 242) in the study of bioterrorism risks in general. He documented this particularly with the 2005 TOPOFF 3 simulation response exercise involving a multi-city terrorist dispersal of plague bacteria, chemical gas, and conventional explosive devices. Planning for the 2003 TOPOFF 2 exercise, involving a radiological terrorist event, included elements intended to highlight affective and sometimes intangible influences on hypothetical victim and public behaviors, but Becker (2005) noted that TOPOFF 2 "did not undertake a systematic effort to capture relevant information and insights" (p. 525) on the handling of psychosocial aspects of bioterror threat perceptions and accompanying public behaviors that were actually built into the scenario at the two hospital sites.

Even some of the existing calls for reflection on risk communication research about terrorism, while acknowledging the uncertainty and limitations of conclusions reached by currently predominant empirical research, further entrench a narrow awareness of potentially valuable theories and methods. For instance, after documenting the inadequacy of attempts to precisely quantify terrorism risks (given the constantly changing variables surrounding any given threat), Haimes (2011) emphasizes the need for "a continuous quantification of the dynamically evolving risk function" regarding terrorism (p. 1184). In other cases, even calls for methodological pluralism are subsequently co-opted by preferences for empirical research.

For example, Lee, Lemyre, and Krewski (2010) state that "it is increasingly recognized that these more qualitative, dreaded, and unknown facets of risk have real consequences on individuals' feelings and behaviors that must be accounted for in risk-management frameworks" (p. 242), but the authors proceed to study those qualitative perceptions of terrorism risks quantitatively with Likert-type surveys.

Sparks et al. (2005) list several areas of communication studies that they argue should be brought to bear on the study of terrorism risk communication, ending with the inclusive final phrase "among other relevant research areas" (p. 3), but notably absent from the list are rhetorical and critical/cultural studies. Given that these areas represent two of the largest divisions of communication inquiry catalogued by the National Communication Association, and a significant amount of research on terrorism has been published by communication scholars using these approaches, their absence from what has been understood to count as risk communication research is troubling. Equally significant is the problematic manner in which some risk communication scholarship treats concepts like rhetoric in ways that would be unrecognizable to the vast majority of rhetoricians today. For example, Fischoff (2011) attempts to acknowledge the significance of rhetoric by announcing that risk "communications must adopt a rhetorical stance that is either *persuasive*, trying to induce some behavior (e.g., stock up, take shelter), or *nonpersuasive*, trying to facilitate informed decision-making (e.g., about how best to use the time until fallout arrives)" (p. 526). However, the notion that information can somehow be segregated from its potentially persuasive implications, as if the content and manner of information dissemination has no effect on its persuasive force, would find little purchase with any contemporary rhetorical theorist.

To be clear, the fact that researchers prefer particular theoretical frameworks, even to the point of privileging some in describing their discipline, is neither a novel observation nor unusual. Merton (1996) observed two decades ago that the "very difference of perspective" in theoretical frameworks "typically leads them to focus on different rather than the same problems" (p. 36). Unfortunately, the tendency of the preference for particular theories to result in the artificial competition, or overt exclusion, of differing theories is also not exactly a new phenomenon. As Merton noted, although "theories are often complementary or unconnected rather than contradictory," the inability or refusal to acknowledge that fact "often results in the mock controversies that recurrently pepper the history of the sciences" (p. 36). Such controversies about theory and method can be found in virtually all academic disciplines, and across them as well; the "science wars" that emerged in debates about the application of humanistic inquiry to natural sciences during the 1990s are especially illustrative (see Slack & Semati, 1997; Sokal, 1996). These intellectual divisions are thus clearly not unique to the study of risk communication. Moreover, the fact that risk is implicated in so many different facets of human life, and that so many different academic fields are impacted by the study and practice of risk communication, itself generates some of this theoretical partisanship.

As Althaus (2005) has noted, "Each discipline applies a particular form of knowledge to uncertainty so as to order its randomness and convert it into a risk proposition" (p. 569). Expanding upon Althaus' claim, Palenchar and Heath (2007) conclude that "each discipline is an epistemological system that focuses on risk matters with a unique set of bifocals and varying interpretive screens" (p. 122). The fact of these different lenses for inquiry in diverse academic disciplines is not itself a point for judgment or blame; as scholars in different fields, even when we study the same phenomenon, we examine it with different interests, from differing angles, and with different assumptions. Medical doctors may be especially interested in the accurate diagnosis of the pathogen deployed in a suspected biological attack, public health officials may be focused on the status of the disease as communicable or not, and health communication experts planning messages about the suspected attack might focus on whether public audiences understand the difference between infectious and communicable disease in order to determine the language used in press releases. Too often, however, the understandable differences in disciplinary focus become not merely different lenses but limits to what researchers consider as relevant or legitimate expertise. One illustration that may be especially striking for communication scholars is Fischoff's (2011) relegation of "communication specialists" to the role of creating "channels for staying in touch" (p. 529) with the public, while it is "psychologists who can study their audience's needs, design potentially effective communications, and evaluate their usefulness" (p. 528). Fischoff's privileging of psychology might merely be a nod to the article's publication venue, *American Psychologist*, yet that would still demonstrate the entrenched fragmentation of diverse disciplines that all have a part to play in risk communication.

The gulf between disciplines is, as noted above, often replicated within academic fields. Sometimes those differences are the result of the necessary specialization that comes with developing expertise on a given subject and attendant inexperience with alternative theories or methods. Other times, the privileging of one theoretical framework has as much to do with implicit attributions of professional status as it does with the explanatory potential of a given theory. As Robert Hariman (1986) observed three decades ago, "theoretical discourse is political discourse—that is, it inevitably establishes relations of dominance and subordination" (p. 45).

The politics of theory manifest in myriad ways. Most people have probably experienced a colleague denigrating theoretical frameworks to which said colleague doesn't subscribe, and not in all cases because of documented inaccurate conclusions or lack of intellectual rigor. The motives are many: the competitive socialization of graduate school, intradepartmental politics, adaptation to a particular journal, and sometimes simply intellectual parochialism. This disciplinary, theoretical, and methodological fragmentation may not be uncommon, but it is singularly unhelpful for advancing the prospects of risk communication, particularly about terrorism.

Interdisciplinary Theoretical and Methodological Pluralism

Consistent with the tendency toward empiricism in terrorism risk communication research described in the previous section, much of the risk and crisis communication literature frames its goal as helping the public understand what experts believe to be the objective truth of a particular danger. Risk communication research has long lamented the disconnect between public attitudes or behaviors and what hazard experts and risk communication scholars see as the "facts" of a given threat. Current risk communication theory is mostly positivist—i.e., focused only on providing objectively provable information to the publics—which is why there is a great deal of emphasis placed on transparency and clarity in such communications. These empirical approaches to the study of risk communication are necessary, but not sufficient to fully analyze risk communication about terrorism (Ayotte, Bernard, & O'Hair, 2009). Groves and Newman's (1990) observation about the need for pluralistic inquiry in criminology offers a useful analogy: "Positivism works well in establishing co-variations between defined variables. But it does not address, nor does it try to address, the 'meaning' crime has for individuals or for society generally" (p. 106). The "meaning" of terrorism risks, and recalling the range of elements Covello (1992) included—"nature, magnitude, significance, or control of a risk" (p. 359)—is helpful here, but will not adequately be assessed exclusively by any one theory or method.

A far more promising approach to studying terrorism risk communication would be one that seeks out and values interdisciplinary theoretical and methodological pluralism. Such an approach emerges logically from the fundamentally uncertain nature of risk. As Beck (2002) postulates, risk as a concept "presumes decision-making" and requires efforts at "calculating the incalculable" (p. 40) that will always fall short of certainty. Similarly, Palenchar and Heath (2007) observe, citing Aristotle's notion that humans think precisely because of the impossibility of certainty in human affairs, that "[t]he very nature of risk prohibits absolute definitions and knowledge" (p. 125). The humility that should follow from the inability to know with objective certainty, from the inevitable incompleteness of human knowledge, can also serve as the impetus for pluralistic research.

First, terrorism risk communication research must demand interdisciplinary perspectives. At the most basic level, research from different fields must be recognized as potentially valuable to understanding the multiple facets of terrorism threats. The nature of a hypothetical bioterrorist threat encompasses the biology of a weaponized pathogen, the physics of the agent's dispersal, and an adversary's motivation to attack. The probability of the risk depends upon a host of factors, all of which might be evaluated by several academic disciplines. Magnitude not only depends upon the pathogen and dispersal but also variables of epidemiology and the success of response efforts. The response implicates the accuracy and feasibility of public health messages, the public's ability to interpret messages given existing cultural discourses about terrorism, the news media's ability and interest in transmitting information without editorializing, and material resources and distribution plans. Thus, rather than assuming that one discipline's approach is superior, Althaus (2005) recommends that we bring to bear on risk communication what we all know *differently*. Disciplinary pluralism in risk communication research will not be helpful, however, if such perspectives remain fragmented. As Groves and Newman (1990) state, "A truly interdisciplinary approach integrates material from various disciplines into a single image. It is not merely additive" (p. 106). Practitioners of many disciplines must talk to each other with the goal of understanding how distinct or even seemingly divergent perspectives contribute to a more robust understanding of a given risk.

Second, taking seriously the uncertain nature of risk requires acknowledging the necessarily limited nature of a given theory or method for studying it; theoretical pluralism is not just a good idea but a necessary compensation for the limits of any given perspective. As an alternative to the hope for unattainable certainty in risk communication, Palenchar and Heath (2007) acknowledge the insights of narrative theory, which posits that people interpret the world and live their lives not as rationally calculating machines but as participants in a story whose events, characters, and plot are *arguments* rather than objective facts. Such a view necessarily recognizes the value of rhetorical theories and methods, among many other frameworks, and not only those focused on narratives. The uncertainty on which risk is based leads Danisch (2011) to conclude that "[t]he very concept of risk serves as a well of probable knowledge from which many different kinds of arguments can be drawn" (p. 238). Sellnow, Littlefield, Vidoloff, and Webb (2009) turned to argumentation theory in a study of risk communication about terrorist hoaxes because of the nature of such hoaxes as false claims in need of refutation, but we should not restrict ourselves to looking at the words of terrorists as arguments. All risk communication could be tested as argumentation for a particular understanding of the threat, as well as recommended preparedness measures, policy responses, and crisis behavior, all of which rely upon "practical reasoning based on the values and norms to which a group or society is already committed" (Sellnow et al., 2009, p. 138).

The terrorist threat assessments by government agencies and other analysts, upon which all subsequent risk communication is based, depend upon an analysis of both an enemy's capabilities and the vulnerabilities of the potential target, the latter of which are often "matters of heated domestic controversy" (Freedman, 2005, p. 384) regarding individual and collective beliefs about various political, social, economic, and philosophical values and institutions. Claims about the nature of enemy capabilities and intentions are also the result of analytic calculations, which are inevitably shaped by ideology, worldview, emotion, and a host of symbolic connections that shape perceptions of the significance and relevance of data. We cannot assume the objective character of any threat or intelligence estimate, since preferences for various policies and hoped-for outcomes can shape analysis at all levels: "advocates of particular strategic choices develop theories of vulnerability to rationalize their preferences and then seek intelligence estimates which add weight to their theories" (Freedman, 2005, p. 384). The cherry-picking of intelligence regarding Saddam Hussein's WMD capability prior to the 2003 Iraq War offers an especially stark example of the consequences for later risk communication about WMD and terrorist threats. We would be better served by taking to heart Burke's (1969) admonition that descriptions of reality are always "*selections* of reality," and therefore necessarily a "*deflection* of reality" (p. 59) as well. If our goal as risk communication researchers is better public understanding of risk and the attendant behaviors for minimizing it, we must actively encourage accounting for many different "selections of reality."

Terrorism, Risk, and the Limits of Parochial Inquiry

This section offers two extended examples of the need for, and value of, interdisciplinary scholarship on terrorism risk communication that is theoretically and methodologically pluralistic. That is, scholarship that takes seriously the contributions of differing disciplines and that both draws from, and is open to, an array of differing theories and approaches to inquiry. The first example considers the role of the media as the primary conduit for risk communication about terrorism, and the second example examines several articles in a special issue of the journal *Terrorism and Political Violence* attacking critical terrorism scholars for allegedly legitimizing terrorism. The goal in each example is not to present an exhaustive case study but rather to demonstrate concretely the consequences of disciplinary, theoretical, and methodological parochialism in specific instances of research on terrorism risk communication.

Mediated Risk

It is a basic fact of terrorism risk communication that "[m]ost Americans must rely exclusively on the media for terrorism-related information" (Nellis & Savage, 2012, p. 751; see also Dobkin, 1992). Luckily, most Americans have no direct experience with terrorism as victims or spectators, much less as participants. Nearly all of our spectatorship, as well as official risk communication about terrorism, is experienced through our television screens and other news media. Although the role of the media in disseminating information about terrorism is generally well recognized, Heilbrun, Wolbransky, Shah, and Kelly (2010) interestingly separate the news media from the government as risk information sources, writing that "[w]hile the media play an important role in providing information . . . , individuals are also likely to depend upon the federal government for ongoing information regarding personal and collective risks of terrorism" (p. 721), as if information from the federal government is not almost always disseminated via the news media. Even when the news media transmit unedited announcements from government sources, those official messages are almost certainly book-ended by interpretive commentary that audiences may not disaggregate when processing the nature of a threat. The point here is not the significance of a single study that fails to understand the ubiquity of media as the fundamental channel through which risk communication flows, but instead the value of fully integrating media theory (which does fully understand the ubiquity of media framing) with this research.

A different problem results from the failure to account adequately for the various ways in which the structural constraints of the news industry, audience reception, and the intertextuality of media messages inevitably shape the meanings of terrorism that are ultimately available to public audiences. The media are often blamed for failures of risk communication (e.g., Murray, Schwartz, & Lichter, 2001; Willis & Okunade, 1997). Heilbrun et al. (2010) note that in addition to "media influences," "irrational fears" and "trouble understanding probabilities . . . may lead people to overestimate and underestimate the seriousness of risk and inappropriately respond to such risks" (p. 719). Although they're a step toward acknowledging the range of variables (not all of them quantifiable) affecting public interpretation of risk communication, the solutions proffered by scholars from outside the field of media studies, or without attention to the insights especially of critical media theory, often simply replicate a positivist hope for the realization of an ideal transmission model of communication. Lowrey et al. (2007), for example, acknowledge that "[n]ews reports of terrorism and natural disasters . . . sometimes have been faulted for inaccurate, incomplete, and sensational coverage that may contribute to public misunderstanding of risks," but emphasize that "[r]esearch suggests journalists are unprepared to cover terrorism and many types of natural disasters, in part because journalists lack sufficient expertise in science and medicine" (p. 2). This leads Lowrey et al. (2007) to call on risk communicators to "[t]ranslate and disseminate the work of experts in health and risk communication" (p. 7) for use by journalists and public information officers. Although that may be part of the solution, whether through training scientists to communicate with lay audiences or training journalists in basic science and research methods, there is also a need for interdisciplinary approaches to the study of risk communication that account for the inherent complexities of mediated communication in the first place, not merely the "translation" of positivist empirical research, as if the mediated channel itself does not shape the message that ultimately reaches public audiences. Even if those deficiencies of science communication were remedied, for instance, it would be inadeqaute to deal with what Mueller (2005) has described as the news media's "congenital incapacity for dealing with issues of risk and comparative probabilities" (p. 226). At least three distinct challenges complicating the media's capacity to serve as the transparent conduit of accurate information about terrorism risks become apparent only when reading across disciplines and with a sincere willingness to consider seriously theoretical and methodological frameworks that may be unfamiliar and perhaps already prejudged with skepticism.

First, a variety of structural factors simultaneously incentivize media exaggeration of risks and disincentivize calmer, more nuanced coverage. In Mueller's (2005) words, "Reporters and politicians mostly find extreme and alarmist possibilities so much more appealing than discussions of broader context, much less of statistical reality" (p. 226), and the reasons are myriad. Experts who may have a financial stake in industry or grant funding tied to terrorism preparedness have an incentive to exaggerate threats, politicians and analysts likely face greater reputational risks for being wrong about a terrorist event than a non-event, and consumers of media and political discourse drive the demand for drama in public culture (see also Dobkin, 1992; Lowrey et al., 2007). Many media scholars have documented the ways in which finite limits on journalists' financial resources and time, against the pressure to meet submission deadlines, lead to the over-reliance on government and other elite sources of information (e.g., Ericson, Baranek, & Chan, 1987; Hall, Critcher, Jefferson, Clarke, & Roberts, 1978; Herman & Chomsky, 2002; Singer & Endreny, 1993; Vincent, 1992). Some of these official sources may have a direct financial incentive to choose alarmism over accuracy, as "[t]here is no surer way for the national labs or the intelligence agencies to receive more money from the Treasury than by hyping the terrorist threat, particularly if the word 'nuclear' can be attached to it" (Weiss, 2015, p. 84). The same was true of federal funding for biodefense research after 2001, and a robust analysis of mediated risk communication about bioterrorism would have to account for incentives at all levels that potentially shape the subjective interpretation of threat information.

Second, the many reasons public audiences have difficulty interpreting probabilities according to the mathematical standards of risk researchers has also been well documented (e.g., Slovic, 1987). One difficulty is that, as Sunstein (2003) explains,

> in the face of ignorance, people assess probabilities through the use of various heuristics, most notably the availability heuristic, in accordance with which probability is measured by asking whether a readily available example comes to mind. . . . In the aftermath of a terrorist act, and for a period thereafter, that act is likely to be both available and salient, and thus to make people think that another act is likely.
>
> (p. 121)

Sunstein's reminder of the need to account for the impact of proximal terrorist events upon interpretations of the probability of future terrorist attacks is important, but greater theoretical scope might help researchers to recognize that a broad range of elements could serve as "available and salient" examples used by audiences to interpret risk scenarios. Hall et al. (1978) describe the news media's reliance upon "cultural 'maps'" through which they "'make sense' for their audiences of the unusual, unexpected and unpredicted events which form the basic content of what is 'newsworthy'" (p. 54; see also Altheide, 2007). Ayotte (2011) documents the news media's inordinate reliance on cultural maps embedded in US popular culture, not just the CDC or the federal government, to explain the 2001 anthrax attacks, which led CNN to turn to novelist Richard Preston as a "bioterrorism expert" (Ayotte, 2011, p. 8). Preston's alleged expertise had already been established by the bestselling status of his novel *The Cobra Event* (1997) and his nonfiction book *The Hot Zone* (1994), such that he had been invited to testify before the Senate in 1998 about the former Soviet Union's bioweapons program—testimony in which he misreported the historical transmission rate of anthrax by a factor of 10 (Ayotte, 2011, p. 11). Thus, the semiotic proximity of popular culture may in some cases be as significant as recent material events in providing available information for public audiences. The key lesson for risk communication researchers is that in the 2001 anthrax attacks and the later SARS outbreak, national news media in some cases turned as often to popular writers as to CDC experts for public information about disease risks, and so our modes of inquiry must draw from a range of theories and disciplines adequate to the complexity of that phenomenon.

Third, Sunstein (2003) also notes that people are likely to engage in "probability neglect" (p. 122), wherein they fail to account for the (un)likelihood of harm for a given risk because of their focus on the horror of the negative impact. Sunstein cites one small study where the vividness of the description of cancer death (as illustrative of the emotional aspect of impact magnitude) seemed to be responsible for substantial effects on participant responses (pp. 124–126). In the context of research in communication studies (Ayotte, 2011; Keränen, 2008) and public policy (Stern, 1999) confirming that visceral revulsion of harms associated with WMD may result in disproportionate feelings of dread and horror, Sunstein's (2003) analysis helps to explain why the news media's tendency to the dramatic may carry very real consequences for the public's interpretation of mediated risk communication.

The various critical media theories drawn upon above—propaganda studies, Marxist political economy, post-structuralist semiotics, and several approaches to cultural studies—demonstrate on-point utility for identifying the gaps in some existing critiques of the media in risk communication research. The conclusions above are reinforced by rhetorical scholarship, as "what is taken to be knowledge of terrorism risks is constructed in significant part by the rhetoric through which those risks are described" (Ayotte et al., 2009, p. 608). Whether the rhetorical characteristics of risk communication emerge in the message development process, the media's dissemination of risk messages, or the audience's interpretation of risk discourse, diverse approaches to risk communication enhance the quality of the overall conclusion. The point is not to disparage empirical research that has not integrated media and rhetorical theory, but rather to emphasize the need to supplement it with awareness of structural, linguistic, and ideological limitations to the transparency, accuracy, and clarity with which the news media will ever be able to communicate information about terrorism risks.

(Un)critical Terrorism Studies

Seeking in part to broaden the theoretical horizons of risk communication scholars to include nuanced questions about the social construction of threats, Palenchar and Heath (2007) argue that "[r]isk communication becomes a tool for communicating values and identities as much as being about the awareness, attitudes and behaviors related to the risk itself" (p. 127). The nature of risk as a potential hazard to something valued necessarily begs the question of how that value came to be established and whose interests are served or threatened by that hazard. Those values and identities, of audiences and risk communicators themselves, are not previously established but rather constituted and reinforced through the discourse in which risks are described and responses prescribed. Questions like this underlie, for instance, Beck's (2002) concern about the phenomenon of "methodological nationalism," which "equates societies with nation-state societies, and sees states and their governments as the cornerstones of a social science analysis. . . . These premises also structure empirical research, as in, for example, the choice of statistical indicators, which are almost always exclusively national" (p. 51). Notable for the current discussion of interdisciplinary, pluralistic inquiry is that critical media and cultural studies scholar Noam Chomsky (1989; see also Herman & Chomsky, 2002) leveled much the same criticism against official US government discourse about terrorism and its omission of violence perpetrated by the United States and ally states.

In the late 1990s, some critical theorists working primarily in departments of international relations and geography began drawing upon a broad array of philosophical, linguistic, and social theories to challenge what they saw as the narrowly positivistic approaches then dominating the discipline of international relations; work in this area came to be referred to under the rubric of Critical Security Studies (see, for example, Campbell, 1998; Krause & Williams, 1997; Shapiro, 1997). A contemporary extension of this critical inquiry regarding the study and representation of international security threats focused specifically on terrorism has emerged under the label of Critical Terrorism Studies (CTS) (e.g., Dixit & Stump, 2016; Jackson, 2007; Jackson, Smyth, & Gunning, 2009; Jarvis, 2009). It is against the backdrop of CTS research, and the sometimes surprisingly visceral and unscholarly reaction to it by other terrorism researchers, that we find another useful example of the opportunity for, and resistance to, theoretical pluralism in risk communication about terrorism.

In 2013, the journal *Terrorism and Political Violence* published a special issue entitled "The Intellectuals and Terror: A Fatal Attraction." Although not exclusively focused on terrorism risk communication, this journal is among the most prominent publishing academic work on the threat of terrorism. If we are to take seriously Covello's (1992) definition of risk communication as including information about the nature of a risk, then the research published in this journal falls squarely under the purview of terrorism risk communication. Recalling Palenchar and Heath's (2007) previously cited observation that risk communication is as much "a tool for communicating values and identities" as it is for describing "the awareness, attitudes and behaviors related to the risk itself," interrogation of the sort of values and identities propounded by this issue of *Terrorism and Political Violence* represents an invaluable exercise in the exploration of theoretical pluralism.

Ranging beyond scholarship specifically associated with the label of CTS, several of the articles in this special issue nonetheless engage lines of argument commonly found in CTS research. Claiming that "[i]ntellectuals have even provided the perpetrators of violence with a legitimacy of sorts at different junctures" (Rimon & Schleifer, 2013, p. 511), the editors provide a platform from which several authors attempt to discredit critical scholarship that asks exactly the sort of questions about the discursive and

219

methodological construction of values and identities in risk communication research called for by Palenchar and Heath (2007) and Beck (2002). The special issue further exemplifies the resistance to theoretical pluralism that is the focus of this chapter. As Hopkins (2014) noted, the special issue of *Terrorism and Policitcal Violence* is "published within a context whereby the editors, the authors and the references they use all have a singular ideological view of terrorism, and where certain assumptions on power and legitimacy are unquestioned" (p. 301). The articles by Landes (2013), Hollander (2013), and Geifman (2013) illustrate the implications of the theoretical parochialism displayed in this journal's special issue.

To begin with, consider this passage from Landes' (2013) article, which establishes the tone of his argument:

> Nothing is more useful to Jihadi ambitions . . . than non-Muslim intellectuals who insist that Islam is a religion of peace; that it is perfectly consonant with democracy; that the terrorists represent a tiny, marginal deviation from true Islam. . . . Historically, no more inane claim can be put forth than that a belligerent (if not the most belligerent) creed . . . could be called "a religion of peace."
>
> (p. 622)

The first thing to note is that Landes does not offer a single piece of evidence to support his claim, not even an asserted contrast to the similarly well-documented bloody history of the Crusades. Landes' (and apparently the editors') assumption of the self-evident truth of such a strident and negative generalization about an entire religion should give any serious researcher pause. By contrast, scholars from various disciplines have disproven the validity, and documented the harms, of the homogenization and vilification of Islam (Ayotte & Husain, 2005; Said, 1994; Said, 1997).

Landes (2013) additionally asserts that postmodern and post-colonial theory are responsible for legitimizing terrorism: "The 'Other' in post-colonial discourse inspired by Levinasian-Derridean post-modernism has come to occupy such a central position that some thinkers actually argue the epistemological priority of the ethnic or national 'Other'" (p. 626). Again, Landes cites no examples, footnoting only his own blog post as evidence, a post whose only mentions of Jacques Derrida consist of secondary references to two conference papers about the late French philosopher. Other scholars have found it similarly acceptable to dismiss the relevance of Derrida's work to the project of Critical Terrorism Studies without bothering to cite a single word of the philosopher's work (e.g., Jones & Smith, 2009). The uncritical caricature of postmodern theory, and particularly of Derrida, reflects a surprisingly widespread comfort with dismissing divergent theoretical frameworks with little expectation of intellectual engagement, which carried over even into the public obituaries (some eulogistic and others bizarrely gleeful) following Derrida's death (Tumolo, Biedendorf, & Ayotte, 2014).

Two other authors in the special issue offer broad indictments of any scholarship that identifies Palestinian suicide bombings and other terrorist violence as a response to Israeli or US foreign policies. Hollander (2013) labels virtually all such critical analyses "rationalizations" (p. 528) of terrorism by "left-of-center" "Western academic intellectuals, especially in the humanities and social sciences" (p. 519). Geifman (2013) goes even further in the special issue, asserting that terrorism scholars who criticize Israeli counter-terrorism policies may be suffering from Stockholm syndrome. She implies that such critical perspectives amount to "redirecting liability from the architects of brutality to its victims," allegedly "[a] common symptom of the Stockholm syndrome" (p. 557). The lengthy history of people, from doctors to demagogues, who have relied upon intimations of insanity to disparage or marginalize those with divergent views has been well-documented (van Voren, 2009). Suffice it to say that Geifman's pseudo-psychiatry should be a less-than-compelling reason to dismiss an entire category of terrorism scholarship that happens to differ from hers.

More importantly, if, as Heath and Waymer (2014) recommend, risk communication researchers and policy makers must ask "what message, value position, identity, or interest are some terrorists attempting to communicate" (p. 242), then contra Hollander (2013) and Geifman (2013), we must include in our analyses the self-described motives of terrorists like Osama bin Laden (2001), who himself identified the alleged violence of Israel and Western powers as the impetus for Al Qaeda's terrorism. To simply describe bin Laden's own rationalizations is not to legitimize them, any more than a prosecutor is rationalizing the motive of a murderer when attempting to win a conviction at trial. The hijackers of TWA flight 847 claimed their motive to be partly retaliation for a CIA-involved car bombing in Beirut targeting Sheik Fadlallah, which failed to get Fadlallah but killed dozens and wounded many more (Dobkin, 1992). Far from the Leftist propaganda imagined by Hollander and Geifman, it was the CIA that coined the term "blowback" to label exactly this phenomenon (Johnson, 2000, p. 8). Military scholars have thusly for decades described terrorism, the proliferation of weapons of mass destruction, and guerilla tactics as "asymmetric" responses to the conventional military superiority of the United States and other countries (e.g., Burrows & Windrem, 1994; Cottam, 1988; Klare, 1995; Sloan, 1998).

Because of the nature of journal special issues, the aforementioned articles by Landes (2013), Hollander (2013), and Geifman (2013) may not have gone through the normal anonymous peer-review process designed to ensure rigor and objectivity of research. But the publication of articles that skimp on even basic expectations of evidentiary documentation, analytical reasoning, and openness to intellectual disagreement does not satisfy our need for robust research that helps us understand the nature of terrorism risks. We cannot rely on *ad hominem* arguments or facile reasoning to discount perspectives that differ from ours, and we should object to scholarship that does so when we encounter it.

Conclusion

As documented by Merton (1996), the call for theoretical pluralism is decades old, spanning the natural and social sciences as well as humanistic disciplines. It is a worthy, if unfinished, project because robust research demands an accumulated diversity of inquiry. The stakes involved in the success or failure of risk communication, particularly that about terrorism, make this an important area for pluralistic research. The inevitably incomplete perspective of any one approach to the study of terrorism risks makes such pluralism necessary, since understanding the "contextual complexity" of terrorism risk communication "requires a multi-dimensional approach that combines different disciplines, methodologies, theories and levels of analysis" (Crelinsten, 2002, p. 110). This chapter has sought, through a review of literature on terrorism risk communication and analysis of extended examples of mediated risk communication and the controversy about Critical Terrorism Studies, to demonstrate the need for, and value of, interdisciplinary theoretically and methodologically pluralistic inquiry. Through the sources cited and the integration of complementary and diverse scholarship on terrorism, this chapter has also attempted to put into practice this call for pluralistic research on terrorism risk communication.

The success of efforts to improve the effectiveness of messages about terrorism risks will depend on researchers' ability to account for the myriad influences on risk interpretations by both the media and public audiences. Although not independently a sufficient approach to terrorism risk communication research, Critical Terrorism Studies, and even the theoretical poverty on display in *Terrorism and Political Violence*'s special issue, may offer new perspectives on terrorism threats of significant value to risk communication scholars. This is not to say that each of us must personally utilize theoretical frameworks or methodological tools with which we are unfamiliar or disagree. Nor should we hesitate to criticize research that we believe lacks theoretical coherence or methodological rigor. But we must cultivate theoretical perspectives that differ from our own, with the expectation that they demonstrate their usefulness to the endeavor of better risk communication, in order to develop the most thorough understanding and response to risk that we are able.

References

Althaus, C. (2005). A disciplinary perspective on the epistemological status of risk. *Risk Analysis*, 25(3), 567–588. doi: 10.1111/j.1539-6924.2005.00625.x.

Altheide, D. (2007). The mass media and terrorism. *Discourse & Communication*, 1(3), 287–308. doi: 10.1177/1750481307079207.

Ayotte, K. J. (2011). A vocabulary of dis-ease: Argumentation, hot zones, and the intertextuality of bioterrorism. *Argumentation and Advocacy*, 48(1), 1–21.

Ayotte, K. J., Bernard, D. R., & O'Hair, H. D. (2009). Knowing terror: On the epistemology and rhetoric of risk. In R. L. Heath & H. D. O'Hair (Eds.), *Handbook of risk and crisis communication* (pp. 607–628). New York: Routledge.

Ayotte, K. J., & Husain, M. E. (2005). Securing Afghan women: Neocolonialism, epistemic violence, and the rhetoric of the veil. *NWSA Journal*, 17(3), 112–133.

Beck, U. (2002). The terrorist threat: World risk society revisited. *Theory, Culture & Society*, 19(4), 39–55. doi: 10.1177/0263276402019004003.

Becker, S. M. (2005). Addressing the psychosocial and communication challenges posed by radiological/nuclear terrorism: Key developments since NCRP Report no. 138. *Health Physics*, 89(5), 521–530. doi: 10.1097/01.HP.0000172142. 89475.d2.

bin Laden, O. (2001, December 27). Transcript: Bin Laden video excerpts. *BBC News*. Retrieved from http://news.bbc.co.uk/1/hi/world/middle_east/1729882.stm.

Burke, K. (1969). *A grammar of motives*. Berkeley: University of California Press.

Burrows, W., & Windrem, R. (1994). *Critical mass: The dangerous race for superweapons in a fragmenting world*. New York: Simon and Schuster.

Campbell, D. (1998). *Writing security: United States foreign policy and the politics of identity* (Rev. ed.). Minneapolis: University of Minnesota Press.

Chomsky, N. (1989). *Necessary illusions: Thought control in democratic societies*. Boston, MA: South End Press.

Cottam, R. (1988). *Iran and the United States: A cold war case study*. Pittsburgh, PA: University of Pittsburgh Press.

Covello, V. T. (1992). Risk communication: An emerging area of health communication research. In S. A. Deetz (Ed.), *Communication yearbook 15* (pp. 359–373). Newbury Park, CA: SAGE.

Crelinsten, R. D. (2002). Analysing terrorism and counter-terrorism: A communication model. *Terrorism and Political Violence*, 14(2), 77–122. doi: 10.1080/714005618.

Danisch, R. (2011). Risk assessment as rhetorical practice: The ironic mathematics behind terrorism, banking, and public policy. *Public Understanding of Science*, 22(2), 236–251. doi: 10.1177/0963662511403039.

Dixit, P., & Stump, J. L. (Eds.). (2016). *Critical methods in terrorism studies*. New York: Routledge.

Dobkin, B. (1992). *Tales of terror: Television news and the construction of the terrorist threat*. New York: Praeger.

Ericson, R., Baranek, P., & Chan, J. (1987). *Visualizing deviance: A study of news organization*. Toronto, Canada: University of Toronto Press.

Fischhoff, B. (2011). Communicating about the risks of terrorism (or anything else). *American Psychologist*, 66(6), 520–531. doi: 10.1037/a0024570.

Freedman, L. (2005). The politics of warning: Terrorism and risk communication. *Intelligence and National Security*, 20(3), 379–418. doi: 10.1080/02684520 500281502.

Geifman, A. (2013). The liberal left opts for terror. *Terrorism and Political Violence*, 25(4), 550–560. doi: 10.1080/09546553.2013.814494.

Grabill, J., & Simmons, W. (1998). Toward a critical rhetoric of risk communication: Producing citizens and the role of technical communicators. *Technical Communication Quarterly*, 7(4), 415–441. doi: 10.1080/10572259809364640.

Groves, W. B., & Newman, G. (1990). Criminology and epistemology: The case for a creative criminology. In D. M. Gottfredson & R. V. Clarke (Eds.), *Policy and theory in criminal justice: Contributions in honour of Leslie T. Wilkins* (pp. 91–112). Aldershot, Hants, UK: Avebury.

Haimes, Y. (2011). On the complex quantification of risk: Systems-based perspective on terrorism. *Risk Analysis*, 31(8), 1175–1186. doi: 10.1111/j.1539-6924.2011.01603.x.

Hall, S., Critcher, C., Jefferson, T., Clarke, J., & Roberts, B. (1978). *Policing the crisis: Mugging, the state, and law and order.* New York: Holmes and Meier.

Hariman, R. (1986). Status, marginality, and rhetorical theory. *Quarterly Journal of Speech*, 72(1), 38–54. doi: 10.1080/00335638609383757.

Heath, R., & Waymer, D. (2014). Terrorism: Social capital, social construction, and constructive society? *Public Relations Inquiry*, 3(2), 227–244. doi: 10.1177/2046147X14529683.

Heilbrun, K., Wolbransky, M., Shah, S., & Kelly, R. (2010). Risk communication of terrorist acts, natural disasters, and criminal violence: Comparing the processes of understanding and responding. *Behavioral Sciences and the Law*, 28(6), 717–729. doi: 10.1002/bsl.940.

Herman, E. S., & Chomsky, N. (2002). *Manufacturing consent: The political economy of the mass media* (Rev. ed.). New York: Pantheon Books.

Hollander, P. (2013). Righteous political violence and contemporary western intellectuals. *Terrorism and Political Violence*, 25(4), 518–530. doi: 10.1080/09546553.2013.814491.

Hopkins, J. (2014). Psychologically disturbed and on the side of the terrorists: The delegitimisation of critical intellectuals in *Terrorism and Political Violence*. *Critical Studies on Terrorism*, 7(2), 297–312. doi: 10.1080/17539 153.2014.906983.

Jackson, R. (2007). The core commitments of critical terrorism studies. *European Political Science*, 6(3), 244–251. doi: 10.1057/palgrave.eps.2210141.

Jackson, R., Smyth, M. B., & Gunning, J. (Eds.). (2009). *Critical terrorism studies: A new research agenda.* New York: Routledge.

Jarvis, L. (2009). The spaces and faces of critical terrorism studies. *Security Dialogue*, 40(1), 5–27. doi: 10.1177/0967010608100845.

Johnson, C. A. (2000). *Blowback: The costs and consequences of American empire.* New York: Metropolitan Books.

Jones, D., & Smith, M. (2009). We're all terrorists now: Critical—or hypocritical—studies "on" terrorism? *Studies in Conflict & Terrorism*, 32(4), 292–302.

Keränen, L. (2008). Bio(in)security: Rhetoric, scientists, and citizens in the age of bioterrorism. In D. Zarefsky & E. Benacka (Eds.), *Sizing up rhetoric* (pp. 227–249). Long Grove, IL: Waveland Press.

Klare, M. (1995). *Rogue states and nuclear outlaws: America's search for a new foreign policy*. New York: Hill and Wang.

Krause, K., & Williams, M. C. (Eds.). (1997). *Critical security studies: Concepts and cases*. Minneapolis: University of Minnesota Press.

Landes, R. (2013). From useful idiot to useful infidel: Meditations on the folly of 21st-century "intellectuals." *Terrorism and Political Violence, 25*(4), 621–634. doi: 10.1080/09546553.2013.814504.

Lee, J., Lemyre, L., & Krewski, D. (2010). A multi-method, multi-hazard approach to explore the uniqueness of terrorism risk perceptions and worry. *Journal of Applied Social Psychology, 40*(1), 241–272. doi: 10.1111/j.1559-1816.2009.00572.x.

Lowrey, W., Evans, W., Gower, K., Robinson, J., Ginter, P., McCormick, L. C., & Abdolrasulnia, M. (2007). Effective media communication of disasters: Pressing problems and recommendations. *BMC Public Health, 7*, 97. doi: 10.1186/1471-2458-7-97.

Merton, R. K. (1996). Theoretical pluralism. In P. Sztompka (Ed.), *On social structure and science* (pp. 34–40). Chicago, IL: University of Chicago Press.

Mueller, J. (2005). Simplicity and spook: Terrorism and the dynamics of threat exaggeration. *International Studies Perspectives, 6*(2), 208–234. doi: 10.1111/j.1528-3577.2005.00203.x.

Murray, D., Schwartz, J., & Lichter, S. R. (2001). *It ain't necessarily so: How media make and unmake the scientific picture of reality*. Lanham, MD: Rowman & Littlefield.

Nellis, A., & Savage, J. (2012). Does watching the news affect fear of terrorism? The importance of media exposure on terrorism fear. *Crime & Delinquency, 58*(5), 748–768. doi: 10.1177/0011128712452961.

Palenchar, M. J. (2009). Historical trends of risk and crisis communication. In R. L. Heath & H. D. O'Hair (Eds.), *Handbook of risk and crisis communication* (pp. 31–52). New York: Routledge.

Palenchar, M., & Heath, R. (2007). Strategic risk communication: Adding value to society. *Public Relations Review, 33*(2), 120–129. doi: 10.1016/j.pubrev.2006.11.014.

Preston, R. (1994). *The hot zone: A terrifying true story*. New York: Random House.

Preston, R. (1997). *The cobra event*. New York: Random House.

Rimon, H., & Schleifer, R. (2013). Who will guard the guardians? Introduction to the special issue on the intellectuals and terror: A fatal attraction. *Terrorism and Political Violence, 25*(4), 621–634. doi: 10.1080/09546553.2013.814484.

Ruggiero, A., & Vos, M. (2013). Terrorism communication: Characteristics and emerging perspectives in the scientific literature 2002–2011. *Journal of Contingencies and Crisis Management, 21*(3), 153–166. doi: 10.1111/1468-5973.12022.

Said, E. (1994). *Orientalism*. New York: Vintage Books.

Said, E. (1997). *Covering Islam: How the media and the experts determine how we see the rest of the world*. New York: Vintage Books.

Sellnow, T., Littlefield, R., Vidoloff, K., & Webb, E. (2009). The interacting arguments of risk communication in response to terrorist hoaxes. *Argumentation and Advocacy, 45*(3), 135–150.

Shapiro, M. J. (1997). *Violent cartographies: Mapping cultures of war*. Minneapolis: University of Minnesota Press.

Singer, E., & Endreny, P. M. (1993). *Reporting on risk: How the mass media portray accidents, diseases, disasters, and other hazards*. New York: Russell Sage Foundation.

Slack, J., & Semati, M. (1997). Intellectual and political hygiene: The "Sokal affair." *Critical Studies in Mass Communication, 14*(3), 201–227. doi: 10.1080/15295039709367012.

Sloan, S. (1998). Terrorism and asymmetry. In L. J. Matthews (Ed.), *Challenging the United States symmetrically and asymmetrically: Can America be defeated?* (pp. 173–193). Carlisle Barracks, PA: Strategic Studies Institute, U.S. Army War College.

Slovic, P. (1987, April 17). Perceptions of risk. *Science, 236*, 280–285.

Sokal, A. (1996). Transgressing the boundaries: Toward a transformative hermeneutics of quantum gravity. *Social Text, 14*(1/2), 217–252. Retrieved from www.jstor.org/stable/466856.

Sparks, L., Kreps, G., Botan, C., & Rowan, K. (2005). Responding to terrorism: Translating communication research into practice. *Communication Research Reports, 22*(1), 1–5. doi: 10.1080/08824090520000343462.

Stern, J. (1999). *The ultimate terrorists*. Cambridge, MA: Harvard University Press.

Sunstein, C. (2003). Terrorism and probability neglect. *Journal of Risk and Uncertainty, 26*(2), 121–136. doi: 10.1023/A:1024111006336.

Tumolo, M., Biedendorf, J., & Ayotte, K. (2014). Un/civil mourning: Remembering with Jacques Derrida. *Rhetoric Society Quarterly, 44*(2), 107–128. doi: 10.1080/02773945.2014.888463.

van Voren, R. (2009). Political abuse of psychiatry—an historical overview. *Schizophrenia Bulletin, 36*(1), 33–35. doi: 10.1093/schbul/sbp119.

Vanderford, M. (2003). Communication lessons learned in the emergency operations center during CDC's anthrax response: A commentary. *Journal of Health Communication, 8*(Suppl 1), 11–12. doi: 10.1080/10810730390224820.

Vincent, R. C. (1992). CNN: Elites talking to elites. In H. Mowlana, G. Gerbner, and H. I. Schiller (Eds.), *Triumph of the image: The media's war in the Persian Gulf* (pp. 181–201). Boulder, CO: Westview Press.

Weiss, L. (2015). On fear and nuclear terrorism. *Bulletin of the Atomic Scientists, 71*(2), 75–87. doi: 10.1177/0096340215571909.

Willis, J., & Okunade, A. A. (1997). *Reporting on risks: The practice and ethics of health and safety communication*. Westport, CT: Praeger.

12

COMMUNICATION ETHICS FOR RISK, CRISES, AND PUBLIC HEALTH CONTEXTS

Shannon A. Bowen and Jo-Yun Li

> By way of introduction, I had defined ethics as a science that teaches, not how we are to achieve happiness, but how we are to become worthy of happiness.
>
> —*Immanuel Kant in his work* On the Old Proverb: That May Be Right in Theory but It Won't Work in Practice (1974, Reprint, p. 45).

The Intersection of Ethical Communication, Risk, Crises, and Public Health

In the modern world, we are surrounded by risk of all kinds. Many of those risks result in crises, and a plethora of health outcomes often follow. For example, the 2016 earthquakes in Japan were a relatively known risk after the 2011 earthquakes and tsunamis that killed tens of thousands. When the 2016 earthquakes hit, that resulted in a public health crisis—not only for first responders and those killed or injured, but for businesses and organizations of all kinds. They had to deal with the resulting lack of electricity, food supplies, transportation, water, and other basic services, along with numerous other implications for survivors.

During and after crises, the number one commodity demanded is communication and the information supplied by that communication. In situations where risk materializes to crisis, people instinctively ask: "What is happening? How bad is it going to get? How long is it going to last? Are my loved ones well?" Whether the crisis is an infectious outbreak or a natural disaster, communication plays the central role and ethical communication is a must.

Theories and principles in risk management and crisis management have been studied from public relations, rhetorical, business, governmental, and financial perspectives. Outgrowths of that study are the specialized fields of risk communication and crisis communication, employed to enhance the effectiveness of communication between publics and the organizations or governments upon which they depend in exigent times. Lives may be at stake during crises, so the goals of ethical communication need to be defined clearly.

Ethical communication can be viewed as providing forthright, candid, honest information (Bowen, 2016). It also entails the concept of contextual disclosure, meaning that relevant information and facts are not withheld, but are provided in a context that helps people make fully informed choices (Bowen, 2016). To provide information that is less than this standard of honesty is unethical, and this chapter explains why. First, we offer a literature review of the current state of research on ethics in risk, crisis, and emergency contexts. Then, we offer an examination of that literature in terms of the evolving media and social media. This chapter then provides an overview of three schools of ethics: utilitarianism, deontology, and virtue ethics. We offer a new, integrated decision-making guideline in which all three of those perspectives are used to examine a risk, crisis, or health problem. A short case study of SARS is offered at the conclusion of the chapter as a means for using the questions in the ethical guideline presented in Figure 12.1. This chapter seeks to offer an understanding of how to use rigorous ethical frameworks to determine the correct course of communication in the face of risk, crises, or public health contingencies.

The State of Risk, Crisis, and Emergency Communication Research Related to Ethics

Risk management entails the collective management and reduction of risk of many kinds, and risk communication facilitates knowledge about that risk. Risk communication in public health has been associated with messages provided by health professionals regarding the potential risks of specific behaviors (Freimuth, Linnan, & Potter, 2000; Witte, Meyer, & Martell, 2001). The messages are expected to alert target audiences to the risks of certain behaviors, such as an unhealthy diet or unsafe sex, and persuade them to adjust their behaviors accordingly.

Crisis communication, on the other hand, is frequently referred to as crisis and disaster management (Barton, 2001; Coombs, 1995). It allows corporations and organizations to follow principles and strategies to repair a damaged reputation after crises and disasters.

Although differences have been recognized, risk communication and crisis communication typically interact at various points (Reynolds &

Seeger, 2005) depending upon the issue at hand. Thus, in order to provide comprehensive communication guidelines, the public health community has merged the two traditions into an integrated approach known as Crisis and Emergency Risk Communication, developed by the Centers for Disease Control and Prevention (Reynolds, Galdo & Sokler, 2002). This five-stage framework includes risk, eruption, clean up, recovery, and evaluation, and it is used to address both risks and urgency of crises or disasters to stakeholders and the general public. Communication challenges can only be overcome when both crisis and risk are covered in the plans. The consideration of ethics is also key to successful communication plans while dealing with crisis and risk, an essential factor in the development and implementation of public health communication (Guttman & Salmon, 2004). From plan purposes to target populations, from message development to effectiveness assessment, and from content consistency to message accuracy, the demands for ethics in public health communication often outweigh their consideration in strategic planning (Guttman & Salmon, 2004).

Findings from emergency communication on ethics. In recent decades, research has focused on the effectiveness and ethical principles of emergency public information (Glik, 2007), as well as the warning messages receivers need in order to receive the words, to understand the words, to realize that the information is related to them, to understand that they need to adopt protective action in order to avoid the risks and, finally, to adopt the assigned action (Mileti & Fitzpatrick, 1991; Mileti & Sorensen, 1990). Transparency, accuracy, and consistency of warning messages play extremely crucial roles in the process of information delivery (WHO, 2003). Transparent public communication allows the public health community and authorities to communicate guidance and suggested protective action effectively; at the same time, it also establishes the authority and credibility of responding sectors (O'Malley, Rainford, & Thompson, 2009).

In 2010, when dealing with one of the largest oil spill crises in the United States, BP management and the local government each drew criticism over a lack of transparency, including delayed disclosure of information and restrictions on media access. The negative perceptions regarding the oil company, reinforced by the outpouring of media reports, reflected a complete failure of private sector crisis management (Kimberly, 2010). Lessons learned from the BP oil spill crisis and similar crises: Rapid, full, and contextual disclosure with honesty and candor are now considered an organization's ethical responsibility, as well as a strategic approach of minimizing the influence of hostile media coverage and fostering relations with customers and stakeholders (Bowen, 2016).

These ethical principles not only apply to crisis and risk management of corporations and organizations but also to the trust-building process between governments, public health professionals, and their publics (Bowen, Hung-Baesecke, & Chen, 2016). While communicable diseases may spread widely, candid, honest, and full communication by the public health community allows authorities to make appropriate decisions and provides sufficient information that targets the audiences that need to adopt protective action. Moreover, transparency is an effective strategy for public health professionals to establish public trust (O'Malley et al., 2009). Particularly when emergencies such as epidemics break out, the effectiveness of restricting individuals' freedom of choices to comply with instructions directly influences public health professionals' crisis and emergency management (Menon & Goh, 2005). The level of mutual trust between authorities and the many involved publics determines individuals' behaviors about whether or not to cooperate with the instructions.

Message consistency, honesty, and public compliance. A lack of ethical public communication could destroy public trust and undermine all phases of emergency management. One infamous example is the management of the 2014 Ebola crisis (Ratzan & Moritsugu, 2014). A day after New York doctor Craig Spencer (who was not required to quarantine himself after returning from treating Ebola patients in Guinea) tested positive for the virus, the New York authorities enforced mandatory quarantines for all travelers from infected areas. However, the policy was revised a few days later to allow home quarantines with monitoring from health professionals. The ambiguous information aroused controversy that greatly damaged public trust and contributed to a national panic about the disease.

In addition to transparency during information delivery, message consistency and accuracy are also key determinants of message recipients' perception and behavior (WHO, 2003). Consistent messages over time are believed to be more effective than inconsistent messages, especially on individuals' understanding and belief regarding risks (Mileti & Sorensen, 1990; Perry, Greene, & Lindell, 1980). For example, inconsistent information from the Centers for Diseases Control and Prevention (CDC) about who were at higher risk of contracting or spreading the Ebola virus caused a serious panic in the United States (Begley, 2014). This lesson was learned not only from Ebola but also from Mad Cow disease, SARS, H1N1, and, more recently, MERS (Middle East Respiratory Syndrome). To communicate with clarity is a crucial ethical obligation for the public health community (Ratzan, 2013). Communication with publics may be significantly different from communication with policy makers and medical professionals. In an era of information overload, consistent information for at-risk publics becomes particularly important.

Moreover, accuracy and certainty of messages can determine peoples' response behavior to the warning messages (Glik, 2007). When an emergency breaks out, the public is eager to know every piece of information that the authorities know. During a public health crisis, every single word counts, whether it is accurate or not (Reynolds & Seeger, 2005). In order to enhance warning efficacy and to persuade the target population to comply with the messages, public health practitioners, authorities, and media often adopt strong motivating appeals (e.g., fear appeals) and attempts to intensify risk (Guttman & Salmon, 2004). Inaccurate and exaggerated information could contribute to unintended adverse effects that negatively influence individual psychological behaviors or cultural beliefs. Unintended negative effects frequently result from such public health interventions (Cho & Salmon, 2007).

The distribution of health or warning messages, particularly messages that limit individual liberty, may motivate message receivers to choose the opposite behaviors that the messages advocate (Dillard & Shen, 2005). Examples include anti-smoking messages, which may trigger an impulse for smokers who are attempting to quit (Stewart & Martin, 1994). Today, media communication may be more persuasive and influential on individuals' behavior than that of medical professionals (Ratzan, 2013), but only when the public health community and authorities disseminate accurate and evidence-based messages, ones where the intended desirable effects and unintended adverse effects are balanced. Overall, public health communication plans that are sensitive to ethical principles are believed to be better implemented and to be more trusted by the public (Guttman & Salmon, 2004).

The Role of a Rapidly Evolving Media in Risk, Crises, and Emergencies

In the era of continual media exposure, the ease of access to information has increased individuals' expectations of instant news reports, particularly when public health crises and emergencies emerge. In the process of information delivery, mass media plays an increasingly decisive role in communicating risks and emergency public information to the public (Bennett, 2010; Reese, Gandy, & Grant, 2001; Stryker, 2003; Stryker, Emmons, & Viswanath, 2007).

In an evolving media environment, messages are ever more fragmented, often poorly sourced, and rapidly moving. These dynamics have given rise to the recent epidemic of "fake news"—essentially misinformation and disinformation that is successful because it is quickly disseminated, rapidly moving, and often difficult to trace or source. As a response to the fake news epidemic, and resulting distrust of information, the implications are heightened for ethical communication. Offering ethical, honest information with transparent sources is more important than ever to help create credibility, trust, and belief among stakeholders and publics.

This is especially true with information about health. More than half of Americans indicate that national, local, and cable television news are their main sources for receiving relevant health information (Kaiser Family Foundation/Harvard School of Public Health, 2001; Newport, 2002). In addition to receiving information passively, individuals have started seeking health information actively and paying more attention to relevant coverage in the news media. Health news trails weather, crime, and sports news in coverage, but has obtained the highest interest (average of 7.8 score) from audiences, using a 0–10 point scale to rate Americans' interest in six issues such as health, science, economy, and politics (National Science Board, 2014).

During health crises or emergencies, the public relies heavily on media and the Internet for updated information (Glik, 2007). Research shows that Internet usage and news website visits after the September 11 attacks were twice as great as the days before the crisis (Glass, 2002). The number of unique visitors to the CNN online news sites increased 23 percent, to 17 million, from the previous week. The Red Cross also received about 400,000 unique visitors every day during the week after the terrorist attacks. The use of media and the Internet by the general public for health information suggested that the public health community must be better prepared for communication with mass media during crises. Otherwise, public health professionals and authorities may fail due to a lack of control of the message during continuous media coverage of the crisis.

Perceptions and frames of issue importance. One aspect of risk management is the relationship between media coverage and individuals' perceptions of issue importance (e.g., McCombs's and Shaw's agenda setting theory, 1972). Previous research shows that there is a high degree of similarity between a prominent agenda in the media and the audiences' priorities (Kim, Scheufele, & Shanahan, 2002). Merely through the amount of coverage, the media tells people what to think about and what to pay attention to (Scheufele, Shanahan, & Kim, 2002). Even though individuals may not understand the specific contents regarding certain issues, they do believe that some are more important than others simply because they see them covered by the media. Thus, the exaggeration and amplification of issues by media may contribute to unintended adverse effects and impede communication plans of the public health community.

Another key idea is media framing of messages. Framing theory says that how the media frames an issue influences how individuals think about an issue (Scheufele, 1999, 2000). The different presentations and frames of the same information can generate different responses. In particular, the media and the public health community possess different perspectives on news relevance during crises (Shoaf & Rottman, 2000). Journalists tend to emphasize conflicts, consequences of crises and emergencies, and attribution of responsibility, while public health professionals attempt to minimize the conflicts and consequences of an issue (Barnes et al., 2008). "The reporter is drawn to the danger and drama, while health professionals emphasize prevention, reassurance and recovery" (Anzur, 2000, p. 197). As a result of the polarizing perspectives of news agenda when crises break out, an ongoing and effective relationship with mass media helps a public health community manage the problem.

Interactivity. Traditional media (i.e., newspapers and television) are still important sources of information between the public health community and the public. But in the past decade, the Internet and social media have become the main sources of information for the general public during health crises (Jones & Salathe, 2009). The user-generated content on the Internet has significantly changed the format of public health communication. The public no longer receives messages passively, but actively participates in the stages of knowledge translation as message generators, transmitters, and sometimes "exaggerators" (Chew & Eysenbach, 2010). Picard (2010) explained:

> In the era of the 24-hour news cycle, the traditional once-a-day press conference featuring talking heads with a bunch of fancy titles has to be revamped and supplemented with Twitter posts, YouTube videos and the like. The public needs to be engaged in conversations and debate about issues of public health, they don't need to be lectured to.
>
> (p. 2)

Given the new interactive format of public health communication, developing effective communication plans is considered just the first stage of crisis and emergency risk communication. In the days before high penetration of the Internet, public health professionals employed traditional evaluation techniques such as surveys and focus groups to measure a target population's perceptions and behavioral responses, in order to examine the success of interventions or communication plans. Now, immediate responses and public expressions on the Internet during crises can be a significant factor in the effectiveness of public health communication. Thus, immediately and consistently assessing information on the Internet and social media is necessary for public health agencies while dealing with emergencies.

Message fluidity and dynamism. When a public health crisis erupts, uncertainty and issue severity usually trigger fast and wide information dissemination that causes anxiety, misinformation, confusion, or even panic. Widespread speculation and rumors occur in the early stage of emergency situations (Samaan et al., 2005; Smith, 2006; Tai & Sun, 2011). Rumors and fake news circulate even faster in the era of participatory social media, which underlines the importance of candid, accurate, factual, clear, transparent public communication. Crisis and emergency information are particularly prone to poorly sourced and exaggerated reporting due to time pressure, fear, and lack of accurate information. Therefore, public health professionals must monitor information and public reaction on the Internet to address problems and speculations carefully.

One example of the influence of social media in crisis and emergency communication is the Ebola quarantine controversy in New York City in 2014. After the New York authorities enforced mandatory quarantines for all travelers from the infected areas, news spread rapidly on Twitter, and promptly drew opposition from some public, who called the policy "inhumane." Under the pressure of public opinion, local governments in New York and New Jersey revised the controversial policy a few days later. The policy change on Ebola quarantines could be considered a demonstration of social media power: attracting attention, mediating the coverage of traditional media, and effectively leading to actual policy changes.

Social media is an increasingly popular forum for the public to obtain information to understand a public health crisis or emergency (Vos & Buckner, 2016). It has the power to clarify incorrect information and stop the message distribution, complying with the requirements in the framework of Crisis and Emergency Risk Communication (Veil, Reynolds, Sellnow, & Seeger, 2008). However, a large proportion of information on social media does not mobilize individuals to adopt protective action, and a great many damaging rumors can be widely disseminated (Vos & Buckner, 2016).

In the 21st century, the evolving media is a double-edged sword. Appropriate coverage and discussion may help public health professionals enhance the public's awareness of crises and emergencies; on the other hand, exaggeration and amplification in the mass media and social media may contribute to negative consequences such as unnecessary anxiety. How to communicate with the public effectively and ethically through media during crises and emergencies has become a primary challenge.

Demands for Ethical Accountability

Ethics is not an optional concern for public and private sector organizations (De George, 2010). Readily available social media channels lead to rising criticism (Li, 2015) and growing public demands for accountability and social responsibility. Infamous cases of governmental wrongdoing, corporate scandals, and failures of ethics have created widespread cynicism. This has resulted in a distrust of corporations, a suspicion of governing bodies, and a dislike for elected officials or leaders. Public trust in both business and government is at an all-time low on a global level (Edelman Trust Barometer, 2015). However, the upside of rapidly evolving media means that organizations can now speak directly to stakeholders and publics to counter rumors, fake news, or inaccurate reports. Doing so with attention to ethics is vital.

234

To create long-term relationships with stakeholders and publics, both internal and external, organizations must be their own best ethical voice, both inside the organization and externally. Employees are exceptionally important to an organization. It has been argued that employees are the most important asset of an organization, giving a competitive advantage when other factors are equal and even acting as ambassadors during times of organizational need. But in order to offer both of those advantages to their employer, employees must have a sense of trust that the organization will treat them with good intent. Ethics builds trust: attention to fairness and integrity builds ethical awareness and creates ethical behavior, and in turn ethical behavior enhances trust.

Research shows that ethics is a vital part of strategic management and organizational decision-making (Bowen, 2008, 2009). Some research perspectives talk about character, others integrity, and others talk about honesty and moral principle. Some perspectives talk about the greater good or public welfare and social justice, while others talk about corporate social responsibility (CSR). When organizations do not attend to creating their own set of ethical values, someone else's values will be imposed upon them. To maintain autonomy and independent decision-making, responsibility seems to be the most morally aware, strategic, and efficient means of creating an ethical framework.

Defining Ethics

Ethical communication requires attention to numerous concerns. Much confusion exists around the terminology of ethics in professional practice (Bowen, 2016), so a concrete definition was sought from moral philosophy. The literature of moral philosophy is the natural place to turn when one seeks to understand ethics. Moral philosophy, or the study of ethics and how we should make decisions, is a discipline that dates back to the beginning of civilization. As an old, rigorous, and formalized study, moral philosophy has much to offer to a younger, applied field such as public affairs or public health. Ethics is defined as rules, principles, or ways of thinking that guide actions, or "systematic study of reasoning about how we ought to act" (Singer, 1994, p. 4). Applied ethics can be defined as determining right from wrong actions.

Ethics is the study of what standards and moral principles apply, and should apply, to our actions or potential actions. The ethical is determined by its intrinsic value in terms of duty, happiness, responsibility, truth, and the ability of the decision to further or to uphold virtues such as integrity. There are three broad schools of normative ethics: utilitarian ethics, virtue ethics, and deontology. Each approach defines what is ethical slightly differently, and each approach has strengths and weaknesses. Therefore, this chapter combines the three classic approaches to normative ethics into a modern, imminently practical decision test offered later in the chapter. A brief review of each type of philosophy offers a basis of understanding that can enhance ethical decision-making on the parts of governmental entities, businesses, NGOs, and citizens.

Utilitarian Ethics

The utilitarian school of ethics, refined and popularized by John Stuart Mill (1861/1957) defined the ethical as that which creates the greatest good for the greatest number of people, while minimizing harm. Although what constitutes "good" may be debatable, the utilitarian ethical framework is applicable in a public health context because the framework seeks to operate in the public interest. In fact, utilitarianism is the basis of the US legal system and is commonly employed in public health contexts (e.g., school vaccination requirements are based on a utilitarian ethos).

Utilitarianism is a consequence-based paradigm, meaning the outcomes, or potential outcomes, of a situation determine the ethical course of action. This framework stands in opposition to other schools of ethics, which consider moral principle, truth, or character as the determinants of ethical behavior. With utilitarianism, consequences carry the day. One must be astute at predicting consequences for the aggregate good, as well as evaluating the potential outcomes of actions.

Utilitarianism begins by requiring a "dispassionate objectivity" in which the decision-maker is "truly impartial" with regard to personal interest and the interests of others (Elliott, 2007, p. 101). Most moral philosophies begin with rationality, requiring objectivity, lack of bias, and an abrogation of selfishness and self-interested concerns that could taint a decision. Engaging in a moral philosophy-based analysis is a rigorous intellectual exercise in logic.

The utilitarian calculus is an estimation of the aggregate number of people who will be positively benefited, in the communitarian sense, by potential action minus the number of negative outcomes or harms created by the action. In other words, decision alternatives and their consequences are weighed against one another. The decision creating the most good and the fewest negatives is the ethical course of action. However, utilitarianism is very specific that rights and justice must be upheld even for those potentially harmed by a decision. Getting to a greater good through unethical actions is specifically forbidden. In other words, one cannot sacrifice ethics in order to create a more ethical consequence in the end. To do so would be illogical and selfish.

Mill believed happiness to be the greater good that should be maximized. He wrote: "The creed which accepts as the foundation of morals, Utility, or the Greatest Happiness Principle, holds that actions are right in proportion as they tend to promote happiness, wrong as they tend to produce the reverse of happiness" (1991, p. 137). Mill maintained that his philosophy must be used to uphold individual rights and to build community, as happiness was found in community and ethic of care, or what is modernly called communitarianism (French & Weis, 2000).

Utilitarianism is a useful theory to help determine what consequences of an action might be in the public interest. However, utilitarianism is often misunderstood and thus has several limitations. The tyranny of the majority can ensue, meaning that minority voices of smaller publics may not be heard. Although Mill was against simply using arithmetic to determine the ethics of actions, that is often how the theory is implemented. Other philosophers protest that human beings and moral ideas cannot be reduced to numbers. In that light, utilitarianism is reductionist in that it measures the outcomes of actions rather than the moral principle of the actions involved. Finally, utilitarianism requires the ability to predict future outcomes, yet we know that many outcomes are unpredictable or even unknowable (e.g., natural disasters, accidents, and so on).

The risks we face in daily living pose challenge enough; predicting potential outcomes of complex situations of risk, crisis, or public health is an intimidating prospect. Some scholars worry that the misapplication of utilitarianism can justify bad behaviors in seeking some greater good outcome. But even when undertaken with the best intentions, to communicate with anything less than honest, full, and contextual disclosure may actually increase the risks people face in the long term. For these reasons, utilitarianism is best used in a combined analysis with other forms of philosophy, as suggested later in this chapter. Combining the relatively common philosophy of utilitarianism with different forms of reasoning allows us to focus on its strength in examining the public interest while compensating for the weaknesses of the philosophy.

Deontological Ethics

Deontology is widely regarded as the most rigorous form of ethical analysis. This approach was developed in the 18th century by the Prussian philosopher Immanuel Kant, who is regarded as the most renowned of the enlightenment philosophers for his masterworks on ethics (1785/1964). He based his work on virtue ethics from ancient Greece but sought to make it more specific and practical. The resulting paradigm of ethics is known as deontology, quite literally the study of duty. Deontology has been studied extensively and applied in professional practice of numerous fields.

Deontology begins with rationality, but perhaps in an even more rigorous form than other moral philosophy. Kantian rationality is based on the equality of all people by virtue of their ability to engage in a rational analysis that is logical rather than aristocratic, well educated, or otherwise privileged (Kant, 1785/1948). One could argue that Kant is the premier philosopher of equality.

Unlike utilitarianism, deontology is not based on consequences; they are simply one factor in a decision no more or less important than other factors. This form of ethics is based on moral principle rather than potential outcomes. It requires a thorough examination of obligations, rights, and duties to a universal moral law that requires all rational people to make decisions without bias. This theory is said to be universal because it is based on equality: it obligates all people to follow moral law through reason alone (Sullivan, 1989).

Deontology also requires a high degree of moral autonomy, meaning independence, objective moral analysis, and decision-making (Kant, 1793/1974). Kant acknowledged that the duty to do something also implies that you can actually implement the change, so some degree of authority to implement an ethical decision may be required. This means that Kantian ethics may be of limited help to those without authority (Bowen, 2004a). Moral autonomy is a form of objectivity that also rules out self-interest, selfishness, societal convention or norms, greed, and other means of introducing bias into an analysis.

Deontology uses three decision tests to guide a moral analysis. Kant termed them categorical imperatives because they are obligations without exception and are not hypothetical, subjective, or conditional, but apply categorically to all rational people. In order to be considered ethical, a decision option needs an affirmative answer to all three tests (Kant, 1785/1948):

1   *Could I will what I'm about to do to be a universal law for all time in all similar situations?* This test examines the universal nature of a decision as well as its reversibility if one were on the receiving end of the action.
2   *Are dignity and respect for publics and stakeholders maintained? Are others involved treated as valuable rational agents in themselves, not as means to an end?* Listening to the needs of publics with dignity and respect is required, and must be coupled with rationality and moral autonomy.
3   *Is the action made from the basis of good will alone or the intention to do the right thing?* Kant held that good will is the ultimate test of ethics because it is the only concept that cannot be corrupted, taken too far, or tainted.

Kant offered the categorical imperative, with its three tests, to help examine a potential decision from multiple viewpoints, such as the perspectives of stakeholders and publics. Kant intended to minimize bias and selfishness with these decision tests. Further, the universal nature of the first test emphasizes the enduring nature of ethical decisions. When competing obligations arise, Kant offered that a deciding factor should guide the decision. The deciding factor is the most important moral principle to be upheld, again speaking to the universal and cross-cultural power of this paradigm. Although it requires a great deal of information or research to understand multiple perspectives, deontology is based on moral principle rather than predicted consequences. Though conducting a deontological ethical analysis is not easy, the outcome is worth the time and effort. Because of the rigorous nature of a deontological analysis, it is thought to create more thorough, defensible, consistent, and enduring ethical decisions than other frameworks (Bowen, 2004b).

Virtue Ethics

The progenitor of deontological ethics, Immanuel Kant, wrote: "I had defined ethics as a science that teaches, not how we are to achieve happiness, but how we are to become worthy of happiness" (Kant, 1793/1974, #357, p. 45). Kant's idea is that worthiness is the ultimate goal, and his definition is derived from virtue ethics. It also shows a eudaimonistic approach, meaning that it accords value to human well-being or a life well lived. The eudaimonistic value of ethics is a tradition established by the ancient Greek philosophers and derived from the Greek term for happiness (Annas, 1993). But ethics cannot be defined through an over-simplified understanding of happiness as self-gratification. Rather, ancient philosophers such as Socrates, Plato, and Aristotle viewed ethics in terms of a life well lived in accordance with achieving the highest or supreme good, based on questioning our conception of what is good through rational examination. This eudaimonistic approach in virtue ethics equates happiness with self-reflection, inner knowledge, truth, peace, and satisfaction from living a life of character, all achieved through practice and rational examination.

Virtue ethics requires reflecting on one's own actions and how they measure up to the ideals of integrity, questioning, arguing for truth, and virtuous moral character, in seeking the life well lived. Virtue ethicists often focus on what they have contributed through living, how they introduced happiness, or how they will be remembered. Modern virtue ethicists (Foot, 2003) have termed these complex goals the pursuit of "human flourishing," enhancing the ability of ourselves and those around us to thrive through the seeking and attainment of high ethical standards. However, this method implies that such judgments require reflection over time and a great deal of life experience, rendering virtue ethics highly impractical. Most issues of risk, crises, and public health emergencies offer little time for reflection, and most of us do not have experience with all of the innumerable possibilities. To make virtue ethics easier to implement, it

239

has been incorporated alongside the supporting deontological theory and utilitarian concepts presented below. When combined with other moral philosophies, the conceptual strengths of virtue ethics can be maintained while compensating for its deficits.

An Integrated Approach to Ethics

Ethics helps to determine the best solution to a dilemma as well as helping to create new options for resolution of complex dilemmas through the analysis of a specific situation. When based on rational analyses, a rigorous consideration of multiple perspectives occurs, resulting in defensible conclusions and well-researched arguments. The more powerful the analysis, the better; so, the three primary forms of moral philosophy have been integrated in this chapter to guide an ethical analysis. Please refer to the Integrated Question Analysis of Ethics in Figure 12.1.

An Integrated Question Analysis of Ethics	
1	Am I as rational as possible?
2	Am I as objective as possible?
3	Am I morally autonomous (i.e., independent) and free of bias?
4	What is the public interest in this case?
5	Are there prior cases to examine?
6	What is the "good" that should be maximized?
7	Can I reasonably predict the consequences in this case?
8	What are the potential consequences that are negative, unlikely, or potentially disastrous?
9	What decision maximizes the good for the greater number of people—while minimizing harms?
10	Could I make this decision a "rule" for all others to follow?
11	What potential crises could result?
12	If my decision were to become universal law for all time, would it still be ethical?
13	What underlying moral principle is the decision based on?
14	Does the decision meet the test of veracity, meaning that it is as honest as possible?
15	What is the deciding factor, i.e., the overriding concern that is more important than others?

16	Is the decision based on true values rather than simply on social norms or conventions?
17	Are dignity and respect maintained, truly hearing and considering multiple points of view?
18	Are dignity and respect maintained, even for the small-in-number publics who comprise the minority?
19	Is disclosure as full as possible, frank or candid, and in context?
20	Does the decision further human flourishing, i.e., improve the human condition in some way?
21	Are there potential negative consequences or alienated publics that taint the decision?
22	What is my intention in making this decision?
23	How does the decision maintain justice, rights, and fairness?
24	If I did not know my role in the decision making process and I could be anywhere, including the receiving end, is the decision still ethical?
25	Have I reflected on the decision from multiple perspectives?
26	To what extent is the potential resolution based on reason, i.e., it is defensible and understandable?
27	What would a leader of exemplary virtue and honest character do in this situation?
28	Is the decision made from a basis of good will?
29	Can I rule out simple legalistic compliance and make an argument based on ethics alone?
30	Looking back on this decision in ten years, will I still be satisfied with it?
31	Have I used discernment and moral courage to determine the right course of action?
32	To what extent does the decision uphold a principle or value that is morally worthy?

Figure 12.1 A question guide to an integrated ethical analysis using virtue, utilitarianism, and deontology

Utilitarian philosophy has a primary strength of considering the effect of actions on publics, pondering the consequences of risk, crises, and public health problems. It is particularly useful for government as it exists to organize and prioritize public interest, but can be employed from any perspective. The shortcomings of utilitarianism are countered by incorporating a powerful principle-based analysis through deontology. That way, public interest is considered as a primary goal, yet tyranny of the majority is not possible because of the rigorous reliance on dignity, respect, and equality for all people.

Deontology is used to introduce a duty-based principled form of ethical decision-making. It maintains a universal perspective, requires dignity and respect for all involved publics, and uses good intention or a morally good will as the ultimate test of an action. A decision is thought to be ethical if it can pass these tests, so all three tests are present in the integrated approach offered here. The concepts of virtue ethics are introduced to enhance ethical goals and fortitude of the analysis while reducing its reliance on hindsight through the more practical questions of utilitarianism and deontology.

Integrating utilitarianism, deontology, and virtue ethics means that multiple definitions of good, duties, rights, and intentions can be examined. Using multiple viewpoints strengthens the intellectual rigor of analysis. Although each of these philosophies may have a different way of defining ethics, they all have in common a reliance on rationality and moral autonomy. That means that these philosophies can be used in conjunction to form an integrated analysis.

The integrated analysis offered below takes the form of questions that are applicable to any situation. These questions can be asked of individuals, groups, or organizations. The beauty of asking questions is that even though answers may not be readily available, decisions are certain to be better analyzed than those undertaken without scrutiny. As many scholars have noted, we grow wise by asking questions. Even questions that remain unanswered may offer insight and fertile new ideas for consideration.

An ethical examination fosters the understanding of complex problems from multiple viewpoints and creates reasoned analyses of difficult situations with numerous implications and competing priorities. Simple yes or no questions rarely need a full ethical analysis to determine the best course of action. The questions presented below are in the chronological order necessary to guide an ethical analysis, and are those best suited to conducting an ethical analysis from each of the three paradigms discussed earlier in this chapter.

SARS Case

Use the following case example to walk through the integrated question analysis.

The Severe Acute Respiratory Syndrome (SARS) epidemic of 2002–2004 offers an excellent case for ethical analysis including elements of risk, crisis, and public health. Interspecies transmission of the SARS virus led to competing narratives from the numerous organizations and countries that were involved. Misinformation resulted from the competing narratives, and insufficient information about the origin of the disease and its modes of transmission were troubling to many. A lack of honesty and candor from the Chinese government were especially troubling. Regional and national health groups in China offered no specifics about the virus outbreak (Bowen & Heath, 2007). The origin and transmission of SARS remained "shrouded in mystery" and exacerbated the health crisis (Bowen & Heath, 2007, p. 74).

The SARS epidemic spread to other countries and concerns of a pandemic of the potentially fatal disease were high. Understanding the origin of the disease was essential to developing a containment protocol and treating cases of SARS. Epidemiologists at the World Health Organization (WHO) and Centers for Disease Control and Prevention (CDC) were heavily involved in researching the SARS virus. The Chinese government remained silent but authorities began to slaughter household pets: dogs and cats were suspected of carrying the SARS virus, but that information was incorrect.

Media coverage of the epidemic was prohibited by the Chinese government after some news reports began to criticize its emergency management (Huang, 2004). Moreover, Chinese authorities avoided communicating with the World Health Organization until a very late stage of the outbreak. The continued information blackout seriously hindered the public from receiving up-to-date information and deterred the authorities from addressing the chaos (Huang, 2004).

In May 2003, Hong Kong researchers identified a wild rodent-like creature called a civet as the source of the coronavirus that led to SARS. Food was scarce in the Guangdong province where SARS originated, so locals had turned to the wild rodent as a food source, resulting in the inter-species contamination that created the SARS epidemic. The Chinese government found this explanation embarrassing and actively worked to suppress information about the source of the disease. It also continued to promote tourism by issuing statements saying that it was safe to visit and tour China. The Chinese government did not recognize any authority of the WHO or CDC. Yet when the Ministry of Public Health quarantined 10,000 Chinese in Nanjing in late May 2003, the crisis could no longer be denied.

Valuable months had been wasted by the Chinese government in an epidemic that caused 8,100 illnesses and 800 documented deaths (Bowen & Heath, 2007).

Where did the Chinese government go wrong? What were their priorities in decision-making? How were the publics, both sick and healthy, considered? Most importantly, what would an ethical analysis using the integrated questioning model have indicated as an ethical resolution to the SARS crisis? What would using the integrated question analysis have you do differently?

[For a detailed discussion and ethical analysis of the SARS case, see Bowen & Heath, 2007.]

Implications

The theoretical implications going forward are many. Using an integrated approach to ethics of virtue, utilitarianism, and deontology offers a robust means of analysis—perhaps stronger than each philosophical approach alone. There are many benefits to using a three-philosophy approach, but also three times more risk. One must be aware of the pitfalls of each philosophy and guard against those entering the analysis: the hindsight and experience needed in virtue ethics can be a hindrance to fast-moving problems in a rapid media landscape. The tyranny of the majority, reducing people's concerns to numbers, and difficulty in predicting future consequences, all inherent in utilitarianism, should be guarded against. The difficulty of finding a universal moral principle that maintains respect for all parties in deontology requires volumes of unbiased research including multiple perspectives.

This process is time-consuming and challenging, involving higher-order reasoning, logic, and critical thinking. This combined moral approach is a new avenue of thought with solid theoretical backing yet scant empirical testing. Combining these forms of moral analysis can offer solid decisions with ethical implications that are based on the most unassailable moral principles. Decisions made in this manner from a basis of good intention should survive the turmoil of a rapidly moving and changing communicative context, assaults from fake news, and challenges from biased opponents. They are defensible based on the most rigorous types of moral analyses yet developed.

In implications for practice, unforeseen hurdles to implementing an integrated virtue-utilitarian-deontological analysis may arise. Decisions are only as good as the data on which they are based, and access to accurate and complete data could be an impediment. The time pressure to communicate during crises, disasters, and public health scares can lead to missteps. Future research could test and study the implementation of this combined moral analysis in various professional settings and situations to refine the theory for practical implementation.

Conclusions

In confronting public mistrust of government and media outlets, organizations now need to be the best and most accurate source of information for stakeholders and publics. That standard requires a high degree of ethical expertise, multiple forms of research and vetted sourcing, and insightful, critical analysis. But in a media environment with accusations of insider collusion and fake news a daily occurrence, organizations face a vacuum of credibility.

Where can stakeholders and publics now turn for truthful, accurate, full, objective, and trustworthy information? The rigorous combined and integrated ethical analysis of virtue-utilitarianism-deontology presented in this chapter offers a means through which that vacuum of credibility can be filled by organizations offering honest and ethical information. The integrated three-philosophy question guide presented in this chapter offers a theoretically strong and analytically insightful way to create better organizations and better communications, one decision at a time.

References

Annas, J. (1993). *The morality of happiness*. Oxford: Oxford University Press.

Anzur, T. (2000). How to talk to the media: Televised coverage of public health issues in a disaster. *Prehospital and Disaster Medicine, 15*(04), 70–72.

Barnes, M. D., Hanson, C. L., Novilla, L. M., Meacham, A. T., McIntyre, E., & Erickson, B. C. (2008). Analysis of media agenda setting during and after Hurricane Katrina: Implications for emergency preparedness, disaster response, and disaster policy. *American Journal of Public Health, 98*(4), 604–610.

Barton, L. (2001). *Crisis in organizations II*. Cincinnati, OH: South-Western College Publishing.

Begley, S. (2014). CDC Chief faulted over confusing Ebola messages. *The Huffington Post*. Retrieved from www.huffingtonpost.com/2014/10/18/cdc-thomas-frieden-ebola_n_6006002.html.

Bennett, P. (2010). *Risk communication and public health*. Oxford: Oxford University Press.

Bowen, S. A. (2004a). Organizational factors encouraging ethical decision making: An exploration into the case of an exemplar. *Journal of Business Ethics, 52*(4), 311–324.

Bowen, S. A. (2004b). Expansion of ethics as the tenth generic principle of public relations excellence: A Kantian theory and model for managing ethical issues. *Journal of Public Relations Research, 16*(1), 65–92.

Bowen, S. A. (2005). A practical model for ethical decision making in issues management and public relations. *Journal of Public Relations Research, 17*(3), 191–216.

Bowen, S. A. (2008). A state of neglect: Public relations as 'corporate conscience' or ethics counsel. *Journal of Public Relations Research, 20*(3), 271–296.

Bowen, S. A. (2009). What communication professionals tell us regarding dominant coalition access and gaining membership. *Journal of Applied Communication Research, 37*(4), 427–452.

Bowen, S. A. (2016). Clarifying ethics terms in public relations from A to V, authenticity to virtue: BledCom special issue of PR review sleeping (with the) media: Media relations. *Public Relations Review, 42*(4), 564–572. doi: 10.1016/j.pub rev.2016.03.012.

Bowen, S. A., & Heath, R. L. (2007). Narratives of the SARS Epidemic and Ethical Implications for Public Health Crises. *International Journal of Strategic Communication, 1*, 73–91. doi: 10.1080/15531180701298791.

Bowen, S. A., Hung-Baesecke, C. J., & Chen, Y. R. (2016). Ethics as a pre-cursor to organization-public relationships: Building trust before and during the OPR model. *Cogent Social Sciences, 2.* doi: 10.1080/23311886.2016.1141467.

Chew, C., & Eysenbach, G. (2010). Pandemics in the age of Twitter: Content analysis of Tweets during the 2009 H1N1 outbreak. *PloS one, 5*(11), e14118.

Cho, H., & Salmon, C. T. (2007). Unintended effects of health communication campaigns. *Journal of Communication, 57*(2), 293–317.

Coombs, W. T. (1995). Choosing the right words for the development of guidelines for the selection of the "appropriate" crisis-response strategies. *Management Communication Quarterly, 8*(4), 447–476.

De George, R. T. (2010). *Business ethics* (7th ed.). Boston, MA: Prentice Hall.

Dillard, J. P., & Shen, L. (2005). On the nature of reactance and its role in persuasive health communication. *Communication Monographs, 72*(2), 144–168.

Edelman Trust Barometer (2015). New York: Edelman public relations. Retrieved from www.Edelman.com/insights/intellectual-property/2015-Edelman-trust-barometer/.

Elliott, D. (2007) Getting Mill right. *Journal of Mass Media Ethics, 22,* 100–112. doi: 10.1080/08900520701315806.

Foot, P. (2003). *Virtues and vices and other essays in moral philosophy.* Oxford: Clarendon.

Freimuth, V., Linnan, H. W., & Potter, P. (2000). Communicating the threat of emerging infections to the public. *Emerging Infectious Diseases, 6*(4), 337.

French, W., & Weis, A. (2000). An ethics of care or an ethics of justice. *Journal of Business Ethics, 27,* 125–136.

Friedman, M. (2002). *Capitalism and freedom: Fortieth anniversary edition.* Chicago, IL: University of Chicago Press. Original publication date 1962.

Glass, A. J. (2002). The war on terrorism goes online: Media and government response to the first post-Internet crisis. *Politics and public policy, Harvard University.* Cambridge, MA: Joan Shorenstein Center for Press.

Glik, D. C. (2007). Risk communication for public health emergencies. The *Annual Review of Public Health, 28,* 33–54.

Guttman, N., & Salmon, C. T. (2004). Guilt, fear, stigma and knowledge gaps: Ethical issues in public health communication interventions. *Bioethics, 18*(6), 531–552.

Huang, Y. (2004). The SARS epidemic and its aftermath in China: A political perspective. In S. Knobler, A. Mahmoud, S. Lemon, A. Mack, L. Sivitz, K. & Oberholtzer (Eds.), *Learning from SARS: Preparing for the next disease outbreak* (pp. 116–36). Washington, DC: National Academies Press.

Jones, J. H., & Salathe, M. (2009). Early assessment of anxiety and behavioral response to novel swine-origin influenza A (H1N1). *PLoS One, 4*(12), e8032.

Kaiser Family Foundation/Harvard School of Public Health. (2001). The health news index. Retrieved from http://kff.org/health-costs/poll-finding/health-news-index-septemberoctober-2001/.

Kant, I. (1785/1964). *Groundwork of the metaphysic of morals* (H. J. Paton, Trans.). New York: Harper & Row.

Kant, I. (1793/1974). *On the old proverb: That may be right in theory but it won't work in practice* (E. B. Ashton, Trans.). Philadelphia: University of Pennsylvania Press.

246

Kant, I. (1785/1948). *The groundwork of the metaphysic of morals* (H. J. Paton, Trans.). New York: Harper Torchbooks.

Kimberly, J. (2010). How BP blew crisis management 101. CNN.com. Retrieved from www.cnn.com/2010/OPINION/06/21/kimberly.bp.management.crisis/.

Kim, S. H., Scheufele, D. A., & Shanahan, J. (2002). Think about it this way: Attribute agenda-setting function of the press and the public's evaluation of a local issue. *Journalism & Mass Communication Quarterly, 79*(1), 7–25.

Li, Z. (2015). *Does power make us mean? An investigation of empowerment and revenge behaviors in the cyberspace.* Unpublished doctoral dissertation, University of Miami.

McCombs, M. E., & Shaw, D. L. (1972). The agenda-setting function of mass media. *Public Opinion Quarterly, 36*(2), 176–187.

Menon, K. U., & Goh, K. T. (2005). Transparency and trust: Risk communications and the Singapore experience in managing SARS. *Journal of Communication Management, 9*(4), 375–383.

Mileti, D. & Fitzpatrick, C. (1991). Communication of public risk: Its theory and its application. *Sociological Practice Review, 2*(1), 20–28.

Mileti, D. S., & Sorenson J. H. (1990). Communication of emergency public warnings: A social science perspective and state of-the-art assessment. *Oak Ridge National Laboratory Rep.* ORNL-6609. Retrieved from http://cires.mx/docs_info/CIRES_003.pdf.

Mill, J. S. (1861/1957). *Utilitarianism.* New York: The Liberal Arts Press.

Mill, J. S. (1991). Utilitarianism. In J. Gray (Ed.), *On liberty and other essays.* New York: Oxford University Press. (Original work published 1863).

National Science Board. (2014). *Science and engineering indicators 2014.* Arlington, VA: National Science Foundation.

Newport, F. (2002). *Americans get plenty of health news on TV, but tend not to trust it.* Princeton, NJ: The Gallup Organization. Retrieved from www.gallup.com/poll/6883/americans-get-plenty-health-news-tv-tend-trust.aspx.

O'Malley, P., Rainford, J., & Thompson, A. (2009). Transparency during public health emergencies: From rhetoric to reality. *Bulletin of the World Health Organization, 87*(8), 614–618.

Perry, R. W., Greene, M. R., & Lindell, M. K. (1980). Enhancing evacuation warning compliance: Suggestions for emergency planning. *Disasters, 4*(4), 433–449.

Picard, A. (2010). What are the public-health lessons of H1N1? Preach less, engage more. *The Globe and Mail.* Retrieved from www.theglobeandmail.com/life/health-and-fitness/what-are-the-public-health-lessons-of-h1n1-preach-less-engage-more/article4323795/.

Ratzan, S. C. (2013). "They say" the next big pandemic is near: Are we prepared? *Journal of Health Communication, 18*(7), 757–759.

Ratzan, S. C., & Moritsugu, K. P. (2014). Ebola crisis—communication chaos we can avoid. *Journal of Health Communication, 19*(11), 1213–1215.

Reese, S. D., Gandy Jr, O. H., & Grant, A. E. (Eds.). (2001). *Framing public life: Perspectives on media and our understanding of the social world.* New York: Routledge.

Reynolds, B. M., Galdo, J. H., & Sokler, L. (2002). Crisis and emergency risk communication: Centers for Disease Control and Prevention. Retrieved from www.bt.cdc.gov/cerc/resources/pdf/cerc_2014edition.pdf.

247

Reynolds, B., & Seeger, M. (2005). Crisis and emergency risk communication as an integrative model. *Journal of Health Communication, 10*(1), 43–55.

Samaan, G., Patel, M., Olowokure, B., Roces, M. C., Oshitani, H., & World Health Organization Outbreak Response Team. (2005). Rumor surveillance and avian influenza H5N1. *Emerging Infectious Diseases, 11*(3), 463–466.

Scheufele, D. A. (1999). Framing as a theory of media effects. *Journal of Communication, 49*(1), 103–122.

Scheufele, D. A. (2000). Agenda-setting, priming, and framing revisited: Another look at cognitive effects of political communication. *Mass Communication & Society, 3*(2–3), 297–316.

Scheufele, D. A., Shanahan, J., & Kim, S. H. (2002). Who cares about local politics? Media influences on local political involvement, issue awareness, and attitude strength. *Journalism & Mass Communication Quarterly, 79*(2), 427–444.

Shoaf, K. I., & Rottman, S. J. (2000). The role of public health in disaster preparedness, mitigation, response, and recovery. *Prehospital and Disaster Medicine, 15*(04), 18–20.

Singer, P. (Ed.) (1994). *Ethics.* Oxford: Oxford University Press.

Smith, R. D. (2006). Responding to global infectious disease outbreaks: Lessons from SARS on the role of risk perception, communication and management. *Social Science & Medicine, 63*(12), 3113–3123.

Stewart, D. W., & Martin, I. M. (1994). Intended and unintended consequences of warning messages: A review and synthesis of empirical research. *Journal of Public Policy & Marketing, 13*(1), 1–19.

Stryker, J. E. (2003). Articles media and marijuana: A longitudinal analysis of news media effects on adolescents' marijuana use and related outcomes, 1977–1999. *Journal of Health Communication, 8*(4), 305–328.

Stryker, J. E., Emmons, K. M., & Viswanath, K. (2007). Uncovering differences across the cancer control continuum: A comparison of ethnic and mainstream cancer newspaper stories. *Preventive Medicine, 44*(1), 20–25.

Sullivan, R. J. (1989). *Immanuel Kant's moral theory.* Cambridge, UK: Cambridge University Press.

Tai, Z., & Sun, T. (2011). The rumouring of SARS during the 2003 epidemic in China. *Sociology of Health & Illness, 33*(5), 677–693.

Veil, S., Reynolds, B., Sellnow, T. L., & Seeger, M. W. (2008). CERC as a theoretical framework for research and practice. *Health Promotion Practice, 9*(4), 26–34.

Vos, S. C., & Buckner, M. M. (2016). Social media messages in an emerging health crisis: Tweeting bird flu. *Journal of Health Communication, 21*(3), 1–8.

World Health Organization (WHO). (2003). Global conference on severe acute respiratory syndrome (SARS): Where do we go from here? *Emerging Infectious Diseases, 9*(9), 1191–1192.

Witte, K., Meyer, G., & Martell, D. (2001). *Effective health risk messages: A step-by-step guide.* Thousand Oaks, CA: SAGE Publications.

13

INOCULATION AS A RISK AND HEALTH COMMUNICATION STRATEGY IN AN EVOLVING MEDIA ENVIRONMENT

Bobi Ivanov, Kimberly A. Parker,
and Lindsay L. Dillingham

Introduction

Communication continues to be at the center of risk and health promotion management strategies (Ivanov, 2012; Ivanov et al., 2016; Pfau, 1995) as many of the processes associated with these activities are "inherently communicative" (e.g., O'Hair & Heath, 2005, p.4). Garnett and Kouzmin, for example, argued that "Hurricane Katrina was and continues to be as much a communication crisis as a natural disaster" (2007, p. 171). As a result, these researchers, in concert with other social scientists (e.g., Degeneffe, Kinsey, Stinson, & Ghosh, 2009; Ivanov, 2012; Pfau, 1995), have called for the design and introduction of effective communication messages to be used as strategic tools in the effort to prevent and manage risk and health issues and crises.

A message strategy that has emerged as an effective tool in managing risk and health promotion is based on the principals of inoculation theory (Compton, 2013; Compton & Pfau, 2005; Ivanov, 2012; Ivanov, in press). As a two-sided message strategy, inoculation has proven to be an effective approach in mitigating the negative effects of politically motivated acts of violence (e.g., Ivanov et al., 2016), underage smoking (e.g., Pfau, Van Bockern, & Kang, 1992; Pfau & Van Brockern, 1994; Szabo & Pfau, 2001), alcohol consumption (e.g., Godbold & Pfau, 2000; Parker, Ivanov, & Compton, 2012), vaccine avoidance (e.g., Wong & Harrison, 2014), and unprotected sex (e.g., Parker et al., 2012), thus prompting

Ivanov to render the "application of the strategy boundless" in the risk and health communication context (Ivanov, 2012, p. 77; Ivanov, in press).

Yet, despite its research longevity spanning over five and a half decades, inoculation scholars have dedicated limited attention to the potential moderating role of communication modality. With very few exceptions that compared traditional media outlets (e.g., Pfau, Holbert, Zubric, Pasha, & Lin, 2000), inoculation has treated modality largely "as a 'neutral' conduit of message content" (Pfau, 1990, p. 195; Dillingham & Ivanov, 2016a). Thus, research on the impact of different traditional and emerging modalities on the process of inoculation and its subsequent message efficacy is largely underdeveloped. In a rapidly evolving multimedia landscape (Dholakia et al., 2010) that features online socializing and digitization of modalities (Zemmels, 2012), for inoculation to remain a relevant strategy in general, and in risk and health promotion and management in particular, scholars have to consider the impact of evolving media on the effectiveness of inoculation as a communication message strategy.

This chapter begins with an introduction of the theory of inoculation. More specifically, the chapter opens with a summary of inoculation's conception and logic, as well as original and newly identified theoretical mechanisms, variables, processes, and boundaries. It then focuses on inoculation's strategic application in risk and health promotion management by reviewing the extant inoculation studies conducted in these contexts. The chapter continues with an examination of the role that modality has played in previous inoculation research and concludes with considerations for future risk and health, but also general inoculation research in an evolving media environment.

Origins and Mechanisms of Inoculation Theory

Eagly and Chaiken labeled inoculation the "grandparent theory of resistance to attitude change" (1993, p. 561). In contrast to reactive strategies that can potentially restore—rather than protect—attitudes, inoculation is a preemptive strategy that works to reduce the effect of future persuasive attempts by motivating individuals to reinforce established attitudes. Inoculation messages are used to strengthen the conviction with which current attitudes are held and prepare individuals for future attacks (McGuire, 1961). The roots of inoculation theory can be found in Lumsdaine and Janis' (1953) seminal study, which examined the persuasive effectiveness of one-sided (i.e., presenting only favorable arguments on one side of the issue) and two-sided (i.e., presenting arguments on both sides of the issue) messages. While both types of messages influenced attitudes and behaviors, two-sided messages emerged as the superior strategy when seeking to generate resistance to future persuasive attacks.

To explain this finding, McGuire (1964) used a biomedical analogy arguing that attitudinal inoculation confers resistance in much the same way as human immunization is stimulated via vaccination. He cleverly observed that through the process of immunization, humans are made resistant to diseases by offering a weakened form of the virus, which stimulates the immune system. The immune system then begins the work of building up resistance to a future viral attack. McGuire (1964) stated that the dosage of the immunization is key to effectiveness; if it is too weak, it may fail to stimulate the immune system and if it is too strong, it may overwhelm it and cause the very disease the immunization aimed to prevent.

Developing his logic from the aforementioned process of immunization, McGuire (1964) argued that attitudinal inoculation can create more resistant attitudes by using persuasive messages designed to threaten, or "shock" (McGuire, 1961, p. 185), the confidence in the established attitude, thus motivating defense preparation. McGuire believed that counterarguing—the process of raising and refuting potential forthcoming attitudinal challenges—is a key component in the defense process, providing practice and confidence in the ability of individuals to withstand attitudinal pressures. As such, McGuire (1964) identified *threat* and *counterarguing* as the key mechanisms of inoculation-conferred resistance.

Unleashing the inoculation process necessitates effective message design, which has traditionally consisted of two message components, *explicit forewarning* and *refutational preemption* (see Ivanov, 2012). The purpose of the explicit forewarning is to demonstrate to individuals that their attitudes are not infallible; but, rather, likely to be challenged and potentially overwhelmed. The refutational preemption component of the message presents individuals with weakened challenges to the current attitudes, and then strongly refutes those relevant challenges. Threat is generated by both message components. While the explicit forewarning does so directly and overtly, the refutational preemption elicits threat more implicitly, or inherently, by introducing individuals to potential forthcoming challenges, thus rendering the danger of attitudinal pressures real. Counterarguing is stimulated by the generated threat and inspired by the guided practice of how to refute forthcoming challenges presented in the refutational preemption component of the inoculation message. According to McGuire (1964), inoculation messages elicit threat, both explicitly and implicitly, which motivates the process of counterarguing—supported by the guided counterarguing practice exemplified in the message—which in turn enhances attitudinal resistance.

Yet, Insko (1967) suspected that the process of inoculation, as originally conceptualized, was incomplete. As such, more recent research has focused on uncovering additional mechanisms to better explain the intricacies and complexities of the inoculation process (see Compton, 2013; Ivanov, 2012; Ivanov, in press). The results have shown that, in addition to, or in combination with, generating threat and counterarguing, inoculation elicits greater levels of issue involvement (e.g., Pfau et al., 2004), self-efficacy (e.g., Farchi & Gidron, 2010; Ivanov et al., 2016; Jackson, Compton, Whiddett, Anthony, & Dimmock, 2015; Pfau et al., 2009), and affect (e.g., Compton & Ivanov, 2014; Ivanov et al., 2012a, 2012b; Miller et al., 2013). Inoculation also boosts attitude accessibility (Pfau et al., 2003, 2004), strengthens the associative networks of those inoculated (e.g., Pfau et al., 2005), and bolsters attitudinal certainty (e.g., Pfau et al., 2004; 2005), all of which enhance attitude resistance. As a result, inoculation messages seem to offer a promising approach to designing successful risk and health promotion strategies.

Theoretical Boundaries

As a theory-based strategy, inoculation functions within specified boundaries. These boundaries are both theoretical and practical. This chapter briefly addresses the three boundaries most relevant to risk and health communication and message design: initial attitudes, issue involvement, and cross-protection.

Initial Attitudes

Ivanov and colleagues suggested that "McGuire's (1964) use of the biological analogy was not merely stylistic, it was explanatory" (2015, p. 220). Inoculation is used to immunize healthy individuals. Conversely, individuals who have already succumbed to the disease are not good candidates for preventive inoculation. Consequently, mirroring the biological analogy, attitudinal inoculation should only be used on individuals with "healthy" (i.e., established) attitudes. Using inoculation as anything but a preventive strategy would diverge from the theoretical undergirding of the biomedical analogy (Ivanov et al., 2016). Yet, from a pragmatic standpoint, a robust message strategy that can simultaneously reinforce desirable established attitudes, but also sway neutral attitudes and influence undesirable established attitudes, may present a preferred message approach to a strategy only designed to protect attitudes.

An inoculation-based strategy can in fact do all of the above (e.g., Ivanov et al., 2017; Wood, 2007). More specifically, the strategy serves an inoculating, preventive function consistent with the tenets of inoculation theory; it also serves a persuasive, rather than resistance, function as it helps create new, and augment-opposing, attitudes (e.g., Ivanov et al., 2017; Wood, 2007). It does so better than a traditional supportive (bolstering or one-sided) strategy (Ivanov et al., 2017), thus providing a strong alternative message approach for usage in risk and health prevention and management.

Issue Involvement

The importance of the topic, or the involvement with the issue, was previously considered the "key to inoculation's terrain" (Pfau et al., 1997, p. 210). Pfau and colleagues first advanced the idea that an inoculation strategy is most effective with topics or issues that are of moderate importance to individuals. The authors reasoned that highly involving issues would render the effectiveness of this strategy limited as individuals would have already fortified their attitudes due to their importance. Conversely, issues eliciting limited interest and involvement, Pfau and colleagues (1997) reasoned, would fail to motivate individuals to enhance their attitudinal defenses. As a result, moderately involving issues should provide the best opportunity for inoculation's success. These findings-supported assertions suggesting a curvilinear relationship between inoculation's effectiveness and issue involvement—although logically sound and empirically supported in Pfau and colleagues' study—did not receive meta-analytic support (Banas & Rains, 2010). Although the unstandardized beta coefficients were in the hypothesized direction, no linear or curvilineal relationship was discovered (Banas & Rains, 2010). Hence, the potential confounding role of issue involvement in the process of inoculation should be considered with caution.

Cross-Protection

Threat-motivated defense building is at the heart of inoculation's success (Pfau et al., 1997). McGuire (1964) contended, and evidenced, that the motivation to shore up defenses allows individuals to extend the attitudinal protection veil beyond the counterarguing content provided in the refutational preemption of the inoculation message. Stated differently, the effectiveness of inoculation messages extends beyond the message-presented arguments by potentially creating an umbrella (or blanket) protection over all arguments within the issue domain (Compton, 2013; Compton & Pfau, 2005; Ivanov, 2012; McGuire, 1964).

Recently, however, Parker and colleagues (2012, 2016) have argued that the umbrella protection may extend beyond the issue domain by creating cross-protection for related attitudes as well. Their results, as well as that of others (Ivanov et al., 2015; Ivanov et al., 2016), have provided early confirmation for the possibility of cross-protection.

The review of the boundaries shows the possibilities of inoculation-based strategies. Inoculation offers the opportunity for design and implementation of effective risk and health communication strategies for reinforcing, creating, and changing both targeted and related beliefs, attitudes, and behaviors.

Application of Inoculation in Risk and Health Communication Settings

In the fifty-five year history of the theory, inoculation-based strategies have been applied, mostly with success, to numerous contexts including: politics (e.g., Pfau & Burgoon, 1988; Pfau et al., 1990), mass media (Pfau et al., 2006, 2008), commerce (e.g., Ivanov et al., 2009; Ivanov et al., 2017), corporate communication (Dillingham & Ivanov, 2015; Haigh & Pfau, 2006), public relations/crises (Burgoon, Pfau, & Birk, 1995; Wan & Pfau, 2004; Wigley & Pfau, 2010), interpersonal communication (Sutton, 2011), cross-cultural communication (Ivanov et al., 2012b), and education (Compton & Pfau, 2008). An additional context that has received significant attention from inoculation scholars is that of risk and health communication. Consequently, the rest of the contextual focus of this chapter will be placed on specific risk and health related attitudes (or behaviors) and policies featured in previous inoculation research.

Smoking Prevention

Preventing smoking onset with young adolescents has generated inoculation interest and research. Using inoculation strategy in a two-year study, Pfau and colleagues (Pfau et al., 1992; Pfau & Van Bockern, 1994) were successful in protecting anti-smoking attitudes and intentions of at-risk middle school students with low self-esteem. Banerjee and Greene (2006, 2007) organized anti-smoking intervention workshops with the same population and also discovered positive inoculation effect.

Drinking Prevention

Duryea (1982, 1983) advocated for inoculation to be employed as an alcohol education prevention strategy. Since then, studies have explored the efficacy of inoculation in this role. Godbold and Pfau (2000) tested the effectiveness of normative inoculation messages in combating the false, inflated perception regarding the number of adolescent peers consuming alcohol. By creating a more realistic perception of the true number of peers who consume alcohol, inoculation was able to help protect adolescents from subsequent pressures to consume alcohol by peers who cited the behavior as normative.

Focusing on a different population, Parker and colleagues (2012) tested cross-protection effects of inoculation on binge drinking attitudes. More precisely, these authors discovered that inoculating college students against the dangers of unprotected sex indirectly created cross-protection that spanned over a related attitude toward another risky behavior. More precisely, the results showed greater resilience of negative attitudes toward binge drinking.

Unprotected Sexual Engagement

Parker and colleagues (2012) conducted a study to test the ability of inoculation to decrease the possibility of college student engagement in the risky practice of unprotected sexual intercourse. These authors designed an inoculation-based message aimed at protecting the positive attitudes toward condom use. The results were encouraging as the message not only protected the targeted attitudes, but as aforementioned, the effect extended to related ones as well, i.e., the negative attitudes toward binge drinking.

Vaccination

In a recent study, Wong and Harrison (2014; also see Wong, 2016) explored the ability of inoculation messages to protect positive attitudes toward HPV vaccinations. In their experiment they tested two different inoculation message approaches. In the first one, they presented participants with inoculation messages designed to directly protect the attitudes toward HPV vaccinations. In the second approach, the messages were not specific to HPV vaccination, but instead focused on the general practice of vaccination. Both approaches were successful in protecting attitudes toward HPV vaccination. These findings are significant as they show that not only is inoculation an effective risk and health strategy in directly defending favorable HPV vaccination attitudes, but also that inoculation can indeed generate umbrella protection. As the results showed, inoculating general pro-vaccination attitudes generated protection for specific attitudes as well, such as those about HPV vaccination. This outcome suggests that targeting global risk and health-related attitudes (e.g., impaired driving) may have a positive effect on multiple specific attitudes (e.g., drinking and driving, prescription drug usage and driving, and even texting and driving).

Risk and Health Policy

Industry-sponsored, anti-policy messages have been effective in subverting efforts to galvanize support for pro-health policies (Niederdeppe, Heley, & Barry, 2015). In order to buffer attitudes toward pro-health policy, Niederdeppe and colleagues (2015) tested the efficacy of inoculation in combating the effectiveness of anti-policy messaging. More specifically, these authors applied inoculation as a strategy to protect against the effect of industry anti-policy messages designed to decrease support for policies aimed at reducing obesity, cigarette use, and pain-killer addiction. The results were encouraging. The findings indicated that inoculation messages had both immediate and delayed success as the messages were effective both instantly, i.e., after their presentation, and a week later.

Inoculation scholars have found equivalent success in their attempts to protect attitudes in support of numerous government policies related to risk and health such as restrictions on televised violence, gambling, marijuana legalization, and sale and distribution of hand guns (e.g., Miller et al., 2013; Pfau et al., 1997, 2005). In fact, these messages have proven equally effective in protecting both sides of the issues above-listed.

Additional Risk and Health-Related Topics

The effectiveness of inoculation-based strategies is certainly not limited to the already-introduced topics and policies. McGuire's (1964) original research, for example, focused on the protection of different health-related beliefs such as: the belief in regular teeth brushing; the belief in the benefits of penicillin; the belief in annual x-ray exams to detect for tuberculosis symptoms; and the belief in annual doctor's visits for regular checkups. His inoculation messages were successful regardless of the belief protected.

In addition, Rosenburg (2004) suggested that inoculation may be a suitable strategy to curb verbal aggression in schools. Matusitz and Breen believed that inoculation may be a promising strategy to help lower the rates of criminal recidivism (Matusitz & Breen, 2013). These authors also proposed that inoculation may assist in deterring young people from joining gangs (Breen & Matusitz, 2008). In addition, Kingsley Westerman and colleagues recommended using inoculation messages to aid safety training for emergencies (Kingsley Westerman, Margolis, & Kowalski-Trakofler, 2011).

Numerous other health and risk prevention topics remain that could be well-served with an inoculation-based strategy, some of which include the promotion and protection of healthy eating habits, positive attitudes toward mammograms, colonoscopies, breastfeeding (see Ivanov, 2012), and regular exercise (see Compton & Ivanov, in press). Inoculation can also be used as a strategy to prevent relapse in individuals recovering from substance abuse (see Ivanov, in press). Furthermore, it can potentially be used as a strategy to promote healthy sunscreen practices, attitudes, and behaviors (see Ivanov, in press).

Beyond Risk and Health Prevention

Although most of the inoculation research in the area of risk and health communication has focused on prevention application, an inoculation-based strategy is not limited to prevention (Ivanov et al., 2017; Wood, 2007). For example, Ivanov, Burns, and colleagues (2016) used inoculation as a risk and health management, rather than purely preventative, strategy. These authors did not use inoculation-based strategy exclusively with individuals with already established desirable beliefs. Instead, they successfully applied the strategy irrespective of the initial belief valence. In their study, the authors used the strategy to enhance the general public beliefs in the ability of the US government agencies to both prevent and minimize the negative effects of a politically motivated act of violence, such as the intentional downing of a commercial airliner on US soil. In addition, using an inoculation-based strategy, the authors were able to enhance the perceived ability of individuals to cope with the aftermath of such an act while at the same time lowering the perceived intensity of the experienced fear elicited by the politically motivated act of violence. Thus, inoculation-based messages offer a promising strategic approach in risk and health communication management, not just prevention.

Application of Inoculation Using Different Modalities

As addressed in the preceding section, health and risk messages employing an inoculation theory-based design have shown consistent efficacy in conferring resistance to persuasion (see Parker et al., 2012, 2016). However, inoculation research focused on understanding the role of communication modality in the inoculation process has been neither as abundant nor as clear with regard to results (Dillingham & Ivanov, 2016a; Pfau et al., 2000). When considering the relatively "boundless" (Ivanov, 2012, p. 77) potential of inoculation theory to inform applied risk and health message strategy, the question of modality becomes paramount. Stated simply, when inoculation messages leave the controlled experimental environment, can practitioners and scholars have confidence that these messages will perform (i.e., create and sustain resistance to persuasion) in a real-world multimodal communication environment?

Inoculation theory designs featuring print-only messages have largely dominated the previous five decades of research (Dillingham & Ivanov, 2016a). In the words of the late inoculation scholar Michael Pfau, modality has been treated as a "neutral conduit of message content" (1990, p. 195) within the boundaries of inoculation theory. Therefore, much of the empirical support demonstrating the superiority of inoculation messages as compared to both supportive and control messages has been founded on comparing participant sentiment after exposure to a print treatment message (inoculation, supportive, or message/no message control) and a subsequent print attack message (Compton & Pfau, 2005).

To date only two studies (Dillingham & Ivanov, 2016a; Pfau et al., 2000) have explicitly explored the role of modality in the inoculation process. However, several authors have embraced the interchangeable modality concept posited by Pfau (1990) and, as a result, used video messages (rather than or in addition to print) in the course of their respective studies. Yet, the purported neutrality of communication modality in the inoculation process is perplexing when reviewing these studies in tandem. For example, when exploring the potential of inoculation theory to deter adolescent alcohol abuse, Godbold and Pfau (2000) overwhelmed the protection created by a video inoculation message with a video attack message. Yet, unlike Godbold and Pfau, Burgoon and colleagues (1978) used a video inoculation/video attack design, but found evidence of inoculation's effectiveness.

To review, inoculation messages have thrived in a print treatment/print attack environment (see Compton & Pfau, 2005), with the results being mixed in studies that have paired a video treatment with a video attack (Burgoon et al., 1978; Godbold & Pfau, 2000). Some researchers—perhaps due to the assumed interchangeability of modalities—have mismatched video and print treatments within an inoculation study, or paired a print inoculation message with video attack or vice versa (e.g., An & Pfau, 2004; Banas & Miller, 2013). While the majority of these studies support print as the more robust medium, the results are not conclusive. For example, An and Pfau's (2004) video attack message reduced the resistance generated by a print inoculation message. In contrast, the print inoculation messages of both Banas and Miller (2013) and Lim and Ki (2007) showed success when faced with a video attack message. The Banas and Miller (2013) work is particularly notable due to the salience of the video attack. They offered that "the movie had the advantage of imagery, narration, music, and length" (2013, p. 198), and also lasted 40 minutes. Nonetheless, the print inoculation message created sustained resistance. More recently, and in the health context, Wong (2016) combined print and video formats in the pro-vaccination inoculation message and the generated resistance sustained persuasive attack presented through video. And, while Pfau, Van Bockern, and Kang (1992) did not include an attack phase in their study, the authors were able to inoculate low self-esteem middle school students against smoking initiation using video inoculation messages.

While scholars have noted (see Dillingham & Ivanov, 2016a) that some of the aforementioned studies (e.g., An & Pfau, 2004; Godbold & Pfau, 2000) demonstrate the potential for video to overwhelm the resistance created by print inoculation treatments, other work has demonstrated differences not just in the presence/absence of multimodal formats (i.e., video), but also in the evocative or engaging nature of the video messages. Nabi (2003), in the context of animal experimentation, explored whether or not inoculation messages presented by a "talking head" (p. 202) news anchor would impact participants as strongly as a video inoculation message that incorporated animal cruelty images. When faced with a video attack message, participants in Nabi's (2003) study showed increased resistance following exposure to the visually evocative inoculation message.

Further support for the strength of imagery was provided by Pfau and colleagues (2006, 2008) who found participants to be more affected (i.e., reporting negative feelings toward war) by a video featuring war footage compared with a video comprised of only news anchor reporting. The impact of video war footage was so salient, in fact, that Pfau and colleagues (2006) did not have success inoculating those participants against anti-war sentiment. Meanwhile, the anchor-only video attack group retained its inoculation-generated resistance, even in the face of a purportedly strong video attack (e.g., An & Pfau, 2004; Godbold & Pfau, 2000). It should be noted that Pfau and colleagues (2006) used print inoculation treatments with both (i.e., footage-inclusive and anchor-only) video attack messages. In a 2008 follow-up study about evocative visuals, Pfau and colleagues found that resistance created by neither print-only nor print-with-photograph inoculation messages could withstand a footage-inclusive video attack.

Despite the aforementioned ancillary findings that modestly suggest the strength of video messages compared to print and, more specifically, the enhanced salience achieved through use of evocative or engaging imagery, the two studies (Dillingham & Ivanov, 2016a; Pfau et al., 2000) that have systematically investigated modality-induced differences in inoculation message processing have not reflected these nuances. When comparing and contrasting the two efforts, Dillingham and Ivanov (2016a) and Pfau and colleagues (2000) share failed hypotheses about the strength of one modality over the other (video versus print) while using engaging (i.e., not news anchor–only) video footage in direct comparison to a print-only message. In both studies, video performed slightly better than print, but fell short of statistical significance. By way of contrast, Pfau and colleagues (2000) explored the impact of varied modality in the inoculation message, while Dillingham and Ivanov (2016a) compared print and video attack messages. The two author groups also hypothesized in different directions (i.e., in favor of a different modality).

Largely based on medium theory's (see Meyrowitz, 1994) supposition that print is a more engaging media form because reading requires active, central processing while television content can be passively (i.e., peripherally) processed, Pfau et al. (2000) hypothesized that participants who read an inoculation message would achieve an enhanced inoculation effect (i.e., greater resistance to persuasion) compared to those who viewed a video inoculation message. Dillingham and Ivanov (2016a), disparately, predicted that a video attack message would damage print-induced resistance in inoculated individuals more than a print attack message. The authors based their hypothesis on video-enhanced findings of Godbold and Pfau (2000), Nabi (2003), and An and Pfau (2004). As both studies (Dillingham & Ivanov, 2016a; Pfau et al., 2000) noted, the failed prediction that modality would alter the inoculation process, while not inherently good for the studies themselves, is actually quite positive for the advancement of inoculation theory. Not only is a large body of inoculation research that has employed a print-only research design still applicable to modern theorizing, as both author groups note, the seeming modality-neutral environment inherent in the inoculation process boosts the applied value of the theory. After all, practitioners using this strategy can only control the format of the inoculation message—and even then both video (Pfau et al., 1992; 2000) and print (Dillingham & Ivanov, 2016a) inoculation messages have withstood subsequent persuasive attack—but intervention designers cannot control or perfectly foresee what attack modalities their target population could face.

To summarize, when directly addressing the issue of modality, Pfau et al. (2000) and Dillingham and Ivanov (2016a) offer support for Pfau's (1990) original suggestion that modalities are interchangeable and simply a "neutral conduit of message content" (p. 195) in the inoculation message. These findings potentially explain consistent confounding results within video and print inoculation experiments and help diffuse empirical hints (e.g., Godbold & Pfau, 2000) that video might alter the inoculation process. The lessened sensitivity to modality suggested by inoculation research (Dillingham & Ivanov, 2016a; Pfau et al., 2000) seems to persist when an interpersonal component is introduced during the process. In addition to the burgeoning literature on post-inoculation talk (PIT) (see next section), where resistance generated via print has protected against persuasive attack even after the participant has discussed the issue within his or her social networks, a recent study (Jackson et al., 2015) showed the efficacy of a health oriented print inoculation treatment even when the persuasive attack was delivered verbally and in-person to a group of research participants by a confederate.

Inoculation Modality and Post-Inoculation Talk (PIT)

To this point, the discussion of the chapter has focused on a modality-controlled distribution of the risk and health strategic inoculation message, or what Rogers (1995) referred to as the linear model of communication. Stated differently, in our discussion the message content, format, timing, and dispersion vehicle were controlled by the strategic communication specialist and flowed one way, directly to the intended message receiver. This process is consistent with the traditional understanding of the mechanisms that elicit and facilitate the inoculation-based effects. To remind, risk and health inoculation messages generate motivation to shore up attitudinal defenses. The motivation is bolstered by the presentation of counterarguing material and guided practice designed to enhance the ability of the individual to counterargue forthcoming attitudinal challenges (McGuire, 1964). The motivated counterarguing practice is credited with the added skill or ability of the individual to withstand challenges (Compton, 2013; Compton & Pfau, 2005; Ivanov, 2012). Until recently, this counterarguing practice was considered to be entirely an internal process (Ivanov, Parker, & Dillingham, 2013), "as though one is having an intrapersonal dialogue with the anticipated attack message source" (Ivanov et al., 2012a, p. 704). Indeed, Brandt (1979) has suggested that counterarguing is "presumed to be [a] subvocal, psychological process" (p. 324). Therefore, if internal counterarguing exists solely, no further dispersion of the risk and health inoculation message is likely to occur and the inoculation process may truly be linear, where the inoculation message information is shared one way—from the strategic communication specialist to the message receiver—which motivates an internal defensive process.

However, in a seminal inoculation essay, Compton and Pfau (2009) theorized that the process of counterarguing is not exclusively *intrap*ersonal, as once anticipated (e.g., Brandt, 1979); but instead, it is *inter*personal as well. They suggested that inoculation message recipients may talk with others about the message content and topic for the purposes of reassuring and/or advocating their own attitudinal positions. If so, the process of risk and health inoculation message diffusion may not exclusively fit the linear model of communication (Rogers, 1995). Instead, the process of inoculation may also fit the convergence model, in which communication participants create and share information in an effort to reach mutual understanding (Rogers & Kinkaid, 1981). Recent inoculation research has provided evidence that the process of counterarguing may be both subvocal and vocal as inoculation message receivers talk to others in an effort to reassure and advocate their positions (Dillingham & Ivanov, 2016b; Ivanov et al., 2015). More specifically, by examining the communication content, Ivanov and colleagues (2015) found evidence that inoculated individuals not only shared the content contained in the inoculation message, but they also introduced novel arguments not present in the inoculation message. The conversations, termed post-inoculation talk, or PIT (Ivanov et al., 2012a), centered on both the topic at hand, as well as related topics, a practice which is closely associated with both the traditional and modern understanding of the inoculation process. Thus, the recent PIT findings suggest that, contrary to previous conceptualizations, inoculation message strategy relies, at minimum, on a dual process of message diffusion. The first is a traditional (linear) one-way controlled diffusion of information in which the message strategist disperses a controlled, prepared-in-advance inoculation message using the desired modality and timing of message transmission (Rogers, 1995). Yet, inoculation may also be diffused as information-exchange among receivers and non-receivers of the inoculation message, a process outside of the communication strategist's control (Rogers & Kinkaid, 1981).

Extant inoculation research that has focused on the traditional or linear process of inoculation message diffusion evidences the effectiveness of one-way communication in shoring up attitudes and combating attitudinal challenges (Compton, 2013; Compton & Pfau, 2005; Ivanov, 2012). However, what effect, if any, does the secondary diffusion process—inoculation as an information-exchange—have on the effectiveness of the inoculation process?

The first and most obvious added effect of PIT is the interpersonal diffusion of inoculation messages along social networks. As research shows (e.g., Ivanov et al., 2015), the content of the information shared via PIT contains the original message components, thus dispersing the intended inoculation message content to individuals not reached by the original presentation of the message. This outcome increases the practical utility of the inoculation-based message strategy due to its increased reach. In addition, in circumstances that provide only limited opportunity for one-way traditional dispersion of messages (e.g., natural or man-made disasters impacting traditional and/or electronic channels of communication), an interpersonal dispersion of the risk and health inoculation message via social networks may prove to be an invaluable asset to a communication specialist. For example, in a country such as Nigeria where per capita distribution of television sets, cellular phones, and other technological devices is low ("Compare Countries," n.d.), the ability to interpersonally diffuse an inoculation message about an Ebola outbreak and management strategies via social networks may be quite useful to a risk and health communication strategist.

The fact that inoculation messages are diffused interpersonally through social networks is quite beneficial for the purpose of risk and health message distribution; however, what effect does the PIT have on the interlocutors? After all, should the inoculation effect be eroded as a result of PIT, then the benefit gained from the process of interpersonal message diffusion would be offset by the diminished inoculation effect. To date, little is known about the effect of the inoculation message on the individuals receiving the message via PIT for the first time. What is clear is that non-recipients of the initial, traditionally distributed inoculation message may receive the inoculation message by talking to inoculated others (e.g., Dillingham & Ivanov, 2016b; Ivanov et al., 2012b, 2015). What effect inoculation has on these individuals is far less clear as, to date, no research has investigated the effect of inoculation when diffused through social networks. This remains an important empirical question.

More is known about the effect of PIT on the initial inoculation message recipients. Ivanov and colleagues (2012b) investigated the attitudinal impact of PIT. Their results suggested that PIT has the ability to enhance attitudes. More specifically, they discovered that inoculation generates threat, which motivates anger against current attitudinal challengers and challenges. Both threat and anger inspire PIT, which enhances the target attitude. Dillingham and Ivanov (2016b) conducted a more nuanced comparison of attitudinal impact of inoculation messages both in the presence and absence of PIT. Their findings indicated that traditional inoculation using subvocal counterarguing moved the attitudes in the desired direction. PIT, on the other hand, enhanced the certainty or conviction with which those attitudes were held. Taken together, the above studies show that PIT not only benefits the strategy by increasing its reach, but also by enhancing the target attitudes.

As traditionally conceptualized, the dispersion of the risk and health inoculation message was considered to be a one-way linear diffusion of a strategist-controlled message. Recent research (e.g., Dillingham & Ivanov, 2016b; Ivanov et al., 2012b, 2015) has suggested that the process of inoculation message distribution may be two-tiered. Risk and health inoculation messages are initially dispensed with a communication strategist–selected modality or modalities using a precise message presented at desired times, frequency, and to a predetermined target audience. In addition, inoculation is also spread via PIT, which is not under direct control of the risk and health communication strategist. Thus, inoculation can be diffused using multiple modalities and, at minimum, in two ways: by direct, controlled, one-way transmission from source to receiver and also as information-exchange among the participants of the PIT process (Rogers, 1995; Rogers & Kinkaid, 1981). The outcome is an overall greater rate of risk and health message diffusion and stronger inoculation effects experienced by the initial message recipients.

The Future of Inoculation as a Risk and Health Communication Strategy in an Evolving Media Context

Different Modalities

While, as previously mentioned, extant research supports the notion that modality does not substantially impact the inoculation message outcome (Dillingham & Ivanov, 2016a; Pfau et al., 2000), some unanswered questions remain. The modality-neutral inoculation environment is encouraging for practitioners, but remains perplexing for scholars. Almost unanimously, leading mass communication theorists (see McQuail, 2010) advance the idea that medium and message have an inextricable inter-play, even to the point of McLuhan's (1964) legendary assertion that "the medium is the message" (p. 1). How, then, can inoculation theory osten-sibly deviate from this norm?

One potential explanation is that print and video inoculation messages generate the same overall outcome (i.e., resistance to persuasion), but do so via different processes. Potentially, differences in processing moder-ate generated resistance in ways that have yet to be explored. Pfau and colleagues (2000) suggested processing differences in their initial study of modality and inoculation, citing abundant support for dual-process models, namely the Elaboration Likelihood Model (ELM) (see Petty & Cacioppo, 1986). More specifically, the authors considered print mes-sages a modality that required central processing and argued that video messages could be processed peripherally. As such, they argued, the print-generated resistance should bear the positive traits of central processing, such as more deeply rooted and longer lasting attitudinal resistance. While the authors' subsequent hypothesis that a print inoculation mes-sage would generate resistance beyond the capability of video was not supported, their idea deserves reconsideration in light of the findings addressed in this chapter. Possibly, the print inoculation message did gen-erate longer-lasting and more thoughtful, or intentional, resistance, but those nuances were not captured in the Pfau et al. (2000) analysis.

Pfau and colleagues (2000) measured attitude toward the attack as the primary dependent variable. As such, video and print inoculation mes-sages did not show significant differences. However, could these results have differed if certainty about the attitude had been measured? Studies (see Dillingham & Ivanov, 2015, 2016a, 2016b; Pfau et al., 2005) that have measured attitude or belief certainty have done so as a separate out-come variable. If Pfau and colleagues' (2000) suggestion that modalities engage different processes to arrive at the same outcome holds merit, pos-sibly print could increase certainty in a way video does not, even though both print and video generate overall resistance. Results from the other study, which explicitly studied modality in inoculation message process-ing (Dillingham & Ivanov, 2016a), do not dampen the idea that print could encourage central processing while video leaves the opportunity for peripheral processing. Dillingham and Ivanov found that participants reported higher levels of beliefs and certainty in those beliefs when their print-generated resistance was attacked with both print and video mes-sages. As such, print inoculation messages could have been processed centrally and yielded enhanced certainty.

Also, as previously discussed, save the work of An and Pfau (2004), several studies that have mismatched print and video messages have demonstrated the strength of print inoculation treatments. These stud-ies do not confound the idea that print leads to central processing and video to peripheral. Banas and Miller (2013), Lim and Ki (2007), and Wong (2016) all failed to erode print-generated resistance with a video inoculation message. In addition, while their study primarily concerned metainoculation (i.e., inoculating against an inoculation treatment), Banas and Miller also suggested the possibility of heuristic and central processing in the inoculation process. Based on their findings, the authors noted that "inoculation . . . can work heuristically as well as through mindful processing" (2013, p. 200). The disparate video inoculation/video attack study results (Burgoon et al., 1978; Godbold & Pfau, 2000) also make more sense when viewed through the lens of processing differences. If video is a modality that is processed peripherally within inoculation theory, then various cues such as imagery, color, or sound, could alter the level of generated resistance. Future studies should explore the central and peripheral processing possibilities within inoculation theory as well as measure attitudinal certainty following print-generated inoculation treatments.

Multimedia Campaigns

The lack of hindrance from modality concerns points to an intriguing future for multimedia risk and health-based inoculation campaigns. As research has shown (Pfau et al., 2000), both print and video inoculation messages can generate resistance, and future research may point to print engaging central processing. If central and peripheral processing are at play, practitioners have an even greater advantage as a print-based inoculation message is more easily controlled and precisely theoretically grounded (see Ivanov, 2012) and, presumably, distributed in a more cost-efficient manner via pamphlets, paper, email, websites, or other text-based media. Also encouraging for practitioners is the resilience of text-based inoculation messages to video attack (Banas & Miller, 2013; Dillingham & Ivanov, 2016a). While gaps in literacy could be an obstacle for practitioners using print-based inoculation risk and health campaigns, research has demonstrated that video inoculation messages can also generate resistance, thereby protecting pro-health attitudes (Burgoon et al., 1978; Pfau et al., 2000).

The notion that modalities can be mixed (in the inoculation message) and matched (with various attack formats) with relative confidence of the overall strategy effectiveness has empirical support (Dillingham & Ivanov, 2016a; Pfau et al., 2000). Video could also accompany the print component similar to the work of Wong (2016). While studies have explored mismatched (print inoculation and video attack and vice versa) treatment effects, to our knowledge Wong has pioneered combining modalities within the treatment condition. The efficacy demonstrated in his study is encouraging for practitioners. The video message does not seem to overwhelm or distract from the print inoculation message; rather, the two seem to work in unison. Future research should explore the impact of multimedia (i.e., combination video and print) attack messages to ascertain the impact of mixing media types in both the inoculation and attack message. Furthermore, in contrast to the modality-neutral results (Dillingham & Ivanov, 2016a; Pfau et al., 2000), support for integrating evocative visuals in inoculation video treatments as a strengthening mechanism is consistent (Nabi, 2003; Pfau et al., 2006, 2008).

Practitioners can assert a reasonable degree of confidence that venturing beyond the traditional format of inoculation message design (see Ivanov, 2012)—i.e., using a degree of creativity in designing the audiovisual components that accompany the inoculation message—would not sacrifice message effectiveness. While at this point suggesting supplanting the print inoculation message with video is unwarranted (Banas & Miller, 2013; Pfau et al., 2000), when working with media-saturated populations such as adolescents, the use of evocative and memorable video should not derail inoculation-generated resistance (Wong, 2016). While still images have not been studied, the modality flexibility evidenced via video study (Dillingham & Ivanov, 2016a; Pfau et al., 2000) could translate to text-accompanied photographs. A recent non-inoculation study (Dixon, 2016) about two-sided (pro and against) health messages demonstrated greater recall and higher risk perception related to negative behavior when photos accompanied text that explained the pros and cons of vaccination. Continued applied experimentation with print, video, photo, and even interpersonal communication is warranted based on the findings here reviewed.

One modality concern not addressed by inoculation research, though probable in a real-world health campaign, is the effectiveness of audio-only messages presented through media such as radio or podcast. Particularly in natural disasters (see Kingsley Westerman et al., 2011), radio waves could be the lone form of communication during the early stages of relief. Could inoculation messages be dispersed via radio that advise victims to follow safety recommendations despite fear or temptation to flee and/or crowd public spaces? Inoculation research has demonstrated the efficacy of one-modality messages, though print has been dominant (Compton & Pfau, 2005). Perhaps the one-modality effectiveness could extend to audio inoculation messages. Future research should explore this possibility to boost use in health and risk contexts.

Social Media

An uncharted territory of inoculation research is continued efficacy in interactive media environments, both synchronous and asynchronous. The modality-neutral likelihood, alongside growing support for the idea that interpersonal conversation can complement, rather than supplant, the internal inoculation process (Dillingham & Ivanov, 2016b) certainly does not discourage the idea that people using the Internet as a communication tool can (co-)create and possibly share inoculation effects. The research and applied potential is considerable. Can a person share an inoculation message on Facebook, for example, have the message attacked via comments, and demonstrate generated resistance with a counter-comment? Can witnessing the entire inoculation attack cycle serve as a threatening—and potentially resistance-instilling—mechanism for standby social media observers? Likewise, can a Twitter retweet of an inoculation message serve the same strengthening function as a PIT conversation (see Dillingham & Ivanov, 2016b)? These and other questions should be addressed with further research. In addition, when considering the possibility of dispersing inoculation messages using social media, the length of messages becomes a key question. More specifically, inoculation messages used in research have tended to be longer than those allowed (e.g., Twitter's 140-character limit), or reasonably expected, in social media environments.

Terse messages. The emergence of new communication technologies and social media are requiring risk and health inoculation scholars to reconsider both the inoculation message structure and delivery (see Compton & Ivanov, 2013). Traditionally, inoculation messages have favored print or audiovisual formats, delivered via traditional modes (e.g., television, newspaper, etc.) and featured extended message length. For example, Parker and colleagues (2012) designed a successful inoculation message aimed at boosting condom use among sexually active college students. The length of that message was 1,378 words. With the emergence of texting and social media as methods of communication that require a terse way of communicating (e.g., Twitter is limited to 140 characters), the question risk and health inoculation scholars face is whether inoculation messages can be adapted to take full advantage of media specialized in dispensing these short message forms. This need is especially pronounced in the context of risk and health communication where emergency alert systems (EAS) distribute important messages using 90 characters or less (Wimberly, 2015). Yet, relatively little data-driven research exists informing effective message design for these media in general, and in the context of health-related warning messages dispersed by public safety officials in particular (Sutton, League, Sellnow, & Sellnow, 2015). So, can risk and health inoculation messages be "fitted" to be applicable with short-form message dissemination media forms?

Compton and Ivanov (2013) suggested that the length of inoculation messages can be considerably reduced without losing their effectiveness. Similar to their political communication example, consider the following health promotion message aimed at recovering addicts and designed to prevent relapse: "They'll tell u 2 use. It might feel good. But, u use even once & u r back on the bottom. Broke. Helpless. Fight back. Don't give in." (132 characters). This message, suitable for distribution via text or Twitter, has all of the features an inoculation message should have. First, it provides threat. It does so explicitly by submitting a forewarning (e.g., "They'll tell u 2 use"). It then proceeds to offer additional threat implicitly (or inherently; McGuire, 1970) by presenting the receivers with real challenges they are likely to encounter in the future (e.g., "It might feel good"). To clarify, threat is a required requisite of inoculation, not explicit forewarning (Compton, 2009). Threat can be elicited explicitly via a forewarning, but also implicitly through the presentations of counterattitudinal arguments as applied in the above example. Thus, even though a forewarning was used in the example, it is not required for the inoculation-based process to be unleashed and can be omitted should message length become an issue. For example, the same message can be pared down to fit the 90-character length used in risk and health EAS messages by dropping the forewarning (e.g., "Using may feel good. But, u use once. U r back on bottom. Broke. Helpless. Don't give in." [89 characters]).

The risk and health terse message exemplified in the previous paragraph also provides receivers with a refutational preemption, by refuting the benefits of performing the behavior (e.g., "But, u use even once. U r back on the bottom. Broke. Helpless."). The message ends with an encouragement to continue to defend the attitude or behavior (e.g., "Don't give in").

Overall, the example terse message provides its recipients with the motivation to bolster their ability to defend their positive attitudes toward, and/or behavior of, staying sober by showing individuals that their newfound sobriety is likely to be assailed. It then provides them with guided practice of how to counterargue attacks on their sobriety. But this example represents just one way that inoculation can take advantage of short format risk and health message dispersion media. The message can be augmented by inserting a hashtag, which could lead the message receiver to additional refutational or attitude consistent information. Furthermore, the risk and health inoculation message could be designed to provide only an explicit forewarning in the terse message with a link that would take the reader to the full-length refutational component of the message. Using the same topic as above, the inoculation message may be worded in the following way "It's been tough. But, U r sober & in recovery. Yet b wary of pride and old habits. U r not safe. Test is coming. Can u pass it? Find out here." (140 characters). The above message provides a forewarning suggesting that despite the person's recent success aimed at long-term recovery, the hard work is at stake. The forewarning is designed to motivate the recipient to press on the link (i.e., represented by the underlined word "here") where the refutational component of the message can be presented in its full length whether as text, audio, video, or a combination thereof.

Consequently, as exemplified in this section, risk and health inoculation messages could be adapted to take full advantage of short text dispersion media. Their rate of success is an empirical question that necessitates further investigation. However, in a modern environment where individuals rely of their technologies, such as smart phones, tablets, and computers, for information gathering and processing, for inoculation to continue to be a relevant risk and health message strategy, its method of dispersion and presentation has to fit the audience preferred modalities and formats of message reception.

Booster messages. Although the extant research has unequivocally shown inoculation to be an effective message strategy in general (Banas & Rains, 2010) and in the risk and health contexts in particular (e.g., Ivanov et al., 2016; Parker et al., 2012; Wong & Harrison, 2014), its effects erode over time (McGuire, 1962; Pfau, 1997; Pfau et al., 1990; Pryor & Steinfatt, 1978). This outcome is likely a result of message (Stiff & Mongeau, 2003) and motivation (Insko, 1967) decay. As Insko suggested, "induced motivation" to accumulate "belief-bolstering material" will decline over time following "the ordinary forgetting curve" (p. 316). To compensate, inoculation strategists have relied on booster shots, or message reinforcements, with some effectiveness (Pfau, 1997; Pfau & Van Bockern, 1994). The main challenges frustrating inoculation strategists when using inoculation boosters have dealt with the proper timing of the booster shots after the introduction of the initial inoculation message, as well as the proper form, length, and frequency (see Ivanov, in press; Ivanov, Parker & Dillingham, 2016).

The form and length of the booster shot is especially relevant when deciding on the modality of risk and health message distribution. With evolving traditional and social media technologies available to the message strategists, booster messages that can be quickly disseminated through these media should be of particular import and interest. These messages may take longer-length form, as traditionally constructed (Pfau, 1997; Pfau & Van Bockern, 1994), or may even be presented in a terse format. For example, a current risk and health intervention campaign using inoculation to combat the risk of relapse among recently sober addicts, as a follow-up to the inoculation message, is dependent on the use of short text messages to reinforce or boost sobriety.

Evolving media technologies in general, and social media in particular, allow for new ways of delivering booster messages that can be done with better timing and frequency (e.g., using preset triggers for text or e-mail messages). Inoculation messages have been shown to be effective in combating complacency and enhancing resilience (Ivanov et al., 2016). Boosters, which can help assail the threat of message and motivation decay, can play a significant strategic role by reaching message recipients quickly and frequently through different social media platforms and mobile devices (e.g., Twitter, mobile phones, Facebook, tablets, etc.). As such, risk and health inoculation strategists have the opportunity and responsibility to take full advantage of these new modes of booster message delivery.

Post-inoculation talk. Up to this point, the chapter's discussion regarding PIT has centered on the questions of whether inoculation message recipients, including those of risk and health messages, engage in such talk and for what reason (i.e., advocacy, reassurance, or both). However, what has received little consideration to date is the understanding of *how* individuals talk. Stated differently, over what conversational vehicle does the talk take place? Do individuals engage in PIT face to face, via telephone, on Twitter or Facebook, or do they use other and/or multiple modes of communication? The preliminary results of an ongoing study suggest that inoculated individuals talk to multiple others about the message topic and content. In some cases they use the same mode (e.g., in person or face to face) with multiple discussion partners, while in other cases they use different modes with different discussants. What is still unknown is whether individuals have multiple conversations with the same partner over different modes and whether the mode of conversation has an impact on, or is impacted by, the conversational channel.

Compton and Pfau (2009) suggested, and Ivanov and colleagues (2015) affirmed, the usage of PIT for the purposes of both reassurance and advocacy. In addition, Ivanov et al. (2015) discovered PIT in the form of advocacy to encounter greater numbers of counter-attitudinal challenges than PIT in the form of reassurance. Due to reduced normative pressures and inhibitions (Bordia, 1997), computer-mediated communication may be more conducive to social debate (Berger, 2014). If so, then social platforms may be better suited for advocacy-focused PIT, where such preference may not be present with reassurance-motivated PIT. As a result, the PIT channel used for message transmission may moderate the approach taken in the discussion (i.e., to advocate or to self-reassure). Alternatively, the primary purpose of the PIT (i.e., advocacy vs. reassurance) may influence the conversational channel selected. Moreover, inoculated people may choose different conversation channels with different individuals based on the primary purpose of the PIT. The referenced study in progress is designed to provide some answers to the above speculations, but more future research is needed to uncover the impact of modality on the purpose and content of PIT. The potential interaction between modality and the purpose of PIT (i.e., advocacy vs. reassurance) may have a significant impact on the effectiveness of risk and health message diffusion and desired outcomes. For example, faced with an Ebola crisis in affected areas lacking technological devices and platforms needed for computer-mediated communication, inoculation recipients may be counted on to advocate the proper risk and health prevention strategies. However, if these inoculated individuals are not likely to engage others face to face to propagate the message, then the social diffusion advantages of inoculation-elicited PIT will be negated.

Overall, PIT extends the utility of risk and health inoculation-based strategies as it boosts the attitudinal (or behavioral) defenses of target message receivers and aids message diffusion along social networks. However, the transmission channel and platform could potentially impact the process of PIT. As such, the impact of evolving technologies and media on the process of PIT must be considered by risk and health inoculation-based strategists.

Conclusion

Effective message design continues to be an important component of successful communication approaches undergirding risk and health prevention and management strategies (Ivanov, 2012; Ivanov et al., 2016; Pfau, 1995). Due to their demonstrated effectiveness (e.g., Ivanov et al., 2016; Parker et al., 2012; Pfau & Van Brockern; 1994; Wong & Harrison, 2014), inoculation-based messages have gained interest and popularity as risk and health communication strategies (see Compton, 2013; Compton & Pfau, 2005; Ivanov, 2012, in press). However, for inoculation-based approaches to remain relevant, viable strategic options, and for them to continue to gain popularity, their practical application using traditional print and video modalities need to be aligned with multimodal realities of today's digital and social media environment. This chapter provided a review of the robust nature of inoculation-based strategies when used with different traditional, single and mixed modalities. In addition, it featured specific suggestions on how risk and health strategists may be able to take advantage of the evolving media environment in order to enhance the effect and practical application of inoculation-based strategies. By providing examples, as well as direct and ancillary evidence, a call to action was extended to test the efficacy of the strategy in a multimodal, digital environment in order for strategists to take full advantage of the evolving communication technologies.

As a multi-level (i.e., linear and information-exchange) dispersion strategy, inoculation shows significant promise for risk and health prevention and management strategists. Its robustness across different modalities demonstrates the opportunity to deviate from inoculation's standard modal form in order to capitalize on the greatest delivery and presentation prospects. As such, it presents a significant advantage as inoculation provides communication strategists with the potential to incorporate terse and booster messages in the campaign design, as well as take advantage of the ability of inoculation messages to be diffused over social networks.

Successful risk and health prevention and management will continue to depend on the effectiveness of communication strategies supporting these activities. Inoculation-based messages can provide the foundation on which such effective strategies can be built. With the potential to be dispersed across different modalities and forms, inoculation messages provide reliable and exciting strategic approaches that may help maximize the diffusion and intended effect of the targeted communication. Thus, if applied properly, the potential of inoculation-based strategies may be "boundless" (Ivanov, 2012, p. 77) in the rapidly evolving media environment supporting effective health and risk communication.

References

An, C., & Pfau, M. (2004). The efficacy of inoculation in televised political debates. *Journal of Communication, 54*, 421–436.

Brandt, D. R. (1979). Listener propensity to counterargue, distraction, and resistance to persuasion. *Central States Speech Journal, 30*, 321–331.

Banas, J. A., & Miller, G. (2013). Inducing resistance to conspiracy theory propaganda: Testing inoculation and metainoculation strategies. *Human Communication Research, 39*, 184–207. doi: 10.1111/hcre.12000.

Banas, J. A., & Rains, S. A. (2010). A meta-analysis of research on inoculation theory. *Communication Monographs, 77*, 281–311.

Banerjee, S. C., & Greene, K. (2006). Analysis versus production: Cognitive and attitudinal responses to antismoking interventions. *Journal of Communication, 56*, 773–794. doi: 10.1111/j.1460-2466.00319.x.

Banerjee, S. C., & Greene, K. (2007). Antismoking initiatives: Effects of analysis versus production media literacy interventions on smoking-related attitude, norm, and behavioral intention. *Health Communication, 22*(1), 37–48.

Berger, J. (2014). Word of mouth and interpersonal communication: A review and directions for future research. *Journal of Consumer Psychology, 24*(4), 586–607.

Bordia, P. (1997). Face-to-face versus computer-mediated communication: A synthesis of the experimental literature. *Journal of Business Communication, 34*(1), 99–120.

Breen, G. M., & Matusitz, J. (2008). Preventing youths from joining gangs: How to apply inoculation theory. *Journal of Applied Security Research, 4*, 109–128.

Burgoon, M., Cohen, M., Miller, M. D., & Montgomery, C. L. (1978). An empirical test of a model of resistance to persuasion. *Human Communication Research, 5*, 27–39.

Burgoon, M., Pfau, M., & Birk, T. S. (1995). An inoculation theory explanation for the effects of corporate issue/advocacy advertising campaigns. *Communication Research, 22*, 485–505.

Compare countries on just about anything! (n.d.). NationMaster Website. Retrieved September 7, 2016, from www.nationmaster.com/au.

Compton, J. (2009, Fall). Threat explication: What we know and don't yet know about a key component of inoculation theory. *STAM Journal, 39*, 1–18.

Compton, J. (2013). Inoculation theory. In J. P. Dillard & L. Shen (Eds.), *The SAGE handbook of persuasion: Developments in theory and practice* (2nd ed.) (pp. 220–236). Thousand Oaks, CA: SAGE.

Compton, J., & Ivanov, B. (2013). Vaccinating voters: Surveying political campaign inoculation scholarship. In E. L. Cohen (Ed.), *Communication yearbook 37* (pp. 250–283). New York: Routledge.

Compton, J., & Ivanov, B. (2014, November). *Inoculation theory and affect: Emotions and moods, mediators and moderators, and new directions for affect-focused resistance scholarship.* Paper presented at the annual meeting of the National Communication Association, Chicago, IL.

Compton, J., & Ivanov, B. (in press). Inoculation messaging. In B. Jackson, J. Dimmock, & J. Compton (Eds.), *Persuasion and communication in sport, exercise, and physical activity.* New York: Taylor & Francis.

Compton, J., & Pfau, M. (2005). Inoculation theory of resistance to influence at maturity: Recent progress in theory development and application and suggestions for future research. In P. Kalbfleisch (Ed.), *Communication yearbook 29* (pp. 97–145). Mahwah, NJ: Lawrence Erlbaum.

Compton, J., & Pfau, M. (2008). Inoculating against pro-plagiarism justifications: Rational and affective strategies. *Journal of Applied Communication Research, 36*(1), 98–119.

Compton, J., & Pfau, M. (2009). Spreading inoculation: Inoculation, resistance to influence, and word-of-mouth communication. *Communication Theory, 19,* 9–28.

Degeneffe, D., Kinsey, J., Stinson, T. & Ghosh, K. (2009). Segmenting consumers for food defense communication strategies. *International Journal of Physical Distribution Logistics Management, 39,* 365–403.

Dholakia, U. M., Kahn, B. E., Reeves, R., Rindfleisch, A., Stewart, D., & Taylor, E. (2010). Consumer behavior in a multichannel, multimedia retailing environment. *Journal of Interactive Marketing, 24*(2), 86–95.

Dillingham, L. L., & Ivanov, B. (2015). Boosting inoculation's message potency: Loss framing. *Communication Research Reports, 32,* 113–121.

Dillingham, L. L., & Ivanov, B. (2016a, November). *Talk while they will listen: Inoculation messages as a pre-emptive crisis communication strategy.* Paper presented at the annual meeting of the National Communication Association, Philadelphia, PA.

Dillingham, L. L., & Ivanov, B. (2016b). Using post-inoculation talk to strengthen generated resistance. *Communication Research Reports, 33*(4).

Dixon, G. (2016). Negative affect as a mechanism of exemplification effects. *Communication Research, 43*(6), 761–784. doi: 10.1177/0093650215579222.

Duryea, E. J. (1982, April). *Application of inoculation theory to preventive alcohol education.* Paper presented at the National Convention of the American Alliance for Health, Physical Education, Recreation and Dance, Houston, TX.

Duryea, E. J. (1983). Utilizing tenants of inoculation theory to develop and evaluate a preventive alcohol education intervention. *Journal of School Health, 53,* 250–256.

Eagly, A. H., & Chaiken, S. (1993). *The psychology of attitudes.* Orlando, FL: Harcourt Brace Jovanovich.

Farchi, M., & Gidron, Y. (2010). The effects of psychological inoculation versus ventilation on the mental resilience of Israeli citizens under continuous war stress. *The Journal of Nervous and Mental Disease, 198*(5), 382–384.

Garnett, J. L., & Kouzmin, A. (2007). Communicating throughout Katrina: Competing and complementary conceptual lenses on crisis communication. *Public Administration Review, 67,* 171–188.

Godbold, L. C., & Pfau, M. (2000). Conferring resistance to peer pressure among adolescents. *Communication Research*, 27, 411–437.

Haigh, M. M., & Pfau, M. (2006). Bolstering organizational identity, commitment, and citizenship behaviors through the process of inoculation. *International Journal of Organizational Analysis*, 14(4), 295–316.

Insko, C. A. (1967). *Theories of attitude change*. New York: Appleton-Century-Crofts.

Ivanov, B. (2012). Designing inoculation messages for health communication campaigns. In H. Cho (Ed.), *Health communication message design: Theory and practice* (pp. 73–93). Thousand Oaks, CA: SAGE Publications.

Ivanov, B. (in press). Inoculation theory applied in health and risk messaging. In R. Parrott (Ed.), *Encyclopedia of health and risk message design and processing*. New York: Oxford University Press. doi: 10.1093/acrefore/9780190228613.013.254.

Ivanov, B., Burns, W. J., Sellnow, T. L., Petrun, E. L., Veil, S. R., & Mayorga, M. W. (2016). Using an inoculation message approach to promote public confidence in protective agencies. *Journal of Applied Communication Research*, 44(4). doi: 10.1080/00909882.2016.1225165.

Ivanov, B., Miller, C. H., Compton, J., Averbeck, J. M., Harrison, K. J., Sims, J. D., Parker, K. A., & Parker, J. L. (2012a). Effects of post-inoculation talk on resistance to influence. *Journal of Communication*, 62(4), 701–718.

Ivanov, B., Parker, K. A., & Dillingham, L. L. (2013). Measuring counterarguing: A review and critique of the most popular techniques. *The International Journal of Interdisciplinary Studies in Communication*, 7, 59–74.

Ivanov, B., Parker, K. A., & Dillingham, L. L. (2016, April). *Inoculation, boosters, and multiple attacks: How much can inoculation withstand?* Paper presented at the meeting of the Kentucky Conference on Health Communication, Lexington.

Ivanov, B., Parker, K. A., Miller, C. H., & Pfau, M. (2012b). Culture as a moderator of inoculation success: The effectiveness of a mainstream inoculation message on a subculture population. *The Global Studies Journal*, 4(3), 1–22.

Ivanov, B., Pfau, M., & Parker, K. A. (2009). The potential of inoculation in protecting the country of origin image. *Central Business Review*, 28, 9–16.

Ivanov, B., Rains, S. A, Geegan, S. A., Vos, S. C., Haarstad, N. D., & Parker, K. A. (2017). Beyond simple inoculation: Examining the persuasive value of inoculation for audiences with initially neutral or opposing attitudes. *Western Journal of Communication*, 81(1), 105–126. doi: 10.1080/10570314.2016.1224917.

Ivanov, B., Sims, J. D., Compton, J., Miller, C. H., Parker, K. A., Parker, J. L., Harrison, K. J., & Averbeck, J. M. (2015). The general content of post-inoculation talk: Recalled issue-specific conversations following inoculation treatments. *Western Journal of Communication*, 79, 218–238. doi: 10.1080/10570314.2014.943423.

Jackson, B., Compton, J., Whiddett, R., Anthony, D. R., & Dimmock, J. A. (2015). Preempting performance challenges: The effects of inoculation messaging on attacks to task self-efficacy. *PLoS ONE*, 10(4), e0124886. doi:10.1371/journal.pone.0124886.

Kingsley Westerman, C., Margolis, K. A., & Kowalski-Trakofler, K. M. (2011, November). Training for safety in emergencies: Inoculating for underground coal mine emergencies. *Professional Safety*, 42–46.

Lim, J. S., & Ki, E. (2007). Resistance to ethically suspicious parody video on YouTube: A test of inoculation theory. *Journalism and Mass Communication Quarterly, 84*(4), 713–728.

Lumsdaine, A. A., & Janis, I. L. (1953). Resistance to "counterpropaganda" produced by one-sided and two-sided "propaganda" presentations. *Public Opinion Quarterly, 17*(3), 311–318.

Matusitz, J., & Breen, G. M. (2013). Applying inoculation theory to the study of recidivism reduction in criminal prison inmates. *Journal of Evidence-Based Social Work, 10,* 455–465. doi: 10.1080/15433714.2012.760929.

McGuire, W. J. (1961). Resistance to persuasion conferred by active and passive prior refutation of same and alternative counterarguments. *Journal of Abnormal Psychology, 63,* 326–332.

McGuire, W. J. (1962). Persistence of the resistance to persuasion induced by various types of prior belief defense. *Journal of Abnormal and Social Psychology, 64,* 241–248.

McGuire, W. J. (1964). Inducing resistance to persuasion: Some contemporary approaches. In L. Berkowitz (Ed.), *Advances in experimental social psychology* (Vol. 1, pp. 191–229). New York: Academic Press.

McGuire, W. J. (1970, February). A vaccine for brainwash. *Psychology Today,* 36–39, 63–64.

McLuhan, M. (1964). *The medium is the message.* New York: Bantam Books.

McQuail, D. (2010). *McQuail's mass communication theory* (6th ed.). London: SAGE.

Meyrowitz, J. (1994). Medium theory. In D. Crowley & D. Mitchell (Eds.), *Communication theory today* (pp. 50–77). Stanford, CA and London: Stanford University Press and Polity Press.

Miller, C. H., Ivanov, B., Sims, J. D., Compton, J., Harrison, K. J., Parker, K. A., Parker, J. L., & Averbeck, J. M. (2013). Boosting the potency of resistance: Combining the motivational forces of inoculation and psychological reactance. *Human Communication Research, 39,* 127–155.

Nabi, R. L. (2003). "Feeling" resistance: Exploring the role of emotionally evocative visuals in inducing inoculation. *Media Psychology, 5,* 199–223.

Niederdeppe, J., Heley, K., & Berry, C. L. (2015). Inoculation and narrative strategies in competitive framing of three heath policy issues. *Journal of Communication, 65,* 838–862. doi: 10.1111/jcom.12162.

O'Hair, H. D., & Heath, R. L. (2005). Conceptualizing communication and terrorism. In H. D. O'Hair, R. L. Heath, & J. A. Becker (Eds.), *Community preparedness and response to terrorism* (pp. 1–12). Westport, CT: Praeger.

Parker, K. A., Ivanov, B., & Compton, J. (2012). Inoculation's efficacy with young adults' risky behaviors: Can inoculation confer cross-protection over related but untreated issues? *Health Communication, 27,* 223–233. doi: 10.1080/10410236.2011.575541.

Parker, K. A., Rains, S. A., & Ivanov, B. (2016). Examining the "Blanket of Protection" conferred by inoculation: The effects of inoculation messages on the cross-protection of related attitudes. *Communication Monographs, 83,* 49–68. doi: 10.1080/03637751.2015.1030681.

Petty, R. E., & Cacioppo, J. T. (1986). *Communication and persuasion: Central and peripheral routes to attitude change.* New York: Springer-Verlag.

Pfau, M. (1990). A channel approach to television influence. *Journal of Broadcasting & Electronic Media, 34,* 195–214.

Pfau, M. (1995). Designing messages for behavioral inoculation. In E. Maibach & R. L. Parrott (Eds.), *Designing health messages: Approaches from communication theory and public health practice* (pp. 99–113). Newbury Park, CA: SAGE Publications.

Pfau, M. & Burgoon, M. (1988). Inoculation in political campaign communication. *Human Communication Research, 15,* 91–111.

Pfau, M., Compton, J., Parker, K. A., Wittenberg, E. M., An, C., Ferguson, M., Horton, H., & Malyshev, Y. (2004). The traditional explanation for resistance based on the core elements of threat and counterarguing and an alternative rationale based on attitude accessibility: Do these mechanisms trigger distinct or overlapping process of resistance? *Human Communication Research, 30,* 329–360.

Pfau, M., Haigh, M., Fifrick, A., Holl, D., Tedesco, A., Cope, J., Nunnally, D., Schiess, A., Preston, D., Roszkowski, P., & Martin, M. (2006). The effects of print news photographs of the casualties of war. *Journalism & Mass Communication Quarterly, 83*(1), 150–168.

Pfau, M., Haigh, M. M., Shannon, T., Tones, T., Mercurio, D., Williams, R., Binstock, B., Diaz, C., Dillard, C., Browne, M., Elder, C., Reed, S., Eggers, A., & Melendez, J. (2008). The influence of television news depictions of the images of war on viewers. *Journal of Broadcasting & Electronic Media, 52*(2), 303–322.

Pfau, M., Holbert, R. L., Zubric, S. J., Pasha, N. H., & Lin, W. (2000). Role and influence of communication modality in the process of resistance to persuasion. *Media Psychology, 2,* 1–33.

Pfau, M., Ivanov, B., Houston, B., Haigh, M., Sims, J., Gilchrist, E., Russell, J., Wigley, S., Eckstein, J., Richert, N. (2005). Inoculation and mental processing: The instrumental role of associative networks in the process of resistance to counterattitudinal influence. *Communication Monographs, 72,* 414–441.

Pfau, M., Kenski, H. C., Nitz, M., & Sorenson, J. (1990). Efficacy of inoculation strategies in promoting resistance to political attack messages: Application to direct mail. *Communication Monographs, 57,* 25–43.

Pfau, M., Roskos-Ewoldsen, D., Wood, M., Yin, S., Cho, J., Lu, K. H., & Shen, L. (2003). Attitude accessibility as an alternative explanation for how inoculation confers resistance. *Communication Monographs, 70,* 39–51.

Pfau, M., Semmler, S. M., Deatrick, L., Ason, A., Nisbett, G., Lane, L., Craig, E., Underhill, J., & Banas, J. (2009). Nuances about the role and impact of affect in inoculation. *Communication Monographs, 76,* 73–98.

Pfau, M., Tusing, K. J., Koerner, A. F., Lee, W., Godbold, L. C., Penaloza, L. J., Yang, V. S., & Hong, Y. (1997). Enriching the inoculation construct: The role of critical components in the process of resistance. *Human Communication Research, 24,* 187–215.

Pfau, M., & Van Bockern, S. (1994). The persistence of inoculation in conferring resistance to smoking initiation among adolescents: The second year. *Human Communication Research, 20,* 413–430.

Pfau, M., Van Bockern, S., & Kang, J. G. (1992). Use of inoculation to promote resistance to smoking initiation among adolescents. *Communication Monographs, 59,* 213–230.

Pryor, B., & Steinfatt, T. M. (1978). The effects of initial belief level on inoculation theory and its proposed mechanisms. *Human Communication Research*, 4, 217–230.

Rogers, E. M. (1995). *Diffusion of innovations* (4th ed.). New York: The Free Press.

Rogers, E. M., & Kincaid, D. L. (1981). *Communication networks: Toward a new paradigm for research*. New York: The Free Press.

Rosenberg, S. (2004). Inoculation effect in prevention of increased verbal aggression in schools. *Psychological Reports, 95*, 1219–1226.

Stiff, J. B. & Mongeau, P. A. (2003). *Persuasive communication*. New York: The Guilford Press.

Sutton, C. A. (2011). *Inoculating against jealousy: Attempting to preemptively reduce the jealousy experience and improve jealousy expression*. Athens: University of Georgia.

Sutton, J., League, C., Sellnow, T. L., & Sellnow, D. D. (2015). Terse messaging and public health in the midst of natural disasters: The case of the Boulder floods. *Health Communication, 30*(2), pp. 135–143. doi: 10.1080/104102 36.2014.974124.

Szabo, E. A., & Pfau, M. (2001). *Reactance as a response to antismoking messages*. Paper presented at the annual meeting of the National Communication Association, Atlanta, GA.

Wong, N. (2016). Vaccinations are safe and effective: Inoculating positive HPV vaccine attitudes against antivaccination attack messages. *Communication Reports, 29*(3), 127–138. doi: 10.1080/08934215.2015.1083599.

Wong, N. C. H., & Harrison, K. J. (2014). Nuances in inoculation: Protecting positive attitudes toward the HPV vaccine & the practice of vaccinating children. *Journal of Women's Health, Issues & Care, 3*(6). doi: 10.4172/2325-9795.1000170.

Wood, M. L. M. (2007). Rethinking the inoculation analogy: Effects on subjects with differing preexisting attitudes. *Human Communication Research, 33*, 357–378.

Wan, H. H., & Pfau, M. (2004). The relative effectiveness of inoculation, bolstering, and combined approaches in crises communication. *Journal of Public Relations Research, 16*, 301–328.

Wigley, S., & Pfau, M. (2010). Arguing with emotion: A closer look at affect and the inoculation process. *Communication Research Reports, 27*(3), 217–229.

Wimberly, R. (2015, April 24). Longer messages are needed for Wireless Emergency Alerts: A DHS study says 90-character WEA messages create a "milling" effect and are insufficient to convince people to take protective action. Emergency Management Website. Retrieved September 7, 2016, from www.emergencymgmt. com/disaster/Longer-Messages-Needed-Wireless-Emergency-Alerts.html.

Zemmels, D. R. (2012). Youth and new media: Studying identity and meaning in an evolving media environment. *Communication Research Trends, 31*(4), 4–22.

Part IV

EXPLORING MESSAGES AND MEDIA DURING EXTREME EVENTS

14

FIRST ALERT WEATHER

Local Broadcasters' Communication During Weather Emergencies

Michael D. Bruce, Chandra Clark, and Scott Hodgson

Introduction

Meteorologists are trained professionals with expertise in weather who typically view themselves as public servants. They have a mission to study the atmosphere and climate and help people prepare for the weather of the day so they can decide whether to take an umbrella, wear warmer clothes, or pull out the sunglasses. In more dangerous situations such as severe weather, meteorologists can be hailed as heroes or failures. Most forecasters have a passion for communicating information and using the best technology possible to help them disseminate critical weather information to their communities. The audience has high expectations for the person who has that power. They are quickly mocked or scorned when they are wrong, but they are deservedly praised if a family walks out safely after a tornado destroyed their home.

Local stations around the country spend millions of dollars each year on the latest weather tools in order to provide their audiences with up-to-the-minute weather information. The management at these stations have developed a business strategy and a hefty budget to buy satellite trucks, cellular-equipped backpacks, community-installed camera systems in multiple cities, and develop phone applications that allow real-time alerts and updates. They make these tremendous capital expenditures in order to maintain audience ratings, but also because the stations are mandated to be community servants. The Federal Communication Commission requires over-the-air broadcasters to serve their communities in the "public interest, convenience, and necessity" in exchange for a broadcasting license.

Even with all the technology we carry around in our hands, the best and most proven way to communicate to the majority of audiences is still radio and television broadcasting. Local news viewership continues to rise in varying timeslots (Matsa, 2015). In a 2013 Gallup poll, Americans said they turned to television news (55 percent), the Internet (21 percent), newspapers and print publications (9 percent), and radio (6 percent) for current event information (Saad, 2013). While a great communication tool, mobile and web-based technologies have also proven less reliable after power fails during a significant weather event (Burger, Gochfeld, Jeitner, Pittfield, & Donio, 2013).

In the last five years, several major tornado outbreaks and a major hurricane along the East Coast highlighted the role meteorologists, weather forecasters, and local broadcasters play in communicating messages to the public before, during, and after a disaster. The situations caused by unpredictable tornadoes, hurricanes, rising water, and wind damage put local radio and television stations in a prime position for communicating weather emergencies across multiple platforms to those in affected areas.

This chapter is an attempt to add to the journalism and mass communication literature related to local broadcasters' roles in communicating weather emergencies. The authors provide an examination, using elements of the Crisis and Emergency Risk Communication (CERC) model, of broadcasters' communication efforts in the midst of three massive US natural disasters occurring within an eighteen-month period. Through personal interviews and research we investigate broadcasters' severe weather communication strategies.

Rationale

Storm Background

In 2011–2012, three major weather events—an EF-4 tornado in Tuscaloosa, Alabama; an EF-5 tornado in Joplin, Missouri; and Hurricane Sandy—proved how important local media are to communities in times of weather crisis. Since these events, meteorologists and local station managers have examined their media messages and business plans for severe weather in order to refine their communication with the public. Self-assessment of weather professionals and their support staff is no different than local and federal government agencies that see how they can improve before the next big event happens.

In the United States and Canada, the National Weather Service now expresses magnitude or strength and severity of tornadoes in terms of the Enhanced Fujita Scale or EF scale. The greater the magnitude of a tornado, the greater the potential for fatalities, injuries, and damage to property, although more people have died from EF0–EF4 tornadoes because EF5 tornadoes occur less frequently (Paul and Stimers, 2011). The National Hurricane Center measures the strength of a hurricane's sustained wind speed based on the Saffir-Simpson Hurricane Wind Scale. The 1–5 scale estimates potential property damage. Hurricanes reaching Category 3 or higher are considered major hurricanes because of potential for significant property damage and loss of life.

EF-4 Tornado, Tuscaloosa, AL: April 27, 2011. A major tornado outbreak happened in Alabama and in several southeastern states on April 27, 2011. As early as a week before, local meteorologists began seeing weather models predicting chances for what could be a devastating severe storm outbreak for the state. While local stations had a week to implement a plan to cover the potential storms, they were not prepared for the more than 60 tornadoes that touched down in Alabama in that one day.

When the storms calmed the startling results of damage to life and property came in, with fatalities in Tuscaloosa (56), Alabama (252), and the region (316). More than 12 percent of property in the city of Tuscaloosa was destroyed. Property damage in the state was estimated at $1.5 billion and debris measured more than 10 million cubic yards (Thompson, 2011). While the numbers are staggering, the mayor of Tuscaloosa and the state's emergency management agency credited the early warning for saving hundreds of lives that day. Despite the lives saved, the severity of this storm reminded the disaster management community that effective communication strategies need to be refined in Alabama—a state hit by more than 900 tornadoes since 2000, accounting for a quarter of all US tornado deaths (Lewis, 2012).

EF-5 Tornado, Joplin, MO: May 22, 2011. Missouri is no stranger to tornadoes. Tornado watches are issued for some part of the state nearly every week in the spring of each year. The forecast for May 22, 2011, called for severe weather, but no one expected an EF-5 tornado would cut a path through the heart of the city. The tornado was on the ground for 22.1 miles, packed sustained winds of 200 miles per hour and was nearly a mile wide at its peak (Wheatley, 2013). The city of Joplin reported over 18,000 vehicles, 8,000 structures, 400 businesses, 7,000 homes, 8 schools, and a major regional hospital severely damaged or destroyed (Reynolds, n.d.). Causing direct insured losses in excess of $1.9 billion, it is one of the most expensive tornadoes on record (Freedman, 2012). There were also 162 fatalities, making it the single deadliest tornado to hit the United States since modern record keeping began in 1950 (Paul & Stimers, 2011).

Hurricane Sandy: October 29, 2012. Hurricane Sandy made landfall as a Category 1 storm on October 29, 2012, on the Jersey shore along the East Coast of the United States. The storm caused 150 fatalities. Residential damage totaled 346,000 homes in New Jersey and 305,000 homes in New York. Damage from Sandy's winds and floodwaters made it the second costliest hurricane in US history behind Hurricane Katrina.

A year after the storm, business losses totaled $8.3 billion in New Jersey and $19 billion in New York City. Those costs included private, public, and indirect costs (Huffington Post, 2013). Overall, in four states and the District of Columbia, the storm swept away $50 billion in damages (Blake, Kimberlain, Berg, Cangialosi, & Beven, 2013).

The costs continue to rise four years later as countless municipalities throughout the region have been forced to cut programs and services that were once funded by property taxes. Two New Jersey counties have seen property values fall by $5 billion as a result of storm damage. The net result has robbed the local governments and schools of an estimated $77 million in revenue (Maxfield, 2013).

Since these three super storms made 2011–2012 one of the deadliest periods of weather disasters in US history, the preparation, and the lack thereof, has received the attention of social scientists and those in the weather industry (Lewis, 2012). A new approach to looking at message appropriateness for given social settings and high-risk situations, with a focus on the messages and how they are communicated, was deemed important by multiple national weather services. Other factors of interest to meteorologists and risk managers alike include the credibility of those delivering the message and how meteorologists and emergency management officials can have an impact on message effectiveness (Steelman & McCaffrey, 2012).

Literature Review

It is universally accepted that media play a key role in many aspects of weather crises and disasters (Houston, Pfefferbaum, & Rosenholtz, 2012). Keeping communities informed before, during, and after weather risks is a normative function of the media. Scholars recognize that media serve as the public's primary introduction to risk, science, and environmental information (Luhmann, 2000; Nelkin, 1995; Peterson & Thompson, 2009; Scanlon, 2007b; Wilson, 1995). Furthermore, studies indicate that trust in the messenger has an essential impact on whether a receiver trusts the message or not. Leveraging personal credibility with the public, including appropriate officials or authority figures, engenders greater trust in the information (Fessenden-Raden, Fitchen, & Heath, 1987). Most recently, Burger et al. (2013) found television and radio were the most trusted sources of information before, during, and after Hurricane Sandy even after controlling for age demographics.

Despite community dependence on media organizations for risk information, scholars like Quarantelli (2006) who researched catastrophes such as Hurricane Katrina have found that local news media organizations are very limited in their preparedness for handling such events. Quarantelli's (2002) field study of media outlets in disaster-prone cities revealed that little attention is paid to emergency and disaster planning. Of the media entities examined, only 33 percent of radio stations, 54 percent of television stations (15 out of 28), and 60 percent of newspapers had any disaster plans (Quarantelli, 2002). One consistent finding following the 1994 Northridge earthquake was that larger businesses are more likely to prepare than smaller ones (Dahlhamer and Reshaur, 1996; Tierney and Webb, 2001). This characteristic is likely to be applicable to larger media outlets as well.

There is substantial scholarly research devoted to media and weather, but little has been published in journalism and mass communication journals. Scanlon (2007a) noted that researchers in the fields of disaster and mass communication rarely reference each other. This disconnect in research between weather/disaster scholars and journalism and mass communication scholars is likely due to the origins and focus of the various disciplines.

Much of the literature on natural and manmade disasters has been located in the domains of emergency management, meteorology, health, and mental health. From a communication perspective, weather and disaster research has largely resided in risk and crisis communication, which emerged within the fields of organizational communication and public relations (Houston et al., 2012). The emphasis within these domains has traditionally been on the development of persuasive public messages concerning potential health and environmental dangers and recommended responses to those dangers, which is risk communication (Reynolds & Seeger, 2005; Witte, 1995), and the protection of an organization's image, which is crisis communication (Houston et al., 2012).

The disaster research that does find its way into journalism and mass communication journals tends to use content analysis methodology and focus on post-disaster media framing like that conducted on Hurricane Katrina (Borah, 2009; Fahmy, Kelly, & Kim, 2007; Houston et al., 2012). Rarely has the weather research within the domain of journalism and mass communication provided a risk-centered approach to improving how weather emergencies are communicated to the public. The Crisis and Emergency Risk Communication (CERC) model does provide that focus on effective risk communication. Health communicators (Reynolds & Seeger, 2005) working with the Centers for Disease Control and Prevention (CDC) developed this integrated model as a tool to educate and equip public health professionals for the expanding communication responsibilities in complex emergency situations. Crises are by definition chaotic situations where uncertainty exists. Therefore, Reynolds and Seeger believe that the five stages of the CERC model—Precrisis, Initial Event, Maintenance, Resolution, Evaluation—provide a basis for systematically reducing uncertainty in communicating risks.

Veil, Reynolds, Sellnow, and Seeger (2008) note the CERC model can be applied as a general theoretical framework for explaining how risk and crisis are approached in other contexts. For example, CERC was used to examine varying strategies for managing wildfires in California,

Montana, and Wyoming and determine whether certain communication approaches can influence desired natural hazard outcomes and prompt more effective communication (Steelman & McCaffrey, 2012).

Method Collection

The current study utilizes a qualitative/ethnographic methodology. The data presented here were collected within a few weeks of each of these three storms by a small team of university faculty and undergraduate students. The teams were part of a video production crew, commissioned shortly after the Tuscaloosa and Joplin storms on June 11, 2011, by the National Association of Broadcasters and the Broadcast Education Association to illustrate the role of broadcasters during weather emergencies through a series of mini-documentaries. The team was led by two of the authors (Hodgson and Clark).

After weeks of researching and planning resources, interviews, and shooting locations, the team began conducting interviews in Tuscaloosa in July 2011. Interviews were conducted with 21 individuals involved in the Tuscaloosa storms, including storm survivors, local and state officials, radio reporters, and meteorologists and station managers from each station in the Birmingham/Tuscaloosa television market. Those interviews were gathered in a week's time.

In early August, the team set up interviews and data collection in Joplin, Missouri, so there would be a notable comparison of data from the Tuscaloosa and Joplin disasters. While the size of the designated media markets differ, organizers wanted to understand how the two cities prepared for the severe weather risk and the role broadcasters played in saving lives. Eleven interviews were conducted in Joplin from the same types of station employees, local and state emergency officials, and survivors.

When Hurricane Sandy appeared imminent, the team began organizing a trip to cover potential damage of the storm. The team began work in Baltimore, Maryland, on November 13, 2012, and then set out for nine days to conduct 33 interviews with reporters, anchors, meteorologists, and news managers in Washington, DC, Baltimore, Philadelphia, New Jersey, and New York. Government officials such as New Jersey Governor Chris Christie and the Mayor of Belmar, New Jersey, were included in the mix of interviews.

Analysis

Releases were gathered along the way for all interviews that were conducted and for any audio/video content that individuals or broadcast stations offered on behalf of the NAB project. No money was exchanged, but releases were gathered in each situation to ensure validity in use for educational purposes.

A group of undergraduate and graduate students from the authors' institutions compiled transcripts for all of the recorded interviews and audio/video materials. The authors examined these transcripts looking for trends that fit the stages of the CERC model. The trending topics and associated quotes were added to the most relevant stage of the CERC model and are discussed in the findings section. The findings represent the attempt to highlight effective risk communication, as well as threats to effective communication.

Findings

Data from the qualitative/ethnographic study were analyzed using Reynolds and Seeger's (2005) five-stage CERC model—Precrisis, Initial Event, Maintenance, Resolution, Evaluation.

Precrisis

During the precrisis stage, agencies and stations work together to promote storm preparedness. That involves radio and television stations working with emergency management staff before a crisis happens, having cooperative agreements with radio stations, and training for staff and storm spotters.

The stations and first alert staff such as meteorologists could not do their jobs through multiple media platforms without partnerships with businesses and city and state governments. In many cases, a station may partner with a local dealership, which may provide a fully equipped SUV or van to serve as a mobile weather studio. In partnership with city and state agencies, stations gain access to traffic cameras, or install their own camera network around the community, which they can access at any time during a weather event.

Policies concerning interruption of programming and advertising should also be reinforced at this stage. Meteorologists we talked to felt that they had the green light to preempt programming at their discretion. Gene Kirkconnell, general manager of WVTM-TV in Birmingham, Alabama, echoed that sentiment.

> It's something we deal with, but there's never a decision made in the face of a crisis, be it a natural disaster or be it another type of threat to the public, where monetary considerations ever come into play in terms of making a decision about whether or not to take the air or do away with programming, or do away with commercial content, and take as much time and as wide a scope as we need to get life-saving information to the public.
>
> (personal communication, July 22, 2011)

287

In conducting interviews with meteorologists, news directors, reporters, and news managers in Tuscaloosa, Joplin, and Baltimore, Washington, DC, Philadelphia, New Jersey, and New York, it became clear that all the members of the broadcast team play an important role in this process, before, during, and after a major weather event. They are the ones their local audience already trusts, so they believe they have major responsibilities to be a source of information on multiple platforms during a crisis. They also recognized that their stations put in many resources to build trust on a daily basis so people will turn to them in severe weather situations. James Paul Dice of WBRC Fox 6 News in Birmingham said,

> Maybe there's not severe weather going on, but maybe you're out talking to a group on how to be safe when the big storm comes. We did those countless times before April 27th. We were out in the community talking to groups about what to do in case of horrific weather. We were programming weather radios, we had a big weather radio campaign, and we were out there going to all these different communities in our viewing area, all 21 counties out there programming those weather radios. And I think April 27th, when those devastating storms hit, that kind of community service really made a difference.
>
> (personal communication, July 21, 2011)

Working in partnership with local emergency management officials prepares media professionals to provide better communication in the midst of a weather crisis. Keith Stammer, Joplin/Jasper County director of emergency management, explained how his office partnered with the media.

> We are very lucky in this town to have a full-time public information officer, our PIO, that's all she does. Those relationships were already established there in times past. Whenever we would have a disaster drill, we'd have a table-top exercise, we would invite the media, radio, television, newspaper, into our meetings so that they could observe and hopefully even participate in the media function of the table top. So, that when this event happened we were able to call on that resource, on the media first name basis, telephone numbers that we had, faxes, and that type of thing. So that we could use them, if I may use that phrase, to help get out the public service announcements and the information that we needed to be able to tell people.
>
> (personal communication, August 9, 2011)

Lonnie Quinn, WCBS-TV meteorologist in New York City felt that being a local broadcaster resulted in better storm coverage.

So when the big national outlets, the Weather Channel, network news, when they're putting their stories out, they're doing it from spots not right in the storm. Now I realize they have some reporters in the storm, but they are based outside the storm. We are living it. We are breathing it with the people who are going through this whole thing. I mean, I'm from this area. I have relatives, I have family, I have friends who were devastated by the whole thing. The difference is we can report on the streets, the blocks; we know them. This is where we live. We're not just protecting the viewers out there; we're protecting our people.

(personal communication, November 19, 2012)

Initial Event

In the Reynolds & Seeger (2005) model, the initial event is the stage when communication occurs directly with the general public in that affected area. For severe weather, this happens through traditional and new media and can happen as early as a week out. More commonly, there is much less warning. During this stage, the tools that are already in place from precrisis planning are utilized. Radio and television stations use their regularly scheduled broadcasts and social media to keep the public informed and updated. Stations also start using the "Be Weather Aware" approach to promote making sure family and friends know and understand the current situation. When a severe threat is imminent, stations use all existing programming and promotional time to make sure people know where to turn for the latest information.

Numerous stories of survival and warnings came out of the Tuscaloosa tornado, which prompted education to Alabamians about what you should do to help others be weather aware as much as yourself. For example, a college minister, listening to the radio in his car, stopped at a Krispy Kreme donut shop to warn the customers when he heard a local meteorologist say "take shelter now!" He then made a frantic call to his brother and a group of college students at his church. The students come face-to-face with the tornado as they fled for shelter. They emerged to see total destruction. Nothing was left of the Krispy Kreme (T. Durden, personal communication, July 19, 2011).

The call from his older brother prompted Caleb Durden and five other college students to listen and take action after hearing that critical information. They took cover in a utility closet inside Central Church of Christ in Tuscaloosa. They walked out safe, but the church was destroyed. Caleb Durden, college student:

We were watching a couple different channels and everybody was saying the same thing, you know, you need to get in your safe place. Tuscaloosa's going to get hit hard, and you need to

289

find shelter quickly. I was watching ABC 33/40 and they had the tower cam going, they had the radar going, and they just kept talking about Tuscaloosa. This is going to be bad, you need to find a safe place to get. The guy on Fox, JP Dice, he said if you're in Tuscaloosa, you're about to get hammered.

(personal communication, July 19, 2011)

In other instances, radio stations also served as partners in live coverage of weather as they allowed the TV stations to take over their signal and rebroadcast over their airwaves. In Tuscaloosa, some of the most descriptive video of the power of the EF-4 tornado crossing a major interstate area was captured by two radio DJs. They shot video of the massive wall cloud passing right in front of their station (T. Delo, personal communication, July 22, 2011).

In Joplin, news managers and their crews were no strangers to severe weather popping up. The manner in which the EF-5 materialized in the afternoon was one that changed their philosophy in how they approached a routine event to one that prompted coverage from all the resources they had on May 22, 2011. They also reinforced the fact that local information was coming from trusted sources they already knew in their community. Caitlin McCardle, KSNF/KODE-TV meteorologist:

Just before we actually saw the tornado in our tower cam, there had been reports coming out from the National Weather Service of some funnel clouds over Galena, which is just to the west of Joplin. And that was the last report that came out until we saw in our tower cam that tornado actually on the ground. I had noticed a little hook echo developing just to the southwest of Joplin and so I asked our weekend director to go ahead and switch the tower cam looking as far southwest as possible, and good thing we did that because we saw that tornado on the ground. And we were warning everybody before the National Weather Service actually came out and said that there was a tornado on the ground then. We basically spotted it the same time as the storm spotters. But then there was that lag between the time they relayed it back to the National Weather Service and the time that got sent out to the public and all the other media outlets. So we caught that tower cam, that tornado in our tower cam, and it was a fearsome sight.

(personal communication, August 8, 2011)

For Hurricane Sandy, stations spent days preparing crews for coverage of the initial impact, including preparations for landfall, evacuations, and eventually damage. John Montone, reporter, 1010 WINS News Radio in New York, NY, described how the staff at his station prioritized the storm coverage.

> A lot of these guys stayed in hotels or they stayed up at the station, they slept on a sofa. We're 24/7 in the best of times. So you can't go more than 24/7, but you can go full force obviously and not running commercials. You're bumping sports; you're bumping the features. It's just wall-to-wall coverage. If you turn on the radio any minute of the hour, any minute of the day, you're going to get useful information, vital information about this particular catastrophe.
>
> (personal communication, November 20, 2012)

Maintenance

Reynolds and Seeger (2005) identified the maintenance stage as communication with the general public that empowers decision-making and identifies misinformation. In most cases, this stage is not active until after the threat of severe weather has dissipated. In the case of the Alabama storms, the meteorologists did not relinquish control of their station's broadcasts to the news department for reporting about damage and recovery until after the last severe weather warning expired around 10 p.m. James Spann, meteorologist at ABC 33/40 in Birmingham, summed up this philosophy: "I do not want to have a news reporter telling a story about damage when somebody's life is at stake in the path of a tornado. So we kept control of the event" (personal communication, July 19, 2011).

In Joplin, there was less warning time before the storms hit so maintenance communication through local broadcasting became even more important. Broadcasters described the period immediately after the storm as a time of shock, with residents wondering what had just happened. Kristi Spencer, KOAM/KFJX-TV, news director in Joplin, described her station's role immediately after the storm.

> I think we were there just to give any basic information out that we could, which is just about all we could give that night because of some of the hurdles that a tornado that wipes out communication brings. So, I think we were just a link to people who were scared and wondering what was going on around them and hearing it from your local newscaster who you hear things from every night is somewhat reassuring, and I think that we were able to give a real local perspective and answering questions that local people would have that national wasn't able to.
>
> (personal communication, August 8, 2011)

Keith Stammer, Joplin/Jasper County director of emergency management, described how essential it was to communicate with the media after a storm that had caused such widespread destruction.

> I don't know how you successfully handle a search and rescue operation in a strike field of six miles long, a half a mile wide, 1,800 acres, without participating with the media. Not only were they the eyes and ears oftentimes in terms of watching what was going on and giving us a report back, they were also able to enable us to communicate with the people that were out there. We could sort of push information back out to them, they could bring information back in to us. I don't know how we would have done it otherwise.
>
> (personal communication, August 9, 2011)

Some media professionals had storm damage to their own property, but kept working to make sure information continued to flow in the affected areas. Glenn Kalina, program director for WJRZ Magic 100.1, kept working at the radio station even after finding out his own home was a loss.

> I'm on the bay side, so when the bay overflowed and the water from the ocean came down, they met by my house. It was 19 days before we were able to get in the house and it was flooded out pretty badly. We will have to start over with everything. I've still yet to deal with that. There's a lot of people who have it worse off than I do. Take care of the community and I'll take care of my end. I'll get to it.
>
> (personal communication, Saturday, November 17)

Resolution

According to Reynolds and Seeger (2005), resolution includes communication with the general public in general about issues that may affect the community as a whole. Following these destructive storms, police and safety agencies established curfews to keep people out of affected areas while protecting storm victim's belongings and securing the area for safety. The media served to inform communities of curfews and also notified victims and clean up volunteers about accessing the areas.

It's not unusual to have the television and radio airwaves turned over to officials to communicate relief efforts and to control the situation. In the aftermath of these three super storms, local media outlets extended open door and open microphone privileges to law enforcement, healthcare, emergency management, and FEMA representatives as an avenue for broad communication with constituents. In each case, these policies of cooperation had been established in a precrisis stage prior to the storms. Keith Stammer, Joplin/Jasper County director of emergency management said,

> We tried to employ multiple means in the media in order to get information out to people. Radio is an excellent example, our local radio stations do a simulcast on all their different radio stations that they have, and so when you talk to one, you've actually talked to upwards of a half a dozen different radio stations. The television stations did the same thing. We gave information to them they helped get out. The media, in terms of the newspaper, was an interesting venue. You have people out in the field who have no Internet, they have no electricity, their batteries have gone dead in the radio. And so one of the things we did was start, the local newspaper published papers, and then we put them in stands for free at various locations just so people could pick them up and take them back to their site where their home was destroyed, and a lot of people did that so they could read and see what was happening. Plus hand bills. Then, when we were able to set up more stations we were able to put up some monitors since people were able to watch the television and see what was going on, that helped a lot.
>
> (personal communication, August 9, 2011)

In Tuscaloosa, where the city's communication systems were completely destroyed, the local radio and television stations were the voice of the city and allowed many local, state, and federal officials to come into their studios to give out crucial information about available resources, recovery efforts, and curfews. While the mayor of Tuscaloosa credits broadcasters with providing early warning that saved hundreds more from dying that day, he also credits the media for stepping up to serve the public after the storms (W. Maddox, personal communication, July 22, 2011). Clear Channel Radio in Tuscaloosa opened up their phone lines and for the next 17 days allowed listeners to use the airwaves nonstop to talk to each other and share what was going on in the way of personal and physical recovery (T. Delo, personal communication, July 22, 2011).

New Jersey Governor Chris Christie hosts a one-hour monthly radio show on New Jersey 101.5 FM called "Ask the Governor" in which he takes calls about any issue from his constituents. He knew this established program was a credible vehicle for communicating during the recovery. "In the immediate aftermath of the storm, my way to communicate to folks in my state was through the broadcasters as I traveled around the state and assessed the damage" (personal communication, November 20, 2012). Like stations in Tuscaloosa and Joplin, the managers at 101.5 in New Jersey felt obligated to preempt normal programming for recovery information, as the station's program director, Eric Johnson, said it was a responsibility to stay on the air 24/7 and allow the community to talk.

> One of the crises that happened after the storm was it was hard to get fuel in New Jersey. We would have listeners call up and say the Exxon Station on Route 1 has no lines right now and within two minutes, there would be 100 cars there.
> (personal communication, November 20, 2012)

Evaluation

Reynolds and Seeger (2005) also refer to the evaluation stage as the "lessons learned" stage. In this stage, all parties involved in the crisis response evaluate the strengths and weaknesses of their crisis communication efforts. There's typically interagency communication and follow-up discussions to develop new action plans that tie back to the precrisis stage.

Evaluation of Hurricane Sandy revealed a number of communication failures. Freedman (2013) noted several failures by just the National Hurricane Center and the National Weather Service, including: failure to issue watches or warnings north of North Carolina, rules in place at the time that restricted the NWS from leaving hurricane warnings in place after a storm had transitioned to a post-tropical storm, reliance on the Saffir-Simpson Wind Scale alone. Sandy revealed that Saffir-Simpson is insufficient for predicting the severity of a storm because it ignores a storm's size and potential storm surge. Hurricane experts are exploring alternatives to the Saffir-Simpson scale—like the Integrated Kinetic Energy scale—for communicating a hurricane's damage potential.

Improving storm tracking is an issue that was constantly talked about when broadcasters evaluated the aftermath of these storms. Leisha Beard, KSNF/KODE news director in Joplin, Missouri, said that citizens in the community don't always take cover until they confirm they are in immediate danger.

> Not that we didn't take them seriously, but it's just a common thing in the four states to hear a tornado siren. You don't immediately jump in the bathtub when you hear a tornado siren. You usually then turn on the TV and look.
> (personal communication, August 8, 2011)

New storm tracking technology, such as the iMap Weather Radio smartphone application, grew out of the evaluation of communication from the Tuscaloosa and Joplin tornadoes and Hurricane Sandy. It is one of several new apps being developed to help determine whether you are in the path of a storm based on GPS coordinates.

There were other issues that came to light during the evaluation of communicating these storms. Meteorologists said they were reminded just how much weather awareness wears off over time. They also noted the need to use specific language and tone in order to get people to take action. James Spann of ABC 33/40 in Birmingham emphasized continued efforts to make more live video and live observations available to the public.

> Most TV stations do a horrible job with live video of tornadoes. You generally see long form coverage featuring mostly radar, and no meteorologist on camera. You have to be on camera for eye contact and body language, and you must have a fixed camera network and dashcams from spotters in the field to be effective. It doesn't really cost much to have volunteers in the field (properly trained, of course) with live dashcams to supplement TV coverage. (John) Oldshue and (Ben) Greer's live stream of the Tuscaloosa tornado, well before it got into the city, no doubt saved many lives.
> (personal communication, April 10, 2016)

While television and radio stations evaluated their crews and staffing, they also looked at the main purpose they needed to serve. The root of their business is to share stories as journalists, and many felt that was needed during a long recovery process. David Friend is the vice president and news director of WCBS-TV in New York. He was proud of his team's coverage during the hurricane's landfall, but he knew they had a continued responsibility. He said,

> Once the storm was over it was time to tell the stories of so many people who suffered in our area and to bring them as much help as we could. Whether it was through direct donations of blankets or food, teaming up with the Red Cross and raising money, but just letting them tell their stories, letting them tell us the incredible misfortune that they suffered and try to help them rebuild their lives.
> (personal communication, November 19, 2012)

Discussion

Since the killer tornadoes in 2011 in Alabama and Joplin, weather experts have ramped up educational efforts because these types of severe weather events pop up frequently. Chief Scientist Kevin Law of the National Weather Service said they are constantly looking at the science of these storms but also at understanding human behavior in the time leading up to a major weather event and how people react to warnings (Morgan, 2014).

Meteorologists, social scientists, and station managers have learned that using certain terms, having more of a video presence over radar graphics, using live video opportunities on social media, and using more first alert weather notifications can really pay off when it comes to saving lives. In several markets now, you also see weather education, storm alert tours, weather radio programming, and detailed web and weather reports. Depending on the level of the severe weather risk, they are also detailing not only the forecast but also where you should be and in what type of safe place at a certain time.

Television stations and meteorologists have taken the lead in partnership with local officials and emergency management agencies to let people know to use them as a resource before anything happens. States are using anniversaries of major events and other designated dates for weather awareness to do training. Joplin has weather education sessions annually within the city. In central Alabama, television stations hold storm spotter sessions and weather alert tours throughout the year. Along the East Coast when hurricane season approaches awareness campaigns are held related to preparations for generators, home repairs, and food safety. While meteorologists visit schools on a weekly basis and do speaking engagements at civic organizations, emergency management planners also do about 20 different individual weather-training sessions with churches, clubs, nonprofit organizations, and governmental entities.

Doctors and meteorologists have also learned from fatalities and injuries. There's now language in warnings for approaching storms encouraging people to wear bicycle or baseball helmets, or even pots, to protect their heads in case of flying debris. Another reminder is to have a whistle to call for help and wear closed-toed shoes so feet are protected if you have to navigate around debris.

One of the frustrations that weather forecasters have is what words to say to ensure that people will listen to them and take action if needed. Some phrases used more frequently now are: "get to the lowest floor away from windows and doors; put as many walls between you and the outside world as possible; don't be in cars or in a mobile home."

While James Spann won numerous national awards for his weather coverage following the April 2011 tornadoes in Alabama, he became a leading advocate for learning from these devastating events. He said,

> The physical science could not have been better April 27, 2011, yet 252 died. We have gone to social scientists to help us better communicate during life threatening weather; that was our big weakness. Terms like "tornado emergency" can be helpful if used properly. Social scientists have also helped us with things like communicating polygon versus county warnings, reducing siren dependency, map colors, graphics, and terms.
>
> (personal communication, April 10, 2016)

Conclusion

While a number of interviews were conducted totaling hundreds of hours of responses, these represent a small fraction of the local broadcasters involved in communicating these storms. Additionally, the current work only represents three storms. These constraints severely limit the ability to generalize conclusions beyond these examples. Another limitation involved the time it took to get into these affected areas following the weather events. It is difficult for researchers and documentarians to gain access to these areas in the midst of the chaos that immediately follows the event. Even so, the authors believe it is critical to begin collecting data, footage, and interviews as quickly as possible after the event. Furthermore, with the ubiquity of social media and mobile communication it is important to document activities on these channels as well.

Some meteorologists still blame themselves for not saving more lives. In the time since these storms, meteorologists from the affected areas have attended national conferences and spoken about what they have learned about getting their audience to act when faced with a potential weather hazard. Solutions have included a push for more live video tools to track the storms instead of displaying weather maps on screen for long periods of time. These experts believe people do not react with urgency to maps they don't understand. They also emphasize public education about utilizing social media during a weather crisis. Social media is an effective tool to verify the safety of friends and family and channel information through hashtags. Future research should examine what broadcasters are doing differently now, and how they are incorporating social media as a result of what they learned from these storms and others.

In conclusion, some form of public remembrance often marks disaster anniversaries. Thus, it is fitting that we mark the fifth anniversary of these three super storms by advancing research aimed at understanding how broadcasters communicate risk in times of severe weather events. In this short time, some of the lessons already learned have made a difference in how all types of severe storms are covered.

References

Blake, E., Kimberlain, T., Berg, R., Cangialosi, J., & Beven, J. (2013). *Tropical cyclone report: Hurricane Sandy*. National Hurricane Center.

Borah, P. (2009). Comparing visual framing in newspapers: Hurricane Katrina versus tsunami. *Newspaper Research Journal*, 30(1), 50–57.

Burger, J., Gochfeld, M., Jeitner, C., Pittfield, T., & Donio, M. (2013). Trusted information sources used during and after Superstorm Sandy: TV and radio were used more often than social media. *Journal of Toxicology & Environmental Health: Part A*, 76(20), 1138. doi: 10.1080/15287394.2013.844087.

Dahlhamer, J. M., & Reshaur, L. (1996). *Business and the 1994 Northridge Earthquake: An analysis of pre- and post-disaster preparedness.* Newark: University of Delaware Disaster Research Center.

Fahmy, S., Kelly, J. D., & Kim, Y. S. (2007). What Katrina revealed: A visual analysis of the hurricane coverage by news wires and U.S. newspapers. *Journalism & Mass Communication Quarterly, 84*(3), 546–561.

Fessenden-Raden, J., Fitchen J. M., & Heath, J. S. (1987). Providing risk information in communities: Factors influencing what is heard and accepted. *Science, Technology, & Human Values, 12,* 94–101.

Freedman, A. (2012). The Joplin tornado: Where does it rank? *Climate Central.* Retrieved from: www.climatecentral.org/news/the-joplin-tornado-one-year-later-where-does-it-rank.

Freedman, A. (2013). Heeding Sandy's lessons, before the next big storm. *Climate Central.* Retrieved from: www.climatecentral.org/news/four-key-lessons-learned-from-hurricane-sandy-15928.

Houston, J. B., Pfefferbaum, B., & Rosenholtz, C. E. (2012). Disaster news: Framing and frame changing in coverage of major U.S. natural disasters, 2000–2010. *Journalism & Mass Communication Quarterly, 89*(4), 606–623. doi: 10.1177/1077699012456022.

Huffington Post. (2013, October 29). Hurricane Sandy impact. Retrieved from: www.huffingtonpost.com/2013/10/29/hurricane-sandy-impact-infographic_n_4171243.html.

Lewis, R. (2012, March 13). Tornado Tech: What if Dorothy had a smartphone? *All Things Considered* [Radio broadcast]. Birmingham: Alabama Public Radio.

Luhmann, N. (2000). *The reality of mass media.* (K. Cross, Trans.). Stanford, CA: Stanford University Press.

Matsa, K. (2015, April 29). Local TV news: Fact sheet. *Pew Research Center, State of the news media 2015.* Retrieved from: www.journalism.org/2015/04/29/local-tv-news-fact-sheet/.

Maxfield, J. (2013, October 26). Hurricane Sandy anniversary: Economic cost. *Daily Finance.* Retrieved from: www.dailyfinance.com/on/hurricane-sandy-anniversary-economic-cost/.

Morgan, L. (2014, April 24). Tornado psychology after April 27, 2011: Persuading people to act. Retrieved from: http://blog.al.com/wire/2014/04/tornado_psychology_persuading.html.

Nelkin, D. (1995). *Selling science: How the press covers science and technology.* New York: Freeman.

Paul, B., & Stimers, M. (2011). *Tornado warnings and tornado fatalities: The case of May 22, 2011 tornado in Joplin, Missouri.* (Quick Response Report #226). Boulder: Natural Hazards Center, University of Colorado at Boulder.

Peterson, T. R., & Thompson, J. L. (2009). Environmental risk communication: Responding to challenges of complexity and uncertainty. In R. L. Heath & H. D. O'Hair (Eds.), *Handbook of risk and crisis communication* (pp. 591–606). New York: Routledge.

Quarantelli, E. L. (2006, June 11). Catastrophes are different from disasters: Some implications for crisis planning and managing drawn from Katrina. Retrieved from: http://understandingkatrina.ssrc.org/Quarantelli.

Quarantelli, E. L. (2002). *The role of the mass communication system in natural and technological disasters and possible extrapolation to terrorism situations.* Newark: University of Delaware Disaster Research Center.

Reynolds, B., and Seeger, M. (2005). Crisis and emergency risk communication as an integrative model. *Journal of Health Communication*, 10, 43–55.

Reynolds, M. (n.d.). The Joplin tornado: The hospital story and lessons learned [PDF document]. Retrieved from: http://c.ymcdn.com/sites/www.leadingagemi ssouri.org/resource/resmgr/annual_conference/wednesday_joplin_tornado_ les.pdf.

Saad, L. (2013, July 8). TV is Americans' main source of news. *Gallup.com.*

Scanlon, J. (2007a). Research about the mass media and disaster: Never (well hardly never) the twain shall meet. In D. A. McEntire (Ed.), *Disciplines, Disasters, and Emergency Management* (pp. 75–94). Springfield, IL: Charles C Thomas.

Scanlon, J. (2007b). Unwelcome irritant or useful ally? The mass media in emergencies. In H. Rodriquez, E. L. Quarntelli, & R. R. Dynes, 2007. *Handbook of disaster research* (pp. 413–429). New York: Springer.

Steelman, T., & McCaffrey, S. (2012). Best practices in risk and crisis communication: Implications for natural hazards management. *Natural Hazards, 65*(1), 683–705. doi: 10.1007/s11069-012-0386-z.

Thompson, J. (2011, August 30). The Tuscaloosa tornado: Lessons to learn outlined at FRI. *FireRescue1.*

Tierney, K., & Webb, G. (2001). *Business vulnerability to earthquakes and other disasters.* Newark: University of Delaware Disaster Research Center.

Veil, S., Reynolds, B., Sellnow, T., & Seeger, M. (2008, October). CERC as a theoretical framework for research and practice. *Society for Public Health Education, 9*(4), 26–34. doi: 10.1177/1524839908322113.

Wheatley, K. (2013, May 22). The May 22, 2011, Joplin, Missouri EF5 tornado. *Tornado History.* Retrieved from: www.ustornadoes.com/2013/05/22/joplin-missouri-ef5-tornado-may-22-2011/.

Wilson, K. M. (1995). Mass media as sources of global warming knowledge. *Mass Communication Review, 22*(1), 75–89.

Witte, K. (1995). Generating effective risk messages: How scary should your risk communication be? In B. R. Burleson (Ed.), *Communication yearbook 18*, (pp. 229–254). Thousand Oaks, CA: SAGE.

15

IT'S NOT PREVENTABLE, YET YOU ARE RESPONSIBLE

Media's Risk and Attribution Assessment of the 2012 West Nile Outbreak

Nan Yu, Robert Littlefield, Laura C. Farrell, and Ruoxu Wang

Health events such as large-scale disease outbreaks naturally attract journalistic attention because of people's general interest in medical events (Pew Research Center, 2009). News media have closely followed these pandemics year after year and shifted their approaches of doing so throughout the decades (Blakely, 2003; Koteyko, Brown, & Crawford, 2008). The news coverage of public health events is important in that, through these reports, people can develop a concept of a disease and prepare for a potential health risk accordingly (Blakely, 2003; Roche & Muskavitch, 2003).

Many disease pandemics have impacted human societies throughout history. Pandemics such as the 1918 Spanish flu, the 1957 Asian flu, the 1958 Hong Kong flu, and more recently the 2003 SARS and the 2009 H1N1 have all caused severe economic, social, and health consequences in various countries (Blakely, 2003; Hume, 2000; Luther & Zhou, 2005; Yu, Frohlich, Fougner, & Ren, 2011). Among these pandemics, West Nile has been a severe health threat in the US for years (Sifferlin, 2015). Over 30,000 American people have been infected with the West Nile virus since 1999—the year that the first case of West Nile was found in New York ("West Nile virus," 2013). The year of 2012 was unique for West Nile because the infected cases were found in 48 states in the country and the disease caused 286 deaths—making it the largest pandemic of its kind since 2003 (CDC, 2013).

Research on news media's portrayal of disease outbreaks has attracted wide scholarly attention (Blakely, 2003; Dudo, Dahlstrom, & Brossard,

2007; Hume, 2000; Roche & Muskavitch, 2003; Yu et al., 2011). Much of the prior research concentrates on whether media has accurately presented health risks in the news or whether the preventive strategies have been communicated properly (Dudo et al., 2007; Roche & Muskavitch, 2003; Yu et al., 2011). This project intends to extend this line of research by examining the portrayal of the 2012 West Nile outbreak in American media with an emphasis on the depictions of risk, preventability, and attribution of responsibility.

Literature Review

Media coverage of disease outbreaks has transformed significantly over the past century. Blakely (2003), through an investigation of influenza coverage during the 1918 Spanish flu, 1957 Asian flu, and 1968 Hong Kong flu, suggests that the development of science in curbing transmitted diseases has modified the ways that pandemics were depicted. When science became a possible solution to pandemics, media started to shift their focus from public anxiety to scientific preventive methods, attempting to provide answers to these dangerous public health issues (Blakely, 2003). Scholars argue that, beyond presenting the risk and magnitude of a pandemic, media should share the responsibility of providing answers to the "so what" question that is commonly raised by general audience and satisfy the need to know how to reduce the chances of being affected by a health risk (Roche & Muskavitch, 2003). Therefore, this project includes the analysis of risk representations as well as the evaluation of attributions of disease and responsibility in the media.

News Media's Risk Assessment

Risk assessment is of great interest to media scholars because journalists' risk assessment of disease outbreaks shapes how dangerous or threatening the outbreak actually is (Dudo et al., 2007; Roche & Muskavitch, 2003; Yu et al., 2011). Inaccurate risk assessment in media portrayals can be problematic: exaggeration of actual risk in media coverage may induce feelings of panic or hopelessness from individuals, whereas underestimating the actual risk can have serious consequences if people do not take the necessary precautions to protect themselves (Dudo et al., 2007; Roche & Muskavitch, 2003).

Some scholars indicate that media coverage on pandemics can lack quality and often present inaccurate or insufficient information (Dudo et al., 2007; Roche & Muskavitch, 2003; Yu et al., 2011). For example, Roche and Muskavitch (2003) examined the precision of the presentation of the 2000 West Nile outbreak in American major newspapers. Their results suggested that the risk information of West Nile was presented with a low degree of contextual precision. Specifically, the risk magnitude of the outbreak was often described by using qualitative words (e.g., dangerous, deadly, a severe outbreak) and when numerical information was presented, it often lacked contextual background (e.g., the population size).

The depiction of *risk magnitude* has often been used to assess the accuracy and precision of risk presentation in the media. Risk magnitude information varies along a continuum of contextual precision: a low degree of contextual precision contains little informational value for the public, whereas a high degree of contextual precision holds greater value because it offers a comparison of risk compared to the general population (Griffin, Dunwoody, & Neuwirth, 1999; Resnik, 2001). Prior research has identified three key strategies news media can use to portray the magnitude of a health risk (Dudo et al., 2007; Roche & Muskavitch, 2003; Yu et al., 2011). These strategies include: 1) qualitative risk, 2) quantitative risk—numerator (e.g., 5 people died), or 3) quantitative risk—number/population (e.g., 0.02 percent of individuals who were infected died).

When depicting the outbreak as a qualitative risk, news reports often use qualitative phrases to portray the severity of the disease such as "a large threat," "a worse outbreak," or "a fatal disease," to name a few. This is seen as the least precise way to depict a health risk because the judgment of these words could be objective (Dudo et al., 2007; Roche & Muskavitch, 2003; Yu et al., 2011). The precision level of risk magnitude depiction can be improved by using numerical information (i.e., numerator, or number/population), such as "two died" or "one out of two hundred people will develop symptoms." The latter is seen as even more accurate because it offers the public a context when analyzing and evaluating the health risk (Dudo et al., 2007; Roche & Muskavitch, 2003; Yu et al., 2011).

As a source of information about health risks, the news media are essential because many members of the public base their impressions about risks on information presented in the media (Fischhoff, 1995; Kitzinger & Reilly, 1997). Accurate risk presentations allow the public to assess risk in a rational manner (Dudo et al., 2007), and help readers make personal decisions required to reduce overall personal risk while minimizing personal cost (Roche & Muskavitch, 2003). Therefore, news media share an important responsibility to report accurate risk assessment of disease outbreaks so the public has a realistic understanding of their susceptibility and relevance to an illness. Therefore, we proposed the following question:

RQ1: How was risk magnitude portrayed in the 2012 West Nile coverage?

Many scholars have suggested that solely presenting risk information related to a disease outbreak without providing a solution is considered insufficient (Dudo et al., 2007, Yu et al., 2011). Thus, it is expected that media also report preventive methods associated with a disease which are important for the enhancement of personal protection (Dudo et al., 2007; Roche & Muskavitch, 2003; Yu et al., 2011). Hence, in this project, in addition to the examination of risk magnitude of the West Nile disease, we intend to investigate how news media have depicted the preventability of the disease, as well as prevention responsibility shared by different parties during the West Nile outbreak.

Preventability of the West Nile Pandemic

Preventability is considered one of the key characteristics of illnesses. It is defined as the degree to which a disease or its consequences can be prevented or predicted and is considered an important concept related to illness attributions (Lucas, Lakey, Alexander, & Arnetz, 2009a; Lucas, Alexander, Firestone, & Lebreton, 2009b).

Some illnesses can be perceived as more preventable than others (Lucas et al., 2009a; Weinstein, 1984). The concept of preventability is vital for a disease pandemic such as West Nile because whether or not a disease is preventable can directly influence the magnitude of public fear and anxiety caused by a transmitted virus. For example, the SARS epidemic in 2003 caused worldwide panic because the disease was mysterious and untreatable with an unknown preventative strategy at that time (Hung, 2003).

When it comes to the issue of West Nile, avoiding mosquito bites is the only way to prevent being infected. Activities that can help avoid mosquito bites, including minimizing outdoor activities and draining standing water around residential houses, are frequently recommended as effective methods in reducing the risk of being infected with the West Nile viruses ("West Nile virus," 2013). However, many have raised questions regarding the possibilities of avoiding mosquito bites completely (Fox, 2013).

When applying the concept of *preventability* to the context of media coverage about the 2012 West Nile outbreak, we tried to identify whether West Nile has been portrayed as *preventable* (e.g., predictable, vaccination option) or *unpreventable* (e.g., not enough information is known, the spread of illnesses is unpredictable). These types of messages may play an integral role in molding people's perception of whether they can or cannot do something to protect against a virus (Lucas et al., 2009a). Therefore, we proposed the following research question:

RQ2: How was disease preventability portrayed in the media coverage of the 2012 West Nile outbreak?

Ascribing Responsibility of the West Nile Prevention

Framing theory has been used as a theoretical guideline for researchers studying the selection and omission of certain aspects of an issue, especially with regard to causes and responsibility (Iyengar, 1991; Kim, 2015). The existing framing literature shows how the ascribing of responsibility has been presented in the media covering a variety of social and health issues, such as trans fats (Jarlenski & Barry, 2013), autism vaccinations (Holton, Weberling, Clarke, & Smith, 2012), depression (Wang & Liu, 2015), lung cancer (Major, 2009), obesity (Kim & Willis, 2007), and poverty (Jang, 2013). When reporting social problems or health problems, it is common for media to attribute responsibility to different parties such as individuals, community, government, and social organizations, just to name a few. The attribution of societal- or personal-level responsibility may affect policy-making process, judgment of others, and social interactions (Weiner, 1995).

Kim and Willis (2007) analyzed over 300 news reports from American newspapers and TV programs and found that while media emphasized personal causes and solutions rather than societal responsibilities for obesity in general, television news was more likely to mention personal solutions than newspapers. In another study, Kim, Carvalho, and Davis (2010) discovered that media were more likely to attribute society to overcome the problem of poverty and less likely to put the burden on individuals. In another study, Holton et al. (2012) discovered that news media focused on ascribing the responsibility to one guilty individual—Andrew Wakefield—when covering the MMR-autism controversy. Yu and Xu (2016) discovered that social media users frequently blamed scientists and government when things went wrong with genetically modified foods.

The different presentations of responsibility attribution can help lead or mislead audience to determine the causes and solutions for social problems (Holton et al., 2012; Iyengar, 1991; Jang, 2013; Kim & Willis, 2007; Yu & Xu, 2016). For example, Ben-Porath and Shaker (2010) found that the images of victims portrayed in the news significantly impacted people's perceptions of government responsibility in the wake of Hurricane Katrina.

Scholars have been concerned that when social issues are reduced to individual-level matters, societal-level responsibility can be neglected (Wallack, Dorfman, Jernigan, & Thema, 1993). For most pandemic-related health issues, individuals are naturally the responsible parties because when getting infected, individual health consequences can be severe or deadly (such as Ebola or SARS). However, for communicative diseases, one's health condition can also affect people nearby. This makes large-scale disease outbreaks more than just a health problem—they are a threat to the entire family, community, and society at large. For example, the 2003

SARS outbreak in China created societal panic and instability, causing nation-wide shutdowns (e.g., schools and shops closed) (Yu, 2004).

In the face of a health pandemic, media coverage may touch on *who* is responsible for taking preventive measures. Therefore, one of our goals in this project is to understand how responsibilities were attributed toward each individual, a community, or a society at large. In addition to the investigation of how responsibility was covered in the news reports of the 2012 West Nile outbreak, we also examined whether the preventability of this disease (i.e., West Nile being preventable or unpreventable) was linked to a call for preventive actions in the media. Individuals are more likely to assume responsibility when an event is preventable, but responsibility is not typically assumed when something is unpreventable (Weiner, 1995).

Thus, the following research question was proposed:

RQ3: What is the relationship between the portrayal of preventability and the depiction of responsibility in the media coverage of the 2012 West Nile outbreak?

Method

Sampling

This study collected local and national media coverage of the 2012 West Nile virus over the progression of the outbreak. Articles were collected daily (at a consistent time of day) by doing a Google News search using keywords such as "West Nile virus," "West Nile outbreak," and "West Nile cases." The top five articles appearing in the search results were selected for each day. The first case of West Nile virus in humans was detected in Dallas County, Texas, on June 20, 2012, denoting the beginning of the epidemic. By December of 2012, the West Nile virus affected a total of 48 states. A total of 15 weeks of coverage was collected between late July and early November of 2012. After the sample was collected, duplicate stories were eliminated prior to coding. The total sample for this study included 450 stories.

About 83 percent of the sample was from local or regional media outlets, 14.7 percent was from US national media outlets, and 2 percent was from international media outlets. Over 46 percent of the sample was newspaper stories, followed by TV stories (32.9 percent), online media stories (14.4 percent), radio stories (4.0 percent), magazine stories (1.8 percent), and news agency stories (0.4 percent). Even though all articles were collected online, we recorded the original media outlet that produced the article. For example, a story that appeared on WFAA.com was coded as an article from a local/regional TV because WFAA-TV is a local TV station that serves the Dallas-Fort Worth area in Texas.

Coding Scheme

Risk Magnitude. The coding of the presentation of risk magnitude related to West Nile followed the coding strategies used in previous research analyzing coverage of infectious disease outbreaks (Dudo et al., 2007; Roche & Muskavitch, 2003; Yu et al., 2011). The presence of qualitative risk was coded based on a set of qualitative words and phrases depicting the health risk of the West Nile virus. Examples of the words include "large threat," "threatening," "severe outbreak," and "fatal disease," to name a few. The presence of quantitative risk depictions was coded as: 1) numerator (e.g., 30 people died); 2) numerator/population (e.g., 30 out of 1,000 people died, or 2 percent developed symptoms). The difference between these two categories is that the latter offers contextual information, which allows readers to put the numbers into a population context when evaluating the health risk.

Preventability. Coders coded West Nile as *preventable* if there was information about the disease being preventable or the risk being predicable. The portrayal of West Nile was coded as *unpreventable* if the article expressed that the disease could not be prevented, predicted, or treated, or the article conveyed that ways to control the situation were uncertain or unknown.

Responsibility. The coding of responsibility was separated into: 1) individual responsibility and 2) community responsibility. *Individual responsibility* was coded when an article mentioned and advocated individual actions, such as: 1) avoiding mosquito bites (e.g., better screening for windows and doors, reducing outdoor activities, water draining, or wearing insect repellents); 2) cooperating with authority (e.g., reporting dead birds or neglected pools, or supporting community preventive actions); and 3) enhancing awareness and knowledge (e.g., seeking for more information about West Nile). *Community responsibility* was coded if an article reported community efforts in combating the disease, such as: 1) resource provision (e.g., preparing chemicals, mosquito traps); 2) mosquito-control actions (e.g., aerial spraying); and 3) surveillance and education (e.g., monitoring and educating the public about the spread of the virus).

Besides coding of these primary variables, sources of the article were also coded (i.e., local/regional or national media) and the media types (i.e., newspaper, TV, radio, magazine, news agency, and online). The coding book was refined and revised by several rounds of discussions and testing using a small portion of the sample.

Inter-Coder Reliability Test and Coding

Once the codebook was completed, two coders were trained through coding practices and discussions. A mutual understanding of codebook was

306

achieved before the inter-coder reliability test. Two coders completed the inter-coder reliability test. The two coders were both female—one was Caucasian and the other was Asian American. The two coders independently coded 10 percent of articles that were *randomly* selected from the sample. For all categories that were mentioned in the coding scheme (i.e., source, media types, preventability, responsibility), the percentages of agreement ranged from 92 percent to 100 percent, Krippendorff's α ranged from .78 to 1, and Cohen's κ ranged from .80 to 1. Therefore, the overall reliability was satisfactory.

After the inter-coder reliability test was completed, three female coders finished the coding of the entire sample. The whole coding process took approximately three weeks.

Results

Depictions of West Nile Risk

About 6.2 percent of news coverage did not contain any information about risk magnitude associated with the West Nile outbreak. About 9.8 percent portrayed the risk used only qualitative depictions of the disease. For example, the 2012 West Nile outbreak was frequently depicted as "one of the worst outbreaks since 2003." Many articles described the disease as "deadly" and "fatal." Coverage using quantitative risk depictions accounted for 84 percent in total (i.e., presence of numerical information). The articles that used numerator (45.7 percent) or number/population (38.3 percent) to depict the mortality or illness exceeded those that used qualitative depictions of risk only (9.8 percent), as well as those that contained no depictions of risk magnitude (6.2 percent), $[\chi^2 \ (3, \ N = 450) = 214.4, \ p < .001]$ (see Table 15.1). The depiction of the risk magnitude with number/population, the most precise and accurate way to portray risk magnitude, appeared in 38.3 percent of the total stories. Slightly more articles (45.7 percent) presented the

Table 15.1 Percentages of Articles Depicting West Nile Virus Risk Magnitude with Different Level of Precision

No Depiction of Risk Magnitude	Qualitative	Number/ Population	Numerator
6.2%$_a$	9.8%$_a$	38.3%$_b$	45.7%$_b$

Note: Percentages with different subscripts differ at $p < .05$; qualitative = qualitative risk without any numerical information; number/population = numbers of individual affected/ size of population potentially affected; numerator = numerical information without a population context

$\chi^2 \ (3, \ N = 450) = 214.4, \ p < .001$

risk with the actual number of people that were affected or died without providing a context of the overall population. This difference is not statistically significant though [χ^2 (1, N = 378) = 3.1, p = .08].

Preventability of West Nile

RQ2 examined how the media portrayed West Nile regarding whether the disease is preventable or not. The analyses found significantly more articles depicting West Nile being unpreventable (41.4 percent) than those portraying it being preventable (6.4 percent) [χ^2 (1, N = 214) = 113.7, p < .001]. About 52 percent of the articles did not mention the preventability of the disease at all. In other words, over 93 percent of the articles analyzed either omitted the discussion of preventability of West Nile or clearly indicated the random nature of this disease—the virus is transmitted by infected mosquitoes and avoiding mosquito bites cannot be easily guaranteed. In the articles depicting West Nile as being unpreventable, some mentioned there are currently no medications that treat West Nile or a vaccination to prevent the disease. Some claimed that it is too early to monitor the epidemic because the factors associated with West Nile remain unclear (see Table 15.2).

Preventive Responsibility

Individual responsibility. About 51 percent of the coverage mentioned individual responsibility. Specifically, the preventive method of avoiding mosquito bites appeared in 42.4 percent of the articles, enhancing individual awareness and knowledge was presented in 20.3 percent of the articles, and cooperating with authority was mentioned in 8.9 percent of the articles.

The preventive methods suggested by the media include reducing outdoor activities at dawn and dusk, eliminating open water surrounding the house, keeping windows or doors shut, wearing long sleeves and long pants, using insect repellent, or seeking more information regarding West Nile. Individuals were also encouraged to report dead birds to authority or support community mosquito-control programs.

Table 15.2 Percentages of Articles Depicting the Preventability of West Nile Virus

No Mention of Preventability	Unpreventable	Preventable
52.4%$_a$	41.1%$_b$	6.4%$_c$

Note: Percentages with different subscripts differ at p < .05

χ^2 (2, N = 450) = 155.08, p < .001

A 2 X 3 chi-square analysis detected a significant relationship between the portrayal of preventability and individual responsibility [χ^2 (2, $N = 450$) = 19.1, $p < .001$, $V^* = .21$]. Among the articles that depicted West Nile as preventable, significantly more stories (72.4 percent) mentioned individual responsibility of preventing West Nile than those that lacked such information (27.6 percent) [χ^2 (1, $N = 29$) = 5.8, $p < .05$].

When analyzing the stories portraying West Nile being unpreventable, the same pattern emerged. Significantly more articles contained individual responsibility of preventing West Nile (70.8 percent) than those with no such information (29.2 percent) [χ^2 (1, $N = 185$) = 32.1, $p < .001$, $V^* = .21$]. This finding suggests that even though the disease was depicted as unpreventable, media still advocated for individuals to take actions to prevent the disease (see Table 15.3).

Community Responsibility. About 44 percent of the coverage presented the community efforts in combating West Nile. Mosquito-control actions (e.g., aerial spraying, encouraging temporarily shutting down of outdoor businesses) appeared in 30.2 percent of the articles. Surveillance and education in the community was presented in 20.4 percent of the articles. Over 8 percent of the stories mentioned community resource provision (e.g. offering test labs, providing chemicals for mosquito control).

A 2 X 3 chi-square analysis detected a significant relationship between the portrayal of preventability and community responsibility [χ^2 (2, $N = 450$) = 7.36, $p < .05$, $V^* = .13$]. Specifically, when the articles contained no information of preventability, significantly more stories mentioned community responsibility (61.4 percent) than those that did not (38.6 percent) [χ^2 (1, $N = 236$) = 12.4, $p < .001$]. The findings revealed that news articles continued to report community actions to prevent the spread of the West Nile virus even when they were unclear about the preventability of the disease (see Table 15.4).

Table 15.3 Percentages of Articles Depicting Individual Responsibility by West Nile Virus Preventability

| | | Preventability | | |
		Preventable	Unpreventable	No Mention of Preventability
Individual	yes	72.4%$_a$	70.8%$_a$	50.8%$_a$
Responsibility	no	27.6%$_b$	29.2%$_b$	49.2%$_a$

Note: Within column, percentages with different subscripts differ at $p < .05$.

χ^2 (2, $N = 450$) = 19.14, $p < .001$

Table 15.4 Percentages of Articles Depicting Community Responsibility by West Nile Virus Preventability

		Preventability		
		Preventable	Unpreventable	No Mention of Preventability
Community	Yes	58.6%[a]	49.2%[a]	38.6%[a]
Responsibility	No	41.4%[a]	50.8%[a]	61.4%[b]

Note: Within column, percentages with different subscripts differ at $p < .05$.

χ^2 (2, N = 450) = 7.36, $p < .05$

Discussion

Precision of Risk Depictions

One of the key questions we investigated in this study was the precision of the risk depiction in the West Nile coverage. Given that the West Nile outbreak in 2012 was referred to as "the worst outbreak in the past decade" (CDC, 2013), media were expected to accurately and precisely convey the severity and the magnitude of this health risk to the public.

Quantitative risk presentation is believed to be more accurate when compared to using just qualitative risk depictions because it offers more numerical information for audiences to make objective evaluations (Dudo et al., 2007; Roche & Muskavitch, 2003; Yu et al., 2011). The results of the present study suggest the majority of the articles (84 percent) adopted this approach. This can be viewed as a significant improvement from the West Nile coverage in 2000 when limited quantitative information was presented in the news coverage (Roche & Muskavitch, 2003).

Roche and Muskavitch (2003) suggested that coverage of the West Nile outbreak in 2000 generally lacked precision because 89 percent of the articles had no information at the number/population level. A slight improvement was detected in this study. Over 38 percent of the articles included the number of people who were at risk or died of the West Nile virus and also provided an overall population context in the coverage (e.g., 1 in 100 people may develop severe symptoms).

We recommend that journalists continue using this approach when covering health risks in the future because providing a precise context of the risk magnitude can offer an integrated, holistic picture of a health risk and allow individuals to make reasonable and accurate judgments of susceptibility (Dudo et al., 2007; Roche & Muskavitch, 2003). This type of improvement is especially meaningful in a quick-changing media environment, in which information of health risks can be spread quickly through digital media platforms such as online news media or social media (e.g. Twitter, Snapchat, or Facebook).

In a recent report released by the Pew Research Center (Fox, 2014), 72 percent of Internet users reported that they have searched online for health information. When a significant health risk (e.g., Ebola, Zika, or West Nile) approaches, individuals will rely on both the mass media and their personal networks (face-to-face or online) to receive reliable health information. Journalists will face the challenge of reporting health risks promptly and accurately through digital media outlets as more and more traditional media are moving toward fully digitized platforms (Risi, 2016). Therefore, the precision of the risk depictions of large-scale pandemics becomes tremendously important because an inaccurate report of the risk may generate unnecessary fear or anxiety. We hope that news reporters can continually improve their coverage of health risks by presenting both the numeric depictions and the context of the population.

Preventability and Responsibility

Our study discovered that the news stories covering the 2012 West Nile outbreak primarily depicted the disease as unpreventable or simply neglected the discussion of the preventability of the disease entirely. Only 6.4 percent of the stories were optimistic about the preventability of West Nile. Given that there is no vaccine or treatment for West Nile at this time, this pattern of coverage seems reasonable. The small amount of articles that portrayed the disease as being preventable or predictable focused primarily on scientific research about developing models to monitor the spread of the virus. Many of these articles emphasized connecting weather conditions to the breeding patterns of the mosquitoes that spread the virus. These articles conveyed a signal that the West Nile outbreaks may be predicted or prevented in the near future.

However, over 52 percent of the articles did not mention the preventability of the disease and 41 percent suggested the difficulties of preventing the West Nile virus. The majority of the coverage revealed that the come-and-go of the virus was largely unpredictable and the disease was generally unpreventable.

Based on the attribution theory, responsibilities are unlikely to be assumed when risks are unpreventable (Weiner, 1986, 2006, 2010). Therefore, the depiction of disease preventability is meaningful because it may influence whether individuals can be motivated to take precautionary actions. For a disease like West Nile, preventability is largely uncertain because there is no vaccine or treatment for the West Nile virus at this time (Sifferlin, 2015); therefore, the call for actions to protect oneself narrowly focused on avoiding mosquito bites. This preventive strategy, however, carries its own natural uncertainty. It is true that exposure to infected mosquitoes may be decreased by preventive actions such as reducing outdoor activities, using insect repellent, draining standing water, or applying aerial spray in the community (CDC, 2016). However, no one can completely avoid or control mosquito bites realistically. The mosquito population can also surge due to warm and humid weather. The complete elimination of mosquitoes seems impossible ("West Nile virus," 2013).

Our study suggested that the media coverage of the 2012 West Nile outbreak represented a theoretical and practical paradox. Based on the attribution theory, an unpreventable risk is unable to motivate preventive actions. But media have suggested otherwise—the West Nile outbreak was largely unpreventable, yet preventive strategies for individuals and communities were encouraged.

Even though the media coverage consistently portrayed the spread of the West Nile virus as unpreventable, a significant portion of the reports frequently advocated individual preventive actions and highlighted community efforts in combating the disease. The media coverage of West Nile conveyed an unrealistic or false hope to the public—the risk may be minimized by certain preventive actions yet the disease is scientifically unpreventable and unpredictable.

Future Directions

Our study has created some new directions for future research regarding the relationship between media, audiences, and large-scale pandemics. First, given that the accuracy assessment of upcoming health risks is essential, it is meaningful to continue evaluating the performance of different types of media outlets in an evolving media environment. Traditional and online news reporters both carry important responsibilities in precisely communicating health issues such as West Nile to the public. Second, it is also important to investigate peoples' attitudes and perceptions about West Nile to understand how individuals will react to a risk when there is no scientifically approved treatment or vaccine. Third, scholars can also experimentally test the persuasiveness of health messages that advocate preventive behaviors with different portrayals of preventability or responsibility of West Nile. Overall, this study provides research findings that may be useful to investigate other national or international pandemics. Future research can also examine how a disease outbreak has been discussed on social media.

Conclusion

Through the lens of media coverage of the 2012 West Nile outbreak, we found that news stories frequently used the quantitative approach to depict the risk magnitude of the West Nile outbreak. The precision of the coverage of the risk was largely improved compared to the previous coverage of West Nile (Roche & Muskavitch, 2003). The findings of this study revealed that West Nile was often portrayed as unpreventable and media frequently encouraged individuals and communities to engage in preventive actions. This type of coverage may create a conflicting image for the West Nile prevention because individuals were encouraged to perform precautionary actions yet their effectiveness or usefulness remained unknown.

We also suggest future reporters should continue to improve their writing by accurately assessing the risk and responsibility of disease outbreaks so that the public can have a realistic understanding of their relevance to an illness and how to protect themselves.

This study has gone beyond the investigation of the traditional media and their role in reporting a disease outbreak and covered an extensive range of media outlets including national, international, print, broadcast, and online news outlets. This research also tested the attribution theory amongst the news coverage of West Nile, an approach that has linked a social-psychology theory to media studies. As a whole, this study provides valuable theoretical and practical implications for an important venue of research in health and risk communication.

References

Ben-Porath, E. N., & Shaker, L. K. (2010). News images, race, and attribution in the wake of Hurricane Katrina. *Journal of Communication*, 60(3), 466–490.

Blakely, D. E. (2003). Social construction of three influenza pandemics in *The New York Times. Journalism and Mass Communication Quarterly*, 80(4), 884–902. doi: 10.1177/107769900308000409.

Centers for Disease Control and Prevention (CDC). (2013, June 28). *West Nile virus and other arboviral disease—United States 2012*. Retrieved from www. cdc.gov/mmwr/preview/mmwrhtml/mm6225a1.htm?s_cid=mm6225a1_e

Centers for Disease Control and Prevention (CDC) (2016). West Nile virus. Retrieved February 27, 2017 from www.cdc.gov/westnile/prevention/.

Dudo, A., Dahlstrom, M., & Brossard, D. (2007). Reporting a potential pandemic: A risk-related assessment of avian influenza coverage in U.S. newspapers. *Science Communication*, 28(4), 429–454.

Fischhoff, B. (1995). Risk perception and communication unplugged: Twenty years of process. *Risk Analysis*, 15(2), 137–145. doi: 10.1111/j.1539-6924.1995. tb00308.x.

Fox, M. (2013, May 13). 2012 was deadliest year for West Nile in US, CDC says. *NBC News*. Retrieved October 3, 2013 from www.nbcnews.com/health/2012-was-deadliest-year-west-nile-us-cdc-says-1C9904312.

Fox, S. (2014). The social life of health information. *Pew Research Center*. Retrieved February 26, 2017 from www.pewresearch.org/fact-tank/2014/01/15/the-social-life-of-health-information/.

Griffin, R. J., Dunwoody, S., & Neuwirth, K. (1999). Proposed model of the relationship of risk information seeking and processing to the development of preventive behaviors. *Environmental Research, 80*(2), S230–S245. doi: 10.1006/enrs.1998.3940.

Holton, A., Weberling, B., Clarke, C. E., & Smith, M. J. (2012). The blame frame: Media attribution of culpability about MMR-autism vaccination scare. *Health Communication, 27,* 690–701. doi: 10.1080/10410236.2011.633158.

Hume, J. (2000). The "forgotten" 1918 influenza epidemic and press portrayal of public anxiety. *Journalism and Mass Communication Quarterly, 77*(4), 898–915.

Hung, L. S. (2003). The SARS epidemic in Hong Kong: What lessons have we learned? *Journal of the Royal Society of Medicine, 96*(8), 374–378.

Iyengar, S. (1991). *Is anyone responsible? How television frames political issues.* Chicago, IL: University of Chicago Press.

Jang, S. M. (2013). Framing responsibility in climate change discourse: Ethnocentric attribution bias, perceived causes, and policy attitudes. *Journal of Environmental Psychology, 36,* 27–36. doi: 10.1016/j.jenvp.2013.07.003.

Jarlenski, M., & Barry, C. L. (2013). News media coverage of trans fat: Health risks and policy responses. *Health Communication, 28*(3), 209–216. doi: 10.1080/10410236.2012.669670.

Kim, S. H. (2015). Who is responsible for a social problem? News framing and attribution of responsibility. *Journalism and Mass Communication Quarterly, 92*(3), 554–557.

Kim, S. H., & Willis, L. A. (2007). Talking about obesity: News framing of who is responsible for causing and fixing the problem. *Journal of Health Communication, 12,* 359–376. doi: 10.1080/10810730701326051.

Kim, S. H., Carvalho, J. P., & Davis, A. C. (2010). Talking about poverty: News framing of who is responsible for causing and fixing the problem. *Journalism and Mass Communication Quarterly, 87*(3–4), 563–581. doi: 10.1177/107769901008700308.

Kitzinger, J., & Reilly, J. (1997). The rise and fall of risk reporting: Media coverage of human genetics research, "false memory syndrome," and "mad cow disease." *European Journal of Communication, 12*(3), 319–350. doi: 10.1177/0267323197012003002.

Koteyko, N., Brown, B., & Crawford, P. (2008). The dead parrot and the dying swan: The role of metaphor scenarios in UK press coverage of Asian flu in the UK in 2005–2006. *Metaphor and Symbol, 23,* 242–261.

Lucas, T., Lakey, B., Alexander, S., & Arnetz, B. (2009). Individuals and illnesses as sources of perceived preventability. *Psychology, Health, & Medicine, 14*(3). doi: 10.1080/13548500802705914.

Lucas, T., Alexander, S., Firestone, I. J., & LeBreton, J. M. (2009). Belief in a just world, social influence, and illness attributions: Evidence of a just world boomerang effect. *Journal of Health Psychology, 14,* 248–256.

Luther, C. A., & Zhou, S. (2005). Within the boundaries of politics: News framing of SARS in China and the United States. *Journalism and Mass Communication Quarterly, 82*(4), 857–872.

Major, L. H. (2009). Break it to me harshly: The effects of intersecting news frames in lung cancer and obesity coverage. *Journal of Health Communication, 14,* 174–188. doi: 10.1080/10810730802659939.

Pew Research Center. (2009). Health news coverage in the U.S. media, early 2009. Retrieved October 3, 2013 from www.journalism.org/2009/07/29/health-news-coverage-us-media-early-2009/.

Resnik, D. B. (2001). Ethical dilemmas in communicating medical information to the public. *Health Policy*, 55(2), 129–149. doi: 10.1016/S0168-8510(00)00121-4.

Risi, J. (2016). Digital didn't kill traditional media. *The Huffington Post*. Retrieved February 26, 2017 from www.huffingtonpost.com/jennifer-risi/digital-didnt-kill-tradit_b_10116548.html.

Roche, J. P., & Muskavitch, M. A. T. (2003). Limited precision in print media communication of West Nile virus risks. *Science Communication*, 24(3), 353–365. doi: 10.1177/1075547002250300.

Sifferlin, A. (2015). Scientists find a way to predict West Nile outbreaks. *Time*. Retrieved February 26, 2016 from http://time.com/3850841/west-nile-mosquitoes/

Torell, U., & Bremberg, S. (1995). Unintentional injuries: Attribution, perceived preventability, and social norms. *Journal of Safety Research*, 26(2), 63–73. doi: 10.1016/0022-4375(95)00007-D.

Wallack, L., Dorfman, L., Jernigan, D., & Themba, M. (1993). *Media advocacy and public health: Power for prevention*. Newbury Park, CA: SAGE.

Wang, W., & Liu, Y. (2015). Communication message cues and opinions about people with depression: An investigation of discussion on Weibo. *Asian Journal of Communication*, 25, 33–47. doi: 10.1080/01292986.2014.989238.

Weiner, B. (1986). An attributional theory of achievement, motivation and emotion. *Psychological Reviews*, 92(4), 547–573. doi: 10.1037/0033-295X.92.4.548.

Weiner, B. (1995). Judgements of responsibility: A foundation for a theory of social conduct. New York: The Guilford Press.

Weiner, B. (2006). *Social motivation, justice, and the moral emotions: An attributional approach*. Mahwah, NJ: Lawrence Erlbaum Associates.

Weiner, B. (2010). The development of an attribution-based theory of motivation: A history of ideas. *Educational Psychologist*, 45(1), 28–36.

Weinstein, N. D. (1984). Why it won't happen to me: Perceptions of risk factors and susceptibility. *Health Psychology*, 3(5), 431–457.

West Nile virus. (2013, October 3). *The New York Times*. Retrieved October 3 from http://health.nytimes.com/health/guides/disease/west-nile-virus.

Yu, N. (2004, January 20). SARS lessons: How to address crises. *China Daily*, p. 5.

Yu, N., Frohlich, D. O., Fougner, J., & Ren, L. (2011). Communicating in a health epidemic: A risk assessment of the swine flu coverage in US newspapers. *International Public Health Journal*, 3(1), 1–14.

Yu, N., & Xu, Q. (2016). Public discourse on genetically modified foods in mobile sphere: Framing risks, opportunities, and responsibilities in mobile social media in China. In W. Ran (Ed.), *Private chat to public sphere, mobile media, political participation, and civic activism in Asia*. New York: Springer.

16

COMPETING AND COMPLEMENTARY NARRATIVES IN THE EBOLA CRISIS

Morgan Getchel, Deborah Sellnow-Richmond,
Chelsea Woods, Greg Williams, Erin Hester,
Matthew Seeger, and Timothy Sellnow

The surprise, threat, and uncertainty of crises create a momentary void of understanding. For at least a moment, those observing the onset of a crisis are not fully able to comprehend the nature of the crisis—the cause, the extent of the impact, and what can be done immediately. This "communication vacuum and meaning deficit of a crisis create a discursive space that is filled by narratives, often multiple and conflicting" (Seeger & Sellnow, 2016, p. 8). Narratives, the stories we tell that both help us comprehend the crisis personally and explain its origin and impact to others, structure the reality surrounding the crisis. Naturally, those whose reputations are at stake create stories where they and the organizations they lead are portrayed in the most positive light that is reasonable, based on the context of the crisis. Other stakeholders and observers tell stories from their perspectives. Often, the stories of external observers portray the organizations at the center of the crisis with a competing and less favorable tone. Over time, these competing stories coalesce or converge in the eyes of the publics that observe them, leading to less competition and divergence. As more evidence is known, some competing stories are discredited and others are verified. If, however, the crisis under consideration is fraught with ongoing controversy, the narrative process becomes increasingly complex before it resolves into a dominant or broadly accepted narrative.

Health-related narratives are particularly prone to such ongoing controversy. Unlike crises where a specific, contained incident leads to momentary calamity that is quickly resolved, health crises such as epidemics and pandemics linger on, punctuated by volatile points where a disease passes borders or surpasses expectations in its mortality as treatment options falter. In a health setting, the crisis narratives can divide repeatedly and unexpectedly as consequences and perceptions of severity shift and intensify. Such was the case with the West Africa Ebola outbreak beginning in 2013. Previous Ebola outbreaks, though devastating and frightening, had been contained to rural areas relatively soon after the initial diagnosis. In 2013, however, the outbreak took root in highly populated areas and began to spread at unprecedented levels. As the disease spanned across borders and continents, the West Africa Ebola narrative evolved in a fractured and contentious manner for nearly a year. Thus, the West Africa Ebola narrative is an exemplar of health-related crises and their narrative complexity.

In this chapter, we begin with an overview of how the narrative space created by crises moves through divergence to convergence. We then further explain how lengthy crises with high levels of visibility and hazard continually expand the narrative space to allow for exceptional clash in the narratives that are generated to explain the situation. We then provide a description of the controversial narrative that wove through the West Africa Ebola crisis. We conclude with theoretical explanations of the narrative convergence process in complex health crises and offer practical explanations for responding to such protracted crisis narratives.

The Natural Cycle of Crisis Narratives

Narrative explanations are inherent to the evolutions of crises. Crises typically move through three stages: pre-crisis, crisis, and post-crisis (Ulmer, Sellnow, & Seeger, 2014). During pre-crisis, warning signs, subtle or obvious, are present. If these warning signs are missed, ignored, or reach beyond human control, crises occur. In the aftermath of the crisis, investigations occur, corrective actions are taken, and retrospective learning takes place. The crisis ends with a return to pre-crisis where risks are monitored and the lessons learned from the crisis are applied (Seeger & Sellnow, 2016). Similarly, the natural cycle of crisis narratives begins with the onset of the crisis, divergence gives way to the convergence process during the post-crisis discussion, and converges into consistent lessons learned and steps toward future resilience in the new pre-crisis stage. During the crisis stage, multiple narratives are generated to explain what is happening, why it is happening, and who is to blame. The quantity of narratives and the magnitude of their impact are intensified when the crisis period is long.

The fact that multiple narratives emerge in response to crises is essentially positive. By their nature, crises create shock and surprise. Thus, multiple interpretations are naturally and spontaneously created by individuals witnessing the crisis based on their distinct observational points. Stifling this interpretive process through attempts to force a single consistent narrative

317

interpretation onto the crisis process would be, at best, inaccurate and, at worst, a violation of free speech. Perelman (1969) explains that such pluralism in interpretation is essential in the public discussion of any contestable issue. He explains that allowing multiple voices to be heard in the comprehension process "refrains from granting to any individual or group, no matter who they are, the exorbitant privilege of setting up a single criterion for what is valid and what is appropriate" (p. 71). Without *narrative plurality*, for example, an organization or agency could impose a narrative that overlooks its transgressions, assigns blame to innocent or irrelevant parties, and dodges the need for change. Narrative plurality ensures that multiple voices are heard so that all those impacted by the crisis are represented in the narrative discussion. Problematically, narrative plurality can be a means for manipulation. Hidden agendas can be introduced into competing narratives, seeking to discredit opponents or as a ploy to distract or divert the discussion from meaningful debate to hostile and unproductive prattle. Over time, however, attempts at distraction are often exposed in a maturing and converging narrative (Seeger & Sellnow, 2016).

Narrative Plurality as Divergence

Multiple narratives appearing early in the crisis often provide distinct and even competing views of crisis (Heath, 2004). These narratives seek to answer consistent questions focusing on intent, responsibility, and evidence (Ulmer & Sellnow, 2000). Questions of intent focus on pre-crisis activities. Simply put, the narrative seeks to answer the question of whether those with some power to prevent or contain the crisis have the best interest of their stakeholders in mind. For example, were warning signals intentionally ignored? If so, what was the potential benefit to those who ignored the warnings? Questions of responsibility ask who is to blame. Did the disease spread at a rate that, given existing knowledge and capacity, could not have been avoided? If so, efforts to assign responsibility are futile. If, however, the response to the disease outbreak included dimensions of incompetence, apathy, or greed, then assigning responsibility is a natural step in resolving the crisis. Finally, answering questions of intent and responsibility involve the constant discovery and interpretation of evidence. Simply locating and sharing evidence is unlikely to resolve narrative divergence. Instead, evidence typically has some ambiguity in how it can be interpreted. Thus, narrative divergence is likely to continue until some degree of consistency is reached on the meaning of the evidence surrounding the crisis.

Moving From Plurality to Convergence

Narrative convergence is based on consistent interpretations, either partial or complete, from multiple sources (Perleman & Olbrechts-Tyteca,

1969; Sellnow, Ulmer, Seeger, & Littlefield, 2009). Those impacted by crises seek information based on intent, responsibility, and evidence from multiple sources. This confirmation of information among sources is a natural process, particularly when individuals are directly impacted by or keenly interested in the crisis (Anthony, Sellnow, & Millner, 2013). As time passes and more is known about the crisis, some diverging interpretations are widely discounted. Elements of other interpretations appear consistently among a variety of sources. Some degree of disagreement may continue, but agreement is often seen on many aspects of the crisis as the narrative evolves. Accordingly, convergence is distinct from dominance or congruence. Dominance is narrative consistency that is based on information deprivation or coercion. A single narrative is dominant because that is all that the storyteller knows or because telling an alternative story results in punishment or a lack of reward. Congruence, which is seldom achieved, exists when agreement is undisputed and the storytellers believe there is no other story to tell. Congruent narratives would likely be so superficial or obvious that they are of limited interest to storytellers.

Narratives achieve congruence incrementally. As convergence begins, previously divergent narratives begin to align on particular assumptions and characterizations. Observers and storytellers see partial agreement among the differing representations of the intent, responsibility, and evidence surrounding the crisis. Complete agreement is unlikely and, based on Perelman's (1969) notion of plurality, undesirable. Converging narratives have enough consistency to achieve probability and fidelity among storytellers and their audiences (Fisher, 1987). Narratives satisfy the criteria of probability when audiences generally believe the narrative is an accurate representation of the crisis. Narrative fidelity is more precise, focusing on the details shared in the narrative. As Table 16.1 indicates, narratives are convergent in the pre-crisis stage, become divergent in the crisis stage, and begin to converge as probability and fidelity are agreed upon by audiences in the post-crisis stages. Plurality should be present in all three stages of the crisis cycle, being most pronounced in the crisis stage, narrowing in the post-crisis stage, and largely focused on dimensions of fidelity in the pre-crisis stage.

Table 16.1 Convergence in Crisis Narratives

Crisis Stage	Degree of Convergence	Plurality
Pre-Crisis	Highly Convergent	Based largely on fidelity
Crisis	Highly Divergent	Diverse
Post-Crisis	Converging	Narrowing with the emergence of probability and fidelity

The West Africa Ebola Narrative

As mentioned above, prolonged crises, such as those created in response to health crises like epidemics, are slower in achieving narrative convergence. As the morbidity and mortality rise, crossing borders and continents, divergent narratives from multiple sources speculate about the peak of the disease and about the best ways to respond to it circulate (see Table 16.2).

Table 16.2 Ebola Outbreak Timeline March 2014 – November 2014

March 25	The CDC issues its initial announcement on a disease outbreak in Guinea, and reports of cases in Liberia and Sierra Leone. Guinea reports 86 cases, including 59 deaths (fatality rate of 68.5%).
March 24	Preliminary results from the Pasteur Institute in France indicate the Zaire strain of Ebola virus.
April 1	Medical charity Médecins Sans Frontières (MSF) warns the epidemic is "unprecedented." A World Health Organization (WHO) spokesman calls it "relatively small still."
April 4	Mob attacks Ebola treatment center in Guinea. Healthcare workers there and in Sierra Leone and Liberia face hostility from fearful, suspicious people. Reported rumor that the outbreak is a hoax.
April 16	*New England Journal of Medicine* suggests that the current outbreak's Patient Zero was a two-year-old from Guinea who died on December 6, 2013.
May 26	WHO confirms first Ebola deaths in Sierra Leone.
June 17	Liberia reports Ebola in its capital, Monrovia.
June 23	MSF says outbreak is "out of control" and calls for massive resources.
July 25	Nigeria confirms its first Ebola case, a man who traveled from Monrovia.
July 29	Dr. Sheik Umar Khan, who was leading Sierra Leone's fight against the epidemic, dies of Ebola.
July 22	Nancy Writebol, an American aid worker for Samaritan's Purse in Liberia, tests positive for Ebola, having been infected while treating patients.
July 24	Patrick Sawyer, a Liberian-American lawyer and a top government official in the Liberian Ministry of Finance, dies at a local Nigerian hospital. He is the first American to die in this outbreak.
July 26	Kent Brantly, medical director for Samaritan Purse's Ebola Consolidated Case Management Center in Liberia, is infected with the virus.

July 29	Dr. Sheik Humarr Khan who oversaw Ebola treatment at Kenema Government Hospital in Sierra Leone dies from complications of the disease.
July 30	The Peace Corps removes its volunteers from Liberia, Sierra Leone, and Guinea.
July 31	CDC raises warning to Level 3 and suggest avoiding nonessential travel to Sierra Leone, Guinea, and Liberia.
August 2	Ebola patient Dr. Kent Brantly is evacuated to Emory University Hospital in Atlanta, Georgia.
August 4	Reports emerge that the experimental drug, "ZMapp," was flown to Liberia to treat Brantly and Writebol.
August 6	Nancy Writebol arrives at Emory in Atlanta for treatment.
August 8	Experts at the World Health Organization declare the Ebola epidemic an international health emergency that requires a coordinated global approach. The outbreak is described as the worst outbreak in the four-decade history of tracking the disease.
August 12	WHO says death toll tops 1,000, approves use of unproven drugs or vaccines. A Spanish priest with Ebola dies in Madrid hospital.
August 19	Liberia's President Ellen Johnson Sirleaf declares a nationwide curfew beginning August 20 and orders two communities quarantined, with no movement in or out of the areas.
August 20	Security forces in Monrovia fire shots and tear gas to disperse crowd trying to break out of quarantine, killing a teen.
August 21	Dr. Kent Brantly is discharged from Emory University Hospital. It is also announced that Nancy Writebol had been released on August 19. Emory staff report that Brantly and Writebol pose "no public health threat."
August 24	Democratic Republic of Congo declares Ebola outbreak, believed separate from West Africa epidemic. Infected British medical worker is flown home from Sierra Leone for treatment.
August 28	WHO puts death toll above 1,550, warns outbreak could infect more than 20,000.
August 29	Senegal reports first confirmed Ebola case.
September 2	MSF president tells UN the world is losing battle to contain Ebola, slams "global inaction."
September 6	The government of Sierra Leone announces plans for a nationwide lockdown from September 19–21 in order to stop the spread of Ebola.
September 8	Britain to send military and humanitarian experts to Sierra Leone to set up treatment center; United States to send field hospital to Liberia to care for health workers.

(continued)

Table 16.2 (continued)

September 12	Cuba announces it will send 165 doctors and nurses to Sierra Leone to treat Ebola patients once they receive special training.
September 13	Liberia appeals to Obama for aid to fight Ebola.
September 16	United States promises to send 3,000 military engineers and medical personnel to West Africa to build clinics and train healthcare workers.
September 16	President Obama calls the efforts to combat the Ebola outbreak centered in West Africa "the largest international response in the history of the CDC." Speaking from the CDC headquarters in Atlanta, Obama adds that "faced with this outbreak, the world is looking to" the United States to lead international efforts to combat the virus. He says the United States is ready to take on that leadership role.
September 20	Liberian Thomas Eric Duncan flies from Liberia to Dallas via Brussels and Washington after trying to help woman with Ebola in his home country.
September 23	U.S. Centers for Disease Control and Prevention (CDC) estimates between 550,000 and 1.4 million people in West Africa may have Ebola by January.
September 25	Duncan goes to Dallas hospital with fever, abdominal pain. He is sent back to apartment where he is staying despite telling a nurse he traveled from West Africa.
September 28	Duncan returns by ambulance to Dallas hospital.
September 30	CDC confirms Duncan has Ebola; first case diagnosed in the United States.
September 30	Dr. Thomas Frieden, director of the CDC, announces the first diagnosed case of Ebola in the United States. The person has been hospitalized and isolated at Texas Health Presbyterian Hospital in Dallas, Texas.
October 1	Liberian government officials release the name of the U.S. patient, Thomas Eric Duncan.
October 6	A nurse's assistant in Spain becomes the first person known to have contracted Ebola outside Africa in the current outbreak. The woman helped treat two Spanish missionaries, both of whom had contracted Ebola in West Africa.
October 6	NBC freelance cameraman Ashoka Mukpo arrives at Nebraska Medical Center for treatment after contracting Ebola in Liberia. On October 21, the hospital says that Mukpo no longer has the Ebola virus in his bloodstream and will be allowed to leave.
October 8	Thomas Eric Duncan dies of Ebola in Dallas. U.S. government orders five major airports to screen passengers from West Africa for fever.

October 11	Nina Pham, a Dallas nurse who cared for the now-deceased Ebola patient Thomas Eric Duncan, tests positive for Ebola during a preliminary blood test. She is the first person to contract Ebola on American soil.
October 15	Amber Vinson, a second Dallas nurse who also cared for Thomas Eric Duncan, is diagnosed with Ebola. Authorities say Vinson flew on a commercial jet from Cleveland to Dallas days before testing positive for Ebola.
October 17	U.S. President Obama appoints Ebola response coordinator.
October 20	Under fire in the wake of Ebola cases involving two Dallas nurses, the CDC issues updated Ebola guidelines that stress the importance of more training and supervision, and recommend that no skin be exposed when workers are wearing personal protective equipment, or PPE.
October 21	MSF says it will start trials of experimental Ebola drugs at its treatment centers in West Africa next month.
October 23	Craig Spencer, a 33-year-old doctor who recently returned from Guinea has tested positive for Ebola. The fourth case diagnosed in the United States.
October 24	The National Institutes of Health announces one of the Dallas nurses, Nina Pham, has been declared free of the Ebola virus. Pham is released from a Maryland hospital on October 24, and Vinson is released from an Atlanta hospital on October 28.
October 24	In response to the New York Ebola case, the governors of New York and New Jersey announce that their states are stepping up airport screening beyond federal requirements for travelers from West Africa. The new protocol mandates a quarantine for any individual, including medical personnel, who has had direct contact with individuals infected with Ebola while in Liberia, Sierra Leone, or Guinea. The policy allows the states to determine hospitalization or quarantine for up to 21 days for other travelers from affected countries. Dallas nurse Nina Pham is free of Ebola and leaves the hospital. New York and New Jersey order the quarantine of all medical workers returning from Ebola-hit West African countries, including a nurse, Kaci Hickox, who tests negative and is not released until two days later.
October 25	Illinois orders the quarantine of all medical workers returning from Ebola-hit West African countries.
October 26	Florida will monitor for 21 days people returning from Ebola-hit countries.

(continued)

Table 16.2 (continued)

October 27	U.S. military begins isolating personnel returning from Ebola missions in West Africa. Australia closes its borders to the areas hardest hit by Ebola. Bans visas for citizens of Sierra Leone, Liberia, and Guinea.
November 5	Nurse's aide Maria Teresa Romero Ramos, believed to be the first person to contract Ebola outside of Africa, is released from the hospital in Madrid, Spain.
November 11	Dr. Craig Spencer, the first person to test positive for Ebola in New York City, is released from Bellevue Hospital. With Spencer free of the virus, all U.S. patients who had Ebola have recovered or died.
November 15	Dr. Martin Salia, who became infected with Ebola while treating patients in Sierra Leone, arrives at Nebraska Medical Center in Omaha. Salia, a native of Sierra Leone, is a legal permanent resident of the United States married to a U.S. citizen.
November 17	Dr. Salia dies at Nebraska Medical Center.

Compiled from CNN: http://www.cnn.com/2014/04/11/health/ebola-fast-facts/Reuters: http://www.reuters.com/article/2014/10/28/health-ebola-idUSL2N0SG2FH20141028

Mapping the Ebola Narrative

Crises are surprising and uncertain events that require interpretation (Sellnow & Seeger, 2013). Meaning is created as more information becomes available and that information is shared in stories, most typically through news accounts, and increasingly through social media. Narratives from multiple sources help explain the threat and risk of the Ebola narrative. In this section, we explain how narrative explanations of the event differed based on many factors, ranging from who was speaking, their standpoint, who was being addressed, and how the risk was framed.

Initially, the Ebola virus became known to science in 1976, following an outbreak in Zaire. Ebola was identified as the source of severe viral hemorrhagic fevers (VHFs) resulting in an intense albeit rapidly contained outbreak. Ebola is a member of the filoviridae family along with the Marburg virus, identified in German commercial laboratory workers in 1967. That outbreak was associated with African green monkeys imported for research (Peters & Peters, 1999).

Although sporadic outbreaks of Ebola have occurred in rural Africa, the disease has largely been a regional concern until the December 2013 outbreak in Guinea, which quickly spread to Liberia and Sierra Leone. Unlike previous outbreaks, the disease spread rapidly in urban centers. The lack of adequate medical infrastructure, cultural practices for burial, and a slow international response have been identified as factors related to the spread of the disease.

The 2014 Ebola Narrative

As the Ebola outbreak expanded in West Africa, it became the focus of media attention in the US. Two underlying questions framed US media coverage. First, questions were asked about how bad the outbreak was in Africa and what could be done to contain it. Second, questions were asked about the possibility of the disease coming to the US. This second question became particularly prominent after the death of Thomas Duncan in March.

Media coverage became much more prominent and included ongoing reports by the US Centers for Disease Control and Prevention to address the heightened concern and interest in Ebola as well as commentaries and opinions from a variety of members of the medical community.

Public narratives about crises and risks tend, over time, to either converge or diverge (Seeger & Sellnow, 2016). Competing crisis narratives evolve toward unity as more information about the crisis is revealed. Technical information can provide understanding of how or why the crisis happened. First-hand accounts of loss and discomfort contribute to the narrative by humanizing the impact of the crisis. Emotional expression helps to reconcile divisions in preliminary and competing crisis narratives. As time goes on and more is known, evidence is validated or invalidated, the intent of those involved in the crisis begins to crystalize, and blame or responsibility is assigned. Through this process, narratives that were initially divided begin to homogenize as they move toward a common understanding of the crisis.

At their best, competing narratives create space for broader understanding and to test assumptions. The ensuing dialogue allows the expression of alternative views as well as functional understanding of the crisis and what steps could, should, or must be taken to manage the threat. At their worst, competing crisis narratives create space for manipulation, promote misunderstanding, and accelerate the harm. Competing narratives may interact with other issues or trends. Understanding the competing and converging narratives is central to understanding the larger narrative space of an event.

The Ebola Narratives

The goal of this project was to understand the public Ebola narrative(s) within the technical sphere and their relationship to one another. By technical sphere we mean those narratives offered by or referencing subject matter experts and grounded in scientific information about the disease, its treatment, risk, and development (Goodnight, 1999).

325

Narratives were tracked and coded as they were reported in the *New York Times* and the *Washington Post* beginning with September 30, 2014, the day the first US Ebola patient, Thomas Duncan, was diagnosed, and running through November. Those tracking the media were provided with a narrative mapping guide specifying the type of information to be gleaned from each article. Coders recorded the media outlet, date of publication, technical sources quoted, the narrative expressed by those sources, and if that narrative converged or diverged with the official narrative expressed by the CDC. An Excel spreadsheet was used to compile the data for further analysis. The specific narrative story line was recorded and the narratives were then assessed as convergent with the official narrative, divergent or both.

A wide variety of narrative sources were reported in the *New York Times* and *The Washington Post*. These included subject matter experts affiliated with government and universities, health care professionals, and organizations, including aid groups such as Médecins Sans Frontières (Doctors Without Borders). Other narrative sources included business spokespersons, survivors, and politicians.

Of the 187 narratives reported in the *NYT* and *WPO*, 119 were convergent with the official narrative that Ebola represented a minimal threat (see Tables 16.3 and 16.4).

Official Narratives

The official narrative regarding the Ebola outbreak was offered by the CDC as the agency designated by federal law for leading infectious disease outbreaks. The CDC's formal message and associated narrative was relatively consistent throughout the outbreak and focused primarily on the limited risk. These narratives came primarily from a science and public health perspective. According to this narrative, the risk to the average American of contracting Ebola was very small, in fact almost nonexistent. Because the disease can only be spread through direct contact with bodily fluids (urine, blood, saliva, feces) it is hard to contact Ebola through what would be considered casual contact. Moreover, people are not contagious unless they are showing symptoms of the disease (CDC, 2016).

In addition, the CDC noted that Ebola could be controlled in the US through established infectious disease management techniques and

Table 16.3 Ebola Narratives in the NYT and WPO

	Narratives	Convergent	Divergent	Both/Neither
NYT	101	59	38	4
WPO	86	60	17	9

Table 16.4 New York Times and Washington Post Ebola Narratives

New York Times *Narratives*	
Convergent Narratives	
Protocols are adequate	8
Health care heroes	7
Need for more information	6
Monitoring is adequate	6
Response is science driven	6
Resources are needed	4
Difficult to contract Ebola	3
Travel ban not effective	3
Vaccine is in the future	1
Stigma has negative impact	1
Management is effective	1
Divergent Narratives	
Guidelines/responses inadequate	14
Trust in CDC is weak	6
Quarantine needed	3
Travel ban needed	3
Privacy is being undermined	2
Fear at high levels	2
Mixed CDC messages	2
Management ineffective	2
Limits of science	1
Both Convergent and Divergent	
Response resources	2
Travel	1
Vaccine	1
Social distancing inadequate	1
Washington Post *Narratives*	
Convergence	
Protocols/Guidances are adequate	15
Fear/rumors unfounded	10
Resources	9
Health care heroes	9
Success in response	7
Surveillance adequate	5

(continued)

Table 16.4 (continued)

Strong science	3
Stigma	3
Reporting is good	3
Divergence	
Response inadequate	5
Management inadequate	3
Communication poor	3
Lack of preparation	2
Limits of science	1
Warnings ignored	1
Resources	1
Both Convergent and Divergent	
Human interest	2
Travel	2
Responsibility	1
Media criticism	1

protocols. Travel bans, quarantines, and containment are not necessary and may be counterproductive by making any surveillance and reporting more difficult. Fear was unfounded and irrational. Established public health monitoring procedures are adequate. Finally, the Ebola outbreak was in West Africa, far removed from the US

Supporting narratives include the science-based nature of the response, and claims that scientific support for protocols and guidance was adequate. A set of narratives about sufficient resources, robust surveillance, sound science, and success in responses complements the protocols and guidance are adequate narrative. Other converging narratives emerged that fears and rumors about Ebola were simply unfounded, that health care workers were heroes, and that stigmatization of people from Africa was dangerous and unfounded.

The official narrative was reiterated in public statements to officials including President Obama and Dr. Thomas Frieden, head of the CDC. On September 16, 2014, President Obama visited the CDC campus in Atlanta and gave a joint statement with Dr. Frieden. He emphasized the low risk:

> First and foremost, I want the American people to know that our experts, here at the CDC and across our government, agree that the chances of an Ebola outbreak here in the United States are extremely low. We've been taking the necessary precautions,

including working with countries in West Africa to increase screening at airports so that someone with the virus doesn't get on a plane for the United States. In the unlikely event that someone with Ebola does reach our shores, we've taken new measures so that we're prepared here at home.

(Obama, 2014, para. 4)

President Obama went on to praise the health care workers who were working to manage the threat in a professional manner.

This narrative that Ebola was not a threat and could be managed effectively was repeated in many media channels. Various accounts picked up the dominant Ebola narrative. This included a variety of subject matter experts (SME), surrogates, researchers, and public health officials. Exceptions to the dominant narrative by the SME community include a small number of researchers and some health workers, especially nurses.

The Divergent Narratives

Despite a dominant narrative supported by official sources, a counter and divergent narrative emerged. The dominant divergent narrative of the 2014 Ebola outbreak centered around statements by other subject matter experts including independent researchers and medical professionals. Political figures also expressed counter narratives based largely on a general distrust of the federal government as well as specific distrust of the Obama administration. In general, this counter narrative was grounded in three views.

First, the questions were raised about what was not known about Ebola. Most of these related to the possibility that Ebola could be transmitted without physical contact. Some suggestions were made that Ebola could be airborne through the aerosolized spread of mucus from sneezed droplets, although this route of transmission was considered very remote. Well-known epidemiologist Michael Osterholm published an opinion article on September 11, 2014, raising the possibility or airborne Ebola through viral mutations:

You can now get Ebola only through direct contact with bodily fluids. But viruses like Ebola are notoriously sloppy in replicating, meaning the virus entering one person may be genetically different from the virus entering the next [sic]. If certain mutations occurred, it would mean that just breathing would put one at risk of contracting Ebola.

(Osterholm, 2014, para. 5)

A second divergent narrative was grounded in claims that the CDC was simply wrong, or that the CDC was intentionally misleading the public or was simply incompetent. The *Washington Post* noted, for example, in an October 15, 2014, article that the CDC had been hedging its statements. The same article quoted a candidate for congress, Eric Williams, who openly asked, "Are we getting the truth?" The *Post* article pointed out that the chances of contracting Ebola in the US were exceedingly low, but went on to reference high levels of public concern.

Still, all over the country, Americans expressed deep anxiety about the threat of Ebola. According to a new *Washington Post*-ABC News poll, two-thirds of Americans were worried about an Ebola epidemic in the United States, and more than 4 in 10 were "very" or "somewhat worried" that they or a close family member might catch the virus (Harlan, 2014). Similar media reports quoted skeptical politicians, primarily Republicans, who suggested that the federal government was underreacting and that travel bans and quarantines were warranted (Barrett & Walsh, 2014). A number of commentators noted that the Ebola threat had become an influential issue for the midterm elections.

A third interpretation was based in a larger critique of science and included the limits of science, the uncertainty associated with emerging science, and the inadequacy of the government's response. Specifically, the National Nurses United (NNU) was vocal in questioning the idea that medical protocols were sufficient. The NNU began to voice concern regarding a lack of preparedness following Duncan's diagnosis. What followed were public challenges to the CDC's recommendations. Following Dr. Frieden's statements about Nina Pham's protocol violation, the narrative shifted and become more critical of the CDC. The evolving narrative included claims that the CDC's original protocols were both insufficient and inconsistent for health care personnel treating Ebola patients.

Once the CDC introduced new guidelines, however, the NNU began to curb its criticism, stating that the CDC's revised actions were an improvement over previous recommendations, though not as strong as they should be to ensure adequate protection for health care workers. The NNU also acknowledged the CDC has no regulatory power and petitioned hospitals, the White House, and Congress to take action.

These narratives essentially critique and counter the CDC's official narrative based on general distrust and fears. They primarily raised questions about the official, dominant narrative and suggested ways in which it was incomplete or did not fit the existing facts, such as the cases that had occurred in the US.

Discussion

The dominant narrative was predictable and familiar. Science can control the disease. Protocols are adequate. The risks are limited, almost nonexistent. This narrative was grounded largely in the credibility of the source—the Obama administration and the CDC. Overall, the divergent narrative emphasized the uncertainty and what remained unknown. Ebola is an exotic disease and the outbreak forced experts to deal with uncharted waters and numerous unknowns, including how the disease could spread. Overly broad assurances early on and changing guidelines—what protective gear to wear, how to wear it, how to dispose of waste, flight restrictions, and isolation measures—fueled the criticism of the CDC. Rather than being seen as responsive to concerns, they implied that the initial response was flawed. These changes in the response were portrayed as evidence that the CDC simply did not have all the answers.

Three additional factors supported the emergence of a divergent narrative. First, risk communication is always difficult with a novel threat where the science is emerging. Because the public did not understand Ebola, there was more room for diverse interpretations and explanations. Modes of transmission were not familiar. As the risks became manifest in ways that were not seen as consistent with the dominant narrative, the uncertainty became an increasingly central theme in the divergent narrative. Mistrust of the CDC came from skepticism about science and a view that expert opinion is elitist and condescending. Second, the journalistic norm of balance in news reports gave the counter narrative more substance than it might otherwise have warranted. Journalistic accounts often turn to alternative views as a way of telling both or multiple sides of the story and achieving objectivity in reporting. Fairness is sometimes achieved by covering multiple sides of any new story. Balance in a journalistic account can also add context and perspective. In some cases, the search for balance can support alternative storylines and competing narratives that otherwise would not have received attention. Balance may even encourage the development of those narratives by creating an outlet. Finally, as with all risks, the threat of Ebola had significant political implications. In this case, Ebola created an opportunity for the opposition to critique the Obama administration's competence. Issues that create questions about public safety and security can be powerful political forces. The Ebola outbreak, occurring within a context so close to the election, enhanced the likelihood that the issue would be politicized.

This analysis provides several practical applications for risk and crisis communicators facing health-related crises. First, the uncertainty in health-related crises is unavoidable. Even the best science available leaves room for speculation regarding the potential for viruses to mutate, for treatments to fail in some individuals, and the potential for diseases to spread despite actions such as vaccination, protective protocols, and quarantines. Spokespersons should acknowledge this inherent uncertainty and take care to avoid over-reassuring the public. Indeed, acknowledging uncertainty is a tenet of effective crisis communication (Seeger, 2006). Had President Obama and Dr. Frieden been less definitive in their establishment of the primary narrative, they would likely have faced considerably less criticism when the first case of Ebola spreading from one person to another on American soil occurred. Second, recognizing plurality in the crisis narrative, in this case, advanced from a right to a necessity. The National Nurses United spoke on behalf of nurses who were genuinely fearful that the existing protocols were not sufficient. This example points to the vital importance of hearing all voices in the evolution of a crisis narrative. Conversely, divergence in crisis narratives can originate from less genuine or sincere concerns. Some argued that much of the controversy emerging about the trustworthiness of the CDC and President Obama to manage the Ebola risk was little more than political manipulation. The challenge for crisis communicators is to acknowledge such criticism during health-related crises, but to do so in a manner that prioritizes the well-being of those at risk. Quarreling publicly without such emphasis on those who are or feel they are at risk is likely to promote rather than resolve narrative divergence.

The surprise, threat, and uncertainty of Ebola created a void of understanding and meaning. This communication vacuum and meaning deficit was filled with narratives about the risk. In June of 2016, the WHO officially declared the West Africa Ebola outbreak over. A total of eight cases were confirmed in the US and six of those contracted the disease in West Africa. Only two cases of infection occurred in the US. These were a consequence of ineffective protection in the treatment of the first case, Thomas Eric Duncan. While the official narrative proved most accurate, the divergent narrative created a great deal of concern, confusion, and uncertainty, and diverted resources and attention. Crisis managers, however, should always anticipate and prepare for divergent narratives, as these appear to be an inevitable part of the crisis story.

Organizations and agencies can take several practical steps to prepare for diverging and highly critical narratives. An initial step in preparing for divergent narratives is to understand in advance of a crisis how to track the emerging narrative accurately and determine how the organization can best assert itself into the evolving narrative. Organizations and agencies might ask the following questions: Who are our critics? Where do these critics typically voice their opposition? What access does my organization or agency have to this forum? Second, organizations can prepare for divergent narratives by following the standard best practice of working with media reporters well before any crisis occurs (Seeger, 2006). Having a network in place that includes reporters, from both legacy and new media sources, who cover the issues relevant to the organization or agency is essential for making a timely response to crises and having a presence in the crisis narrative from the outset. Third, organizations should be prepared to determine when and if a diverging narrative is significant. Not all divergent narratives warrant a response (Coombs & Holladay, 2012). If a critical narrative is emerging, but the audience is limited or the source is highly questionable, responding to the criticism may only draw attention to a nonissue. These manageable steps can help organizations plan for crises. As is so often the case in crisis communication, failing to develop a comprehensive crisis communication plan can cause devastating delays and diminish the ultimate effectiveness of a response.

Competing narratives are an inherent element of the sense-making process that occurs during and after crises. The Ebola crisis simultaneously created public alarm and uncertainty. Combined, these conditions created an atmosphere where diverging narratives could thrive. Additionally, the Ebola crisis dramatically revealed that planning and resources did not account for many risks with the disease. When cases moved from Africa to the United States, this lack of preparation was distressingly clear. The hope is that this dramatic crisis will inspire organizations and agencies to collaborate and coordinate their efforts and to dedicate sufficient resources in their preparations for such fear-provoking disease outbreaks in the future.

References

Anthony, K. E., Sellnow, T. L., & Millner, A. G. (2013). Message convergence as a message-centered approach to analyzing and improving risk communication. *Journal of Applied Communication Research, 41*(4), 346–364.

Barrett, T., & Walsh, D. (2014, October 3). Ebola becomes an election issue. *CNN. com*. Retrieved from www.cnn.com/2014/10/03/politics/ebola-midterms/.

Centers for Disease Control and Prevention (2015, December 10). What you need to know about Ebola. Retrieved from www.cdc.gov/vhf/ebola/pdf/what-need-to-know-ebola.pdf.

Coombs, W. T., & Holladay, J. S. (2012). The paracrisis: The challenges created by publicly managing crisis prevention. *Public Relations Review, 38*, 408–415.

Fisher, W. R. (1987). *Human communication as narration: Toward a philosophy of reason, value, and action.* Columbia: University of South Carolina Press.

Goodnight, G. T. (1999). The personal, technical, and public spheres of argument. In *Contemporary Rhetorical Theory: A reader*, 251–264. New York: The Guilford Press.

Harlan, C. (2014, October 15), An epidemic of fear and anxiety hits Americans amid Ebola outbreak. *The Washington Post*. Retrieved from www.washingtonpost. com/business/economy/an- epidemic-of-fear-and-anxiety-hits-americans-amid-ebola-outbreak/2014/10/15/0760fb96-54a8-11e4-ba4b-f6333e2c0453_story. html?utm_term=.7f954f9c6b80.

Heath, R. L. (2004). Telling a story: A narrative approach to communication during crisis. In D. Miller & R. Heath (Eds.), *Responding to crisis: A rhetorical approach to crisis communication*, 167–188. Mahwah, NJ: LEA.

Obama, B. (2014). Remarks by the President on the Ebola outbreak. The White House. Retrieved from www.whitehouse.gov/the-press-office/2014/09/16/remarks-president-ebola-outbreak.

Osterholm, M. (2014). What we are afraid to say about Ebola. *The New York Times*. Retrieved from www.nytimes.com/2014/09/12/opinion/what-were-afraid-to-say-about-ebola.html.

Perelman, C., & Olbrechts-Tyteca, L. (1969). *The new rhetoric: A treatise on argumentation*. Trans. John Wilkinson and Purcell Weaver. London: University of Notre Dame Press, 31, 33.

Peters, C. J., & Peters, J. W. (1999). An introduction to Ebola: the virus and the disease. *Journal of Infectious Diseases, 179*(Supplement 1), ix–xvi.

Seeger, M. W. (2006). Best practices in crisis communication: An expert panel process. *Journal of Applied Communication Research, 34*, 232–244.

Seeger, M., & Sellnow, T. (2016). *Narratives of crisis: Telling stories of ruin and renewal* (Vol. 19). Stanford, CA: Stanford University Press.

Sellnow, T. L., & Seeger, M. W. (2013). *Theorizing crisis communication* (Vol. 4). New York: John Wiley & Sons.

Sellnow, T. L., Ulmer, R. R., Seeger, M. W., & Littlefield, R. S. (2009). *Effective risk communication: A message-centered approach*, 19–31. New York: Springer.

Ulmer, R. R., & Sellnow, T. L. (2000). Consistent questions of ambiguity in organizational crisis communication: Jack in the Box as a case study. *Journal of Business Ethics, 25*, 143–155.

Ulmer, R. R., Sellnow, T. L., & Seeger, M. W. (2013). *Effective crisis communication: Moving from crisis to opportunity*. Thousand Oaks, CA: SAGE Publications.

Venette, S. J., Sellnow, T. L., & Lang, P. A. (2003). Metanarration's role in restructuring perceptions of crisis: NHTSA's failure in the Ford-Firestone crisis. *The Journal of Business Communication, 40*(3), 219–236.

INDEX

Willis, L. A. 304
Wilson, K. 129, 131
Winkler, Carol 209
Witte, H. Joe 123–155
Wolbransky, M. 215
Woloshin, S. 161, 169
Womble, F. E. 10
women 39
Wong, N. C. H. 255, 258, 265
Woods, Chelsea 316–334
workplaces 7, 97–122
World Cancer Research Fund
  (WCRF) 169
World Health Organization (WHO)
  243, 320, 321, 332
World Wide Web *see* Internet
Wu, F. 86

Xi Jinping 84
Xie, W. 83

Xu, Q. 304
Xu, Y. C. 85

Yale, R. N. 159
Yan, Y. 80–81
Yao, L. 82
Young, T. J. 158, 160
YouTube 19, 233
Yu, G. 89
Yu, Nan 9–10,
  300–315

Zaire 320, 324
Zhang, L. 88
Zhang Wuben 80
Zhang, Zhian 7,
  78–94
Zhao, X. Z. 150
Zhu, X. 87
Zika virus 311

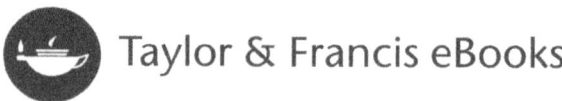

Taylor & Francis eBooks

Helping you to choose the right eBooks for your Library

Add Routledge titles to your library's digital collection today. Taylor and Francis ebooks contains over 50,000 titles in the Humanities, Social Sciences, Behavioural Sciences, Built Environment and Law.

Choose from a range of subject packages or create your own!

Benefits for you

>> Free MARC records
>> COUNTER-compliant usage statistics
>> Flexible purchase and pricing options
>> All titles DRM-free.

Benefits for your user

>> Off-site, anytime access via Athens or referring URL
>> Print or copy pages or chapters
>> Full content search
>> Bookmark, highlight and annotate text
>> Access to thousands of pages of quality research at the click of a button.

REQUEST YOUR **FREE** INSTITUTIONAL TRIAL TODAY

Free Trials Available
We offer free trials to qualifying academic, corporate and government customers.

eCollections – Choose from over 30 subject eCollections, including:

Archaeology	Language Learning
Architecture	Law
Asian Studies	Literature
Business & Management	Media & Communication
Classical Studies	Middle East Studies
Construction	Music
Creative & Media Arts	Philosophy
Criminology & Criminal Justice	Planning
Economics	Politics
Education	Psychology & Mental Health
Energy	Religion
Engineering	Security
English Language & Linguistics	Social Work
Environment & Sustainability	Sociology
Geography	Sport
Health Studies	Theatre & Performance
History	Tourism, Hospitality & Events

For more information, pricing enquiries or to order a free trial, please contact your local sales team:
www.tandfebooks.com/page/sales

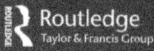 Routledge
Taylor & Francis Group

The home of
Routledge books

www.tandfebooks.com